Recommendations by Professionals

"Dr. Karlinsey is an Oral Health Care Ninja Warrior. His passion for the topic is manifest in this amplified work on how foods, drinks, and toothpaste impact the teeth. *Demin/Remin in Preventive Dentistry* is a comprehensive resource that provides a mouthful of great information. This is a must-read for any Oral Health Care Professional and those focused on oral health and overall wellness."

—**Rich Christiansen**, National Bestselling Author (*Wall Street Journal, USA Today*), Prolific Entrepreneur, and Philanthropist, Utah, USA

"*Demin/Remin in Preventive Dentistry* is well-thought-out, has good flow, is full of scientific research spanning more than 100 years, and can certainly expand on a clinician's knowledge of demineralization and remineralization. I loved the historical tidbits (especially the early 20th century advertisements for toothpaste). This is a fine work, and I'm impressed with the depth of knowledge Dr. Karlinsey provides, not to mention his motivation to become engaged in preventive dentistry."

—**Dr. Dylan Yung**, Aevitas Dentistry, Auckland, New Zealand

"Dr. Karlinsey has an amazing talent of explaining a sometimes confusing or misunderstood topic in an easy-to-understand way. As a practicing dentist for 15+ years, I have seen first-hand a lot of dental demineralization and disease in a real-world clinical setting. *Demin/Remin in Preventive Dentistry* provides some real world applications and up-to-date solutions, and encouraged me to circle back and revisit my understanding of demin/remin processes in order to better combat these ongoing struggles."

—**Dr. Chris Hardin**, Hardin Cosmetic & Family Dentistry, Indiana, USA

"As our overall health begins in the oral cavity, this is an excellent book on demineralization, including the effects of various foods and drinks on the dentition. *Demin/Remin in Preventive Dentistry* should not only be required reading for health care providers, especially dentists, hygienists and pediatricians, but should also be a part of education in all dental and hygiene schools!"

—**Dr. Greg Hardin**, Hardin Cosmetic & Family Dentistry, Indiana, USA

"*Demin/Remin in Preventive Dentistry* has the potential to augment the standard of education in dental schools. Additionally, I believe it can change a dental patient's life and is a great contribution to preventive dentistry!"

—**Dr. Makoto Asaizumi**, Asaizumi Orthodontic Practice, Mobara, Japan

"Based on my clinical perspective, I refer to the mouth as a dynamic chemical laboratory consisting of minerals, compounds, acids, buffers, etc. Furthermore, dental decay results from an imbalance of demineralization/remineralization processes. In order to tip the scale to a caries-free state, a clinician needs to assess not only the oral environment but also the functioning of the body as a whole. The factors that influence the oral environment need to be understood, and in *Demin/Remin in*

Preventive Dentistry, Dr. Karlinsey has explained all these aspects so beautifully with references and cross-references. He has systematically detailed the dental caries process, remineralization approaches, and so much more; in doing so, it is now well-understood that there is more to dental caries than what we previously knew, and there is more to prevention than just brush, use fluoride, and do not eat sugars. *Demin/ Remin in Preventive Dentistry* is a marvelous book, is much needed by dental clinicians, and could become the bible of preventive dentistry!!"

—**Dr. Rajeev Thaper**, Thaper Dental Clinic,
Rajasthan, India

"*Demin/Remin in Preventive Dentistry* brings to light the wide variety of acid types that patients encounter daily that lead to demineralization, while putting emphasis on food and beverage items we may not necessarily expect. Dr. Karlinsey explains the processes behind demineralization, as well as efforts we, as clinicians, can take to provide better quality dental health not only through education but also in-office fluoride formats to promote remineralization."

—**Vanna Murphy**, Registered Dental Hygienist,
North Carolina, USA

"*Demin/Remin in Preventive Dentistry* is well-written and very informative. In particular, the dynamics of dental caries and the role of saliva are beautifully explained."

—**Dr. Meenu Bhola**, Professor and Head of the Dept. of Pediatric Dentistry at the Dasmesh Institute of Research and Dental Sciences, Faridkot, Punjab, India

Demin/Remin

in

Preventive Dentistry

Demin/Remin

in

Preventive Dentistry

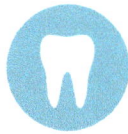

Demineralization
BY FOODS, ACIDS, AND BACTERIA,
AND HOW TO COUNTER USING
Remineralization

Robert L. Karlinsey, PhD

Published by RLK Ventures, LLC
7750 Centerstone Drive, Indianapolis, Indiana 46259

Library of Congress Control Number: 2018905810

ISBN:
Print: 978-0-9995599-0-1
E-book: 978-0-9995599-1-8

Printed in the United States of America

I dedicate this book to Tami and Teegan, two very special, loving, and supportive people in my life.

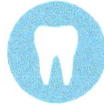

Table of Contents

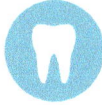

Table of Figures

Chapter 7

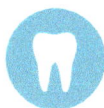

List of Tables & Short Captions

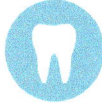

Foreword

Despite significant progress in the management of oral health, tooth decay remains stubbornly widespread and resilient; in fact, tooth decay is the single most preventable disease affecting children. Complicating this further, there remain gaps in clinical use and knowledge involving fluoride and remineralization therapies. While there are plenty of books, reports, and research papers that highlight this ongoing problem, this book is not meant to highlight the fact there is a problem. The problem is well-known and typical solutions involve abstaining from sugar, encouraging more responsible manufacturing of foods, and shifting third-party reimbursement systems (e.g., incentivizing) away from restoration and toward minimal intervention. While efforts to attain a critical mass of each of these stakeholders remains challenging, tooth decay continues to present worldwide problems. Therefore, in a bid to stimulate better oral health today, new approaches and perspectives are in demand now.

To contribute to the fight against tooth decay, *Demin/Remin in Preventive Dentistry* explores demineralization and remineralization processes by synthesizing a variety of data and research to produce a fresh perspective from one who has devoted significant effort to improving remineralization therapies in preventive dentistry. Supporting prevention, stimulating thought, and inspiring change are the major goals of this book, since the decay statistics demand the need for improved oral health strategies. After all, as my good friend and colleague, Dr. Rajeev Thaper, has said to me *you have to have passion for preventive dentistry to make things work.* Well, I'm following Dr. Thaper's advice and the result is this book.

In addition to sharing my perspectives, I'm literally revealing a part of myself to you. I admit it: I have a history of dental decay, ever since I was a young boy. I've had so many cavities that I had been predisposed to thinking that cavities were a part of growing up; strangely, my brother didn't get cavities and I always found this confusing as we ate nearly the same foods and he didn't appear to take better care of his teeth than I did (in fact, it might have been worse!). But many years later and after completing my graduate studies in chemistry and physics, I learned I was harboring a cracked molar, and that it would need to be crowned. Indeed, this proved to be a 'crowning' moment, and I promptly shifted my research focus to dental research and prevention, with the hope I could somehow contribute to improving topical dental products and help others reduce the risk of aggressive intervention. And, through the course of my research, I developed innovative forms of calcium phosphate for enhanced remineralization benefits, and these are presently found in several topical 3M Oral Care products, such as Clinpro™ 5000 and Clinpro™ Tooth Crème.

Therefore, a primary motivation for writing this book is to share my in-depth knowledge and understanding of preventive dentistry, which includes highlighting the benefits of remineralization as part of a minimally invasive dentistry approach. Still, this is not a compilation of my own research as this would be a much shorter read! Rather, I utilized research from around the world and used my best efforts to avoid hashing over timeworn concepts that can be found elsewhere. In doing so, this book provides fundamental, fascinating, and instructive information, underscoring several aspects not addressed in other dentistry books.

For purposes of scope and perspective, each chapter in this book contains rich information dedicated to several key aspects alluded to above. For more in-depth information the reader is respectfully pointed to the relevant references (and the references within those references), especially since there exists a number of very well-researched and well-documented efforts by scientists and agencies worldwide. Many of the references in the bibliography are 'open access' and hyperlinks are provided in such instances.

Here is a brief overview of the book chapters:

✓ Chapter 1 acknowledges and reminds us that tooth decay remains problematic. Just about everyone can relate to the effects of dental decay, which can ultimately lead to the sequela of invasive procedures commonly used to stabilize the condition. Some statistics are shared that underlines this ongoing problem of dental decay that affects either you or someone you know, including perhaps your family, friends, clients, or patients.

✓ Chapter 2 introduces some of the key players in the mouth starting with basic information about the teeth. A more detailed look at the oral flora and the associated acids is then presented, with an emphasis on the mixed ecology of microbes. The value of saliva, which is the most critical part of remineralization, is reviewed.

✓ Chapter 3 reviews micro- and ultrastructural characteristics of sound enamel in order to gain insight into how acids may lead to enamel demineralization. In doing so, crystallite size and morphology is discussed, as is the nature of the water and protein content residing in enamel. Additionally, the existence of microscopic voids is presented.

✓ Chapter 4 explores the structural characteristics of the hard and soft components of the tooth when demineralized by acids. In addition to some clinical observations, simulated caries and erosive lesions are considered, along with demineralization of dentin. Perspectives on microscopic-level demineralization mechanisms are also presented.

✓ Chapter 5 probes why and how some acids are more damaging to the teeth than others based on a variety of characteristics including acid strength, diffusion and size of undissociated and dissociated acids, and stability with calcium complexes. The purpose of this important chapter is to establish the chemical basis for the acid-susceptibility of tooth structure. The information presented here helps establish a foundation for the discussion on the nature of acids found in foods as well as those produced by microbes. A novel perspective of acetic acid is shared, and the chapter closes with a point-by-point generalized perspective of dental demineralization by acids.

✓ Chapter 6 takes a close look at the demineralization risks of various foodstuffs and drinks. Besides the many foods that may have the potential to elicit caries-based (i.e., plaque-based) decay, which includes those rich in cereal grains (e.g., wheat, rice, corn), sugar, or other fermentable substrates, there exist others that present erosive risks. Even further, behavior (including purposeful and otherwise) drives much of the resultant damage to tooth structure. The causative factors in these instances include pH and small organic/inorganic acids, and unlike plaque-based decay, do not require the microbial middleman to destroy the dentition. As such, this chapter emphasizes the role of pH and acid in demineralization. Other factors besides pH and acid type certainly contribute to demineralization risk, such as the titratable or neutralizing acidity, degree of saturation, viscosity, surface tension, salivary stimulus, and so on. But irrespective of acid type, a low (i.e., acidic) pH is required to effect dental softening or demineralization (and pertains to both caries and erosive processes), and thus serves as a primary determinant. Secondly, based on the information presented in Chapter 5, the nature of the small organic/inorganic acid also bears on demineralization and varies according to the food or drink. To gain further insight, in this chapter I present an extensive series of figures that highlight the pH and/or small acid composition of many foods (including fruits, vegetables, and plant-derived foods) and beverages (freshly prepared or ready-to-drink). Though much effort has been made to include as many foods and drinks as possible, these lists are not complete due to the myriad foodstuffs available throughout the world, let alone those subjected to analyses and available in the public literature. Importantly, it is my hope that this information can facilitate healthier choices for foods and/or drinks when several options are available, while also bringing awareness to potentially unhealthy behavior. Three helpful options are presented, and 11 strategies are provided at the end of this chapter to help encourage better dietary choices and behavior.

✓ Chapter 7 provides a glimpse into some historical approaches used in preventive dentistry, including antiquated approaches as well as near-modern use of anti-enzyme, ammonia, and chlorophyll 'actives' introduced in the 20th century. This treatment is meant to be informative and enjoyable, and helps lay the foundation for why fluoride has been welcomed as a primary agent in the management of tooth decay. This is a must-read chapter.

✓ Chapter 8 is all about fluoride, including its anticaries history, the multipronged mechanistic underpinnings of its anticaries benefits, and features of several popular topical fluoride formats. Discussion is centered on fluoride's ability to accelerate remineralization and impact microbial activity. The relative antidecay efficacy of various fluoride modalities, including varnishes, gels, toothpastes, and more are covered. To help illustrate remineralization characteristics from different fluoride levels, two dentifrices comprising fluoride and functionalized tricalcium phosphate are compared.

✓ While fluoride accelerates remineralization, calcium and phosphate comprise the basis for mineral formation and is a key function of saliva. Chapter 9 is, therefore, devoted to remineralization. Although saliva is the natural remineralization system, other calcium phosphate systems are also used but work in different ways. But how do remineralization systems work and are all supersaturated systems the same? To help answer these questions, remineralization processes in general are reviewed. Additionally, solubility calculations are performed that estimate fluoride and/or calcium phosphate phases from supersaturated systems, including specific examples using varnish and dentifrice formats comprising different fluoride and calcium phosphate systems.

✓ A discussion on minimal intervention dentistry is presented in Chapter 10 and rounds out this book. This includes commentary and insights regarding the clinician-patient relationship, along with other factors including nutrition and age-related health concerns. The tone of this chapter touts progress, and supports those research activities dedicated to improving oral health for people everywhere around the globe.

The source material for this book is fairly diverse, with more than 900 references called forth (and many more left out for purposes of redundancy) from various fields of study, including medicine, dentistry, chemistry, biology, materials science, food science, along with reports from journalists, nonprofit foundations, and government organizations.

It is my hope that this work inspires students, researchers, or anyone working in the wellness fields who frequently engages with patients.

Thus, this is intended for those studying cariology or preventive dentistry, including students in dental or hygiene school; dental hygienists, therapists and assistants; general, pediatric, and specialty dentists (especially orthodontists); dietitians and nutritionists; researchers in the dental and life sciences; pediatricians, physicians, nurses, nurse practitioners, and assistants; those working in private or public dental practices; those working with populations prone to or experiencing significant health-related problems; and, this book is also geared toward those with special interests in the demineralization and remineralization of enamel.

In summary, a motley of historical timelines, food and drink data, past and present research into aspects of demineralization and remineralization, and elements of minimal intervention dentistry, which runs counter to the dreaded 'drill-and-fill' prognosis, are presented. *Demin/Remin in Preventive Dentistry* is not only intended for those with a 'prevention-first' mind-set but also for those researchers and clinicians passionate about delivering or improving oral health benefits to those of us (both young and young at heart) most susceptible to tooth decay.

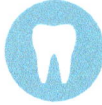

CHAPTER ONE

Tooth Decay is Still Problematic

THE CHANCES ARE UNFORTUNATELY HIGH that if you were born in the United States and you're reading this book, you have had at least one decayed, missing, or filled tooth. If so, then your situation is similar to most of the global population—in fact, tooth decay remains the most prevalent disease affecting children [1–3]. Some common factors contributing to tooth decay include biological makeup, behavior, environment, and lifestyle. While lower socioeconomic status increases risk for tooth decay, dental caries still affects those who are educated and/or affluent. In a frustrating twist, however, the disease is manageable and largely preventable but requires a consistent multi-pronged approach involving professional services and recommendations, along with patient education, habits, and compliance. Of course, ignoring the disease or hoping it will "go away on its own" can be detrimental to overall health and, in extreme albeit rare situations, can even lead to death [3]. While this may seem like a dramatic statement, consider

Some common factors contributing to tooth decay include biological makeup, behavior, environment, and lifestyle.

that more than 830,000 emergency room visits in 2009 were caused by preventable dental conditions—and this statistic represents an *increase* of 16% compared to visits in 2006 [4]!

To set the stage for further discussions on addressing tooth decay, this chapter introduces the motivation for improved preventive approaches by touching on some key statistics relating to tooth decay.

So who is affected from tooth decay and when it does it begin? Personally, my dental history is decorated from relatively benign gingiva-margin measurements to evidence of aggressive intervention marked by fillings and crowns. But this isn't an adult disease that one naturally matures into; rather, risks begin within the first year of a newborn's life.

The American Academy of Pediatric Dentistry (AAPD) defines early childhood caries (ECC) "as the presence of one or more decayed (noncavitated or cavitated lesions), missing (due to caries), or filled tooth surfaces in any primary tooth in a child under the age of six" [5]. Basically, any child with at least **one** decayed tooth surface meets this criterion. To help thwart the onset of ECC, the AAPD published guidelines with respect to "anticipatory guidance and preventive counseling, for infants, children, and adolescents", and recommends establishing a "dental home" beginning with the first tooth eruption and no later than the first 12 months of the child's life [5,6]. This call for a dental home is not without merits: in 2008, less than half of US children between the ages of 2 and 17 had ever received advice from a health care provider about the need for timely checkups [7]: and within this age range, children between the ages of 13 and 17 actually received the least advice. This troubling statistic encompasses the teenage demographic who, exploring emerging independence, begin to assume greater stewardship (or lack thereof) in dietary selections and oral hygiene. Separately, the aforementioned statistics consider children having public, private, or no insurance assistance, and reveal that children from families with greater education and/or income were more likely to make a routine visit to the dentist at least once a year; but even with relatively higher socioeconomic standing, only 63% of children from these families saw the dentist at least once a year [7]!

Given the fact that families well above the poverty level strain to achieve consistent routine dental care for their children, one can imagine the statistics that might arise for resource-strapped families. Approximately 37 million children from low-income families in the United States are primarily served by the government-funded Medicaid mechanism for coverage and access to dental care [2]. Though it may seem these children are covered, evidence indicates otherwise: not only are there deficiencies in the number of Medicaid-participating dentists but also the Medicaid coverage failed to support the requisite services established by the AAPD. For instance, among four states (California, Indiana, Louisiana, and Maryland) which represent nearly one-fifth of all Medicaid-enrolled children, 78% (or, about 2.9 million) failed to receive AAPD-recommended services, including biannual oral exams, dental cleanings, and fluoride treatments over a two-year period (2011 and 2012), with more than 25% of the children *never* having received any dental service during this time [2].

Why is this so? Of course, the answers are many: lack of nearby access to a dentist; poor patient compliance due to myriad reasons; shortage of dental providers due, in part, to ponderous administrative burdens, concerns over low reimbursement rates, or simply misalignment with career aspirations; unethical dental providers with questionable billing practices; or, even the Centers for Medicaid & Medicare Services reluctance to or absence of improving outreach or oversight by, for example, tracking child-specific services on a quarterly basis. Whatever the reason, endemic problems exist, and may contribute—at least in part—to the estimated several million other children living with untreated tooth decay. Hence, it is understandable how deficiencies in such programs can lead to greater oral health problems that, in turn, morph into emergency room visits, the costs of which are estimated to be about 10x that of standard preventive services delivered by a dentist [4].

In 2008 an oral health report was published by the United States Department of Health and Human Services based on data collected from the National Health and Nutrition Examination Surveys [8]. This report provides exceptional detail into prevalence of caries-related tooth decay confronting children and adults at several socioeconomic levels over two separate periods: 1988–1994 and 1999–2004. This included the number of people manifesting some aspect of caries, as well as those experiencing gingival recession or tooth loss. In addition to a most surprising result from this report was the *increase* in caries from children ages 2 to 5 years old from 24% (1988–1994) to 28% (1999–2004), there are other troubling trends that deserve special consideration.

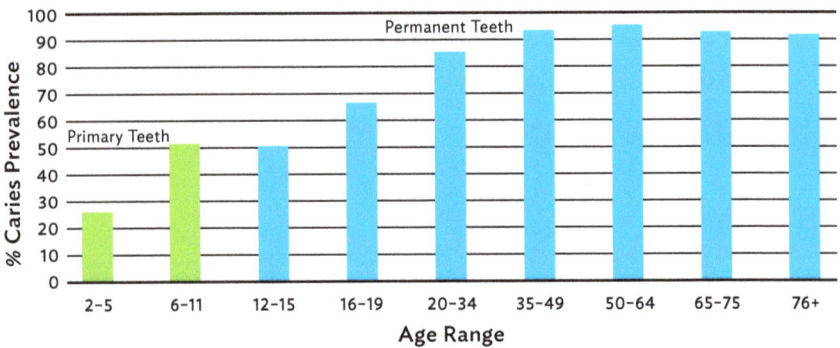

Figure 1.1. Mean percent caries prevalence in children and adults (across all socioeconomic groups) from ages 2 thru 64 surveyed between 1999 and 2004. This chart was constructed from tabulated data [8]. Green and blue bars correspond to primary and permanent teeth, respectively.

Firstly, the trend in developing tooth decay over the course of one's life is eye-opening: by the time a child is entering kindergarten, his/her risk for developing tooth decay is already 28%—this means almost three out of 10 children will have experienced caries, and underlines the importance of establishing a "dental home" as recommended by the AAPD. Of those affected, 72% have decayed surfaces, while the remainder received restorations. From the time when the child enters primary schooling and nearly through fifth grade—which are some of the most formative and enjoyable years in a person's life—one-half (51.2%) exhibit caries, with almost 70% of those affected having received restorations. This not only affects the child's psyche about dentistry (discussed in Chapter 10), but it presents an economical burden on the caretakers (i.e., parents, guardians, etc.) and the insurance system. Furthermore, a major source of subsequent decay arises from pre-existing intervention (i.e., 'secondary caries'), and children exhibiting ECC bear significantly higher risks in developing future caries in their permanent dentition [9].

But the data in **Figure 1.1** demonstrate nearly one out of every two children in middle school and within the first couple years of high school are affected by caries: thus, caries experience has begun in the relatively young permanent dentition. Once the teenager achieves driving age, the rate of decay accelerates, affecting nearly seven out of 10 high-schoolers. Concomitant with the maturation into young adulthood is the further risk for additional decay (almost nine out of 10!) as the individual matures into specific lifestyle and stewardship choices. Decay risk continues to increase until the ages where tooth loss becomes common: after age 64, one can expect to lose (on average) four teeth by the age of 75.

But decay risk over the course of one's life is only a part of the story: what about the actual number of affected teeth? While dental caries can affect all teeth, it is most common for the posterior teeth to be especially affected, with prevalence especially on occlusal molar surfaces [9], as well as interproximal and proximal coronal surfaces [1]. Survey results between 1999 and 2004 reveal the number of decayed (D), missing (M, due to disease), or filled (F) teeth (T) in the permanent dentition compounds with age as shown in **Figure 1.2**. Initially, the number of diseased teeth increases by one tooth every five years from age 9 thru 13; then, the number increases by 4 more teeth by the age of 49; finally, another 5 teeth by age 64 are affected, resulting in an average total of 15 teeth subject to caries. Contributing to these statistics is the fact that many adults simply don't visit the dentist: for example, the Commonwealth Fund reported about 16% (or, about 36 million) of adults in the United States failed to visit the dentist in 2014 [10], and despite improvements in access to healthcare, this was an increase from 15% in 2012!

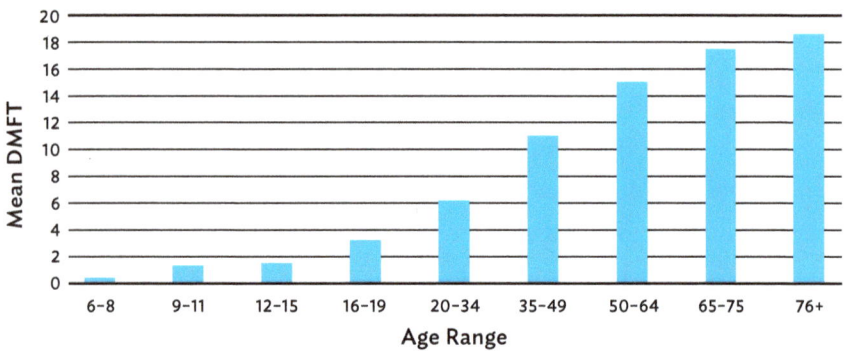

Figure 1.2. Mean decayed (D), missing (M), filled (F), teeth (T) for age groups (across all socioeconomic groups) surveyed between 1999 and 2004. This chart was constructed from tabulated data [8].

With such decay, it is not surprising that those between ages 65 and 75 have, on average, 19 remaining teeth (compared to the original set of 32, including four 'wisdom' teeth). Separate studies also reveal in both 2012 and 2014 about 10% (or, almost 30 million people) of US adults between the ages of 18 and 64 have six or more missing teeth due to tooth decay, gum disease, and infection [10]. What's amazing about these statistics is that dental caries is largely a preventable and manageable disease—so such loss doesn't have to occur!

Such evidence demonstrates tooth decay remains a global health concern and this warrants ongoing attention and fresh perspectives. For those interested in further information, consider the referenced reports and publications cited in this chapter. Over the next several chapters, the oral environment is discussed with special emphasis on bacteria, saliva, and enamel structure as these bear directly on dental caries, erosion, and hypersensitivity. As we progress in our review of tooth decay, however, we are reminded of the words of Dr. Willoughby Miller, one of the great pioneers of dental research: *"there is no doubt that a deterioration of the teeth accompanies the progress of civilization* [11]". And, we should observe that dental caries has long been a problem in the history of man [12–14].

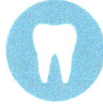

CHAPTER TWO

Key Components in the Mouth: Teeth, Bacteria and Bacterial Acids, and Saliva

TO BETTER UNDERSTAND TOOTH DECAY, it's important to explore the nature of the tooth and the oral environment. This chapter introduces some basic components including tooth composition and structure, bacteria, and saliva. Additional detail on enamel structure is reserved for Chapter 3, while demineralized enamel structure is presented in Chapter 4.

The mammalian tooth is an interesting bioengineered structure comprising layers of a soft inner media underneath a hard outer crown.

About teeth

The mammalian tooth is an interesting bioengineered structure comprising layers of a soft inner media (i.e., dentin) underneath a hard outer crown (i.e., enamel). The inner media encompasses and protects the pulp chamber (which maintains blood and nerve supply), and attenuates shock or pressure experienced during mastication or trauma. Vintage sagittal sketches of maxillary and mandibular tooth structure are shown in **Figure 2.1**, and an idyllic arrangement of the 32 permanent teeth is shown in **Figure 2.2**.

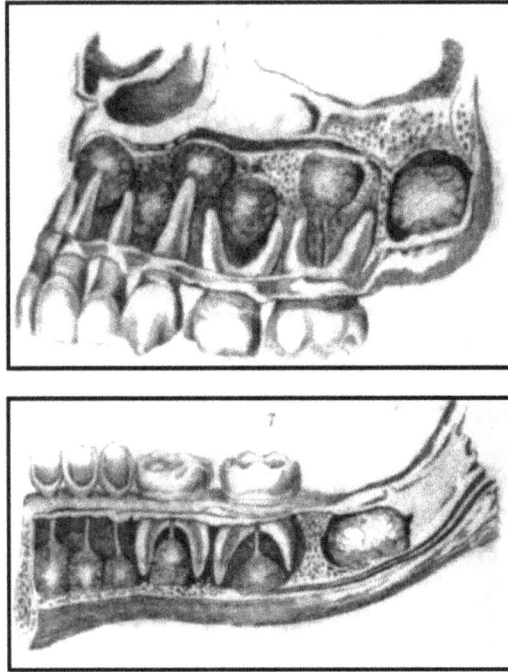

Figure 2.1. 19th century sagittal sketches of model maxillary (top) and mandibular (bottom) tooth structure and arrangement (from [24]). The mandibular sketch reveals distinct regions of the tooth including the enamel crown, the softer media within the crown, along with a perspective of the root environment, replete with stem-like nerves, below the alveolar ridge. Also shown are the nebulous beginnings of the supernumerary molars (or, 'wisdom' teeth) in the alveoli pockets.

Compositionally, dentin is comprised of both organic and inorganic constituents; however, the inorganic fraction in dentin is quite low compared to enamel. For example, calcium weight fractions in dentin are about 28% lower relative to enamel [15,16]. The relatively lower mineral content of dentin is balanced with an elevation in organic content (e.g., 28%) [16]. Although the calcium-to-phosphate ratios in both enamel and dentin are about 2.1 and 2.0, respectively

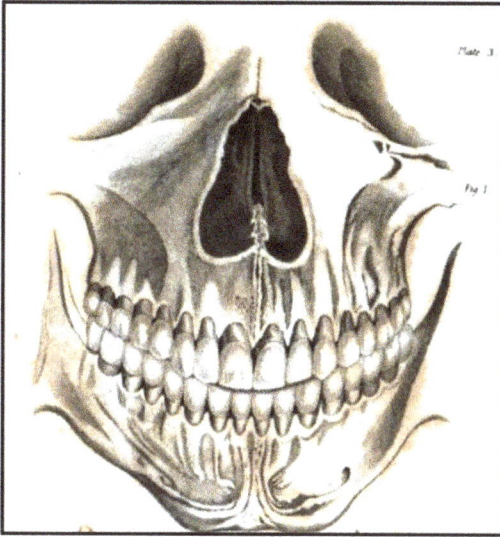

Figure 2.2. 19th century frontal sketch depicting the presence and idyllic arrangement of the 32 permanent teeth (from [24]).

[15], the average specific surface areas differ markedly: 77 m^2g^{-1} and 94 m^2g^{-1} for enamel and dentin, respectively [17]. The relatively higher surface area of dentin may be attributed to the geometry of the collagen tubules manifested within the dentin matrix, which help provide structure and support [18,19].

Enamel can be up to several millimeters thick and is comprised of a heterogeneous arrangement of inorganic mineral and organic substances, including proteins and collagen [20]. With respect to minerals, enamel is comprised of hydroxyl and/or carbonate apatites [21], and may also have magnesium, strontium, and sodium substituted for calcium [22]. Defects and chemical deficiencies are also common in dental enamel [23]. Although advances have facilitated improved specificity in the nature of the inorganic material, remarkably, the approximate percentage of organic components has remained nearly constant since at least 1830 [24]! Enamel microstructure reveals apatite crystals in a hexagonal arrangement, although the actual unit cell pertaining to hydroxyapatite is likely comprised of two different sets of monoclinic crystal arrangements, with one monoclinic arrangement arising from two hexagonal cells [25]. Scanning and transmission electron microscopies have been used with much success for over 30 years to reveal intricacies of enamel ultrastructure, including the identification of defects manifest in dental apatite (e.g., point defects, edge defects, screw dislocations, small angle boundary defects, and variations during amelogenesis) [26–30]. Transmission electron microscopy experiments reveal lath-like crystallites of varying widths (e.g., between 15 nm and 65 nm) that are approximately 2.5x larger relative to thickness [31]; however, lengths (e.g., at least 20 nm) are more difficult to assess due to errors introduced during sample preparation, as well as intra- and inter-tooth orientation differences [31]. These crystallites are separated by thin substances comprised of organic and inorganic matter, which appear more resistant to caries formation [32,33].

This brief overview introduces an important substrate that is sensitive to both bacterial and salivary action. As demineralization and remineralization of enamel is the focus of this book, additional detail regarding sound and demineralized enamel structure is presented in Chapters 3 and 4. Later, aspects of remineralization will also be discussed (Chapters 8 and 9).

Role of bacteria in tooth decay

Dental caries can be described as a disease involving the destruction of tooth structure arising from acids produced by cariogenic bacteria existing in the dental plaque [11,23,34]. But to further explore the etiology of decay, we must recognize the natural abundance of myriad microorganisms living in and on our person: our bodies inherently support beneficial and harmful bacteria, with this delicate balance tipping between 'good' and 'bad' according to vacillations of our health [35,36]. (Note: ref [36] has a fascinating 3D mapping of our skin-residing microbes.) The mouth represents just one of the many microhabitats comprising many specific niches, including cells, enzymes, minerals, proteins, fungus, bacteria, and more. Among these constituents, both commensal and pathogenic bacteria coexist and are responsible for much of the activity in the mouth [11,37–40]. With respect to bacteria, the mouth has among the greatest diversity of all the microhabitats existing in the human body, and trails only the distal gut in the sheer number of bacterial 'operational taxonomic units' (or, OTUs) or species-level phylotypes [35].

Given the mouth hosts an impressive amount of bacteria and that dental caries is a bacterial disease, it follows that further questions would be asked, including how many OTUs (or, species-level bacteria) does a person have? Do all people have the same OTUs? Do people without evidence or history of caries (denoted 'caries-free') host different bacterial makeup compared to a 'caries-active' individual? What are the most beneficial or harmful bacteria? Can the microflora be affected, and if so, how?

Existing and emerging research provides some fascinating answers. First, the number of specific species-level bacterial types (i.e., OTUs) depends on the sensitivity of the refinement procedures selected in the experimental protocol; for this reason, there are ranges in published values [35–43]. In general, those affected by caries typically have greater diversity: in one study, 1,014 and 984 OTUs were identified in caries-active and caries-free primary teeth, respectively [40]. In another study assessing permanent teeth from adolescents, those in the higher caries prevalence group that received no dental care (rural Romanian adolescents with little to no access to professional visits or daily preventive care, including lack of routine toothbrushing) exhibited significantly higher OTUs relative to Swedes with and without caries [43]. Thus, "healthier" mouths seem to harbor slightly less bacterial diversity.

Within the oral environment, specific sites host very diverse OTUs, including the palatine tonsils, hard palate, subgingival or supragingival plaque, tongue, cheeks, and hard tooth surfaces [35,41,42]. After 24 hours of toothbrushing in two unrelated caries-free adult men (between 20 and 30 years old), unstimulated saliva appears to host a greater bacterial diversity compared to stimulated saliva and the tongue (the latter two of which are comparable), while the lingual gingiva hosts less bacterial diversity relative to vestibular gingiva [42]. These results contrast with results from three unrelated caries-free adult men (ages 29, 39, and 45) obtained after 12 hours of toothbrushing, where bacterial diversity was higher in the teeth compared to saliva [41]. Even among healthy, caries-free individuals, both studies demonstrate the dynamism of the oral environment.

In addition to differential diversity, healthier mouths exhibit differential microbial makeup [40]. The Romanian-Swedish study demonstrated that despite consumption of sugary snacks, engagement in professional and daily preventive dental care programs significantly affects diversity: despite the Firmicutes family that naturally thrives in our mouths and is dominated by the *Streptococcus* genus [35,40,41,43], Romanian adolescents had a significantly higher fraction of *Streptococcus* OTUs (i.e., *Streptococcus sobrinus* and *mutans*) compared to the Swedish adolescents [43]. Still, between caries-free and caries-active groups, there exists significant microbial overlap: among the 626 OTUs common to both caries-free and caries-active groups, 87 of these were significantly overrepresented, with, for example, *Streptococcus infantis* and *Veillonella criceti* were dominant in the caries-free group, while *Streptococcus sanguinis* and *Veillonella parvula* were dominant in the caries-active group [40]. These phylotype examples also highlight that an entire genus cannot unequivocally be marked either as benign or pathogenic. For instance, although *Streptococcus* phylotypes are known to ferment lactic acid through digestion of sugar and other fermentable carbohydrates, *Streptococcus mutans* imparts a significant role in deep dentin caries [44,45], while *Streptococcus cristatus* appears healthful [37,38], providing benefits against the gingivitis-causing pathogen *Porphyromonas gingivalis* [46], and inhibiting replication of human immunodeficiency virus type 1 (HIV-1) [47].

At this point it is clear the mouth hosts a large and diverse amount of bacteria, some of which appear virulent while others seem healthful. To understand the bacterial interplay that gives rise to dental caries from today's perspective, we must also acknowledge historical pioneering views.

Dr. Miller's published theory on dental caries was postulated in 1890 based on the relative abundance of bacteria: if there were significant numbers, then conditions favored dental decay of some kind [11]. Specificity was attributed to bacteria that, for instance, fermented carbohydrates, alcohol, fatty acids, and dead tissue. Morphological observations (rods, spheres, crescents, threads, chains, etc.) were made and bacterial terms were described (often using the Latin term 'bacillus' for 'bacteria'), inspired by Pasteur's pioneering research on production of lactic acid by yeast [48]. By 1885, Miller personally identified about 22 cultivatable bacterial species in the mouth, while admitting the overwhelming nature of this enterprise [11], especially since original published observations on oral bacteria influenced Leeuwenhock to declare these *"Animals . . . are so many that I believe they exceed the number of Men in a kingdom"* [49]. And, it was Miller, based on his own as well as his contemporaries' research, who presented the parasitico-chemical theory of parasites (i.e., bacteria) producing acids originating from fermented carbohydrates and imparting loosening of the enamel prisms [11].

Advancements in the 20th century, however, enabled improved sensitivity to detect pathogenic bacteria. In addition to the groundbreaking study that fluoride can inhibit the growth and acid production of oral bacteria (including 11 strains of *Streptococcus* and 12 strains of *Lactobacillus*) [50], additional studies gave rise to a plaque-specific theory that among the 300 or so bacterial species identified, *Streptococcus mutans* was considered the prime pathogen leading to dental caries [44].

Now, in the 21st century, the understanding of dental decay has evolved, aided in no small part to powerful experimental methodologies. Building on elements gleaned since Miller's parasitico-chemical process, the 'extended caries ecological process' returns to a nonspecific approach and emphasizes the diversity and adaptability of the oral microbiome as championed by Nyvad and Takahashi [45,51], including, for example, the sensitive ecology manifest in supragingival plaque as described in **Figure 2.3** and summarized below:

1. The dynamic equilibrium existing prior to initial tooth decay, with ever-present acid-generating and acid-neutralizing activities; and,

2. an acidogenic environment in the initial stages of tooth decay where an acidic plaque pH intermittently dominates; and,

3. an acidophilic environment where an acidic plaque pH consistently dominates and progresses the caries process.

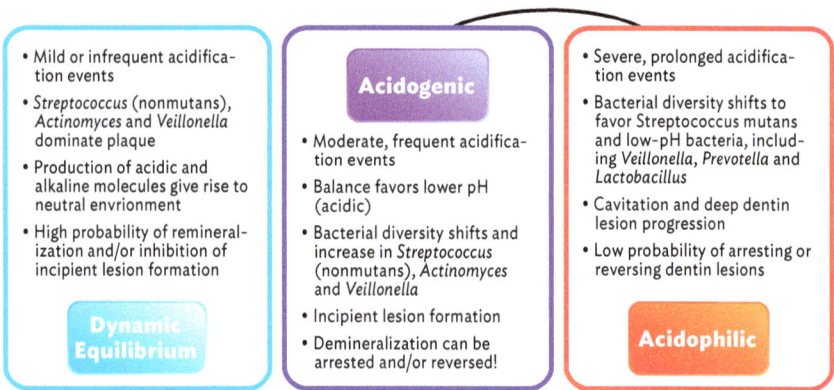

* Mild or infrequent acidification events
* *Streptococcus* (nonmutans), *Actinomyces* and *Veillonella* dominate plaque
* Production of acidic and alkaline molecules give rise to neutral envrionment
* High probability of remineralization and/or inhibition of incipient lesion formation

Dynamic Equilibrium

Acidogenic

* Moderate, frequent acidification events
* Balance favors lower pH (acidic)
* Bacterial diversity shifts and increase in *Streptococcus* (nonmutans), *Actinomyces* and *Veillonella*
* Incipient lesion formation
* Demineralization can be arrested and/or reversed!

* Severe, prolonged acidification events
* Bacterial diversity shifts to favor Streptococcus mutans and low-pH bacteria, including *Veillonella*, *Prevotella* and *Lactobacillus*
* Cavitation and deep dentin lesion progression
* Low probability of arresting or reversing dentin lesions

Acidophilic

Figure 2.3. Detail regarding the nonspecific ecologies existing in supragingival plaque based on the nonspecific caries hypothesis [45,51], and expanded to include recent microbiological research [38–43].

Dental plaque is a constantly adapting ecological system that includes the many energetic, quiescent, or dead microbial species (e.g., bacteria, cells, fungus, etc.), salivary constituents (e.g., proteins, minerals, enzymes, etc.), and networks of saccharide secretions produced from fermentations [52–54]. Plaque pH is affected by the acidic and alkaline products generated by microbial action as contemplated in **Figure 2.4**. Though in dynamic balance, there remains abundant microbial activity, including competition among the diverse bacterial species for dominance. In a near neutral pH environment, the acidic and alkaline molecules are offset and the risk for tooth decay is low. When this balance is tipped to slightly more alkaline or acidic, the ecology is correspondingly affected and the risks for dental decay increase. With respect to an acidic pH, the bacterial milieu adjusts and results in net demineralization of tooth structure; with respect to an alkaline pH, the ecology shifts and presents greater risks to gingival tissue. Ergo, it is important to explore the nature of acidic and alkaline molecules to better understand what it means to have a 'healthy mouth'.

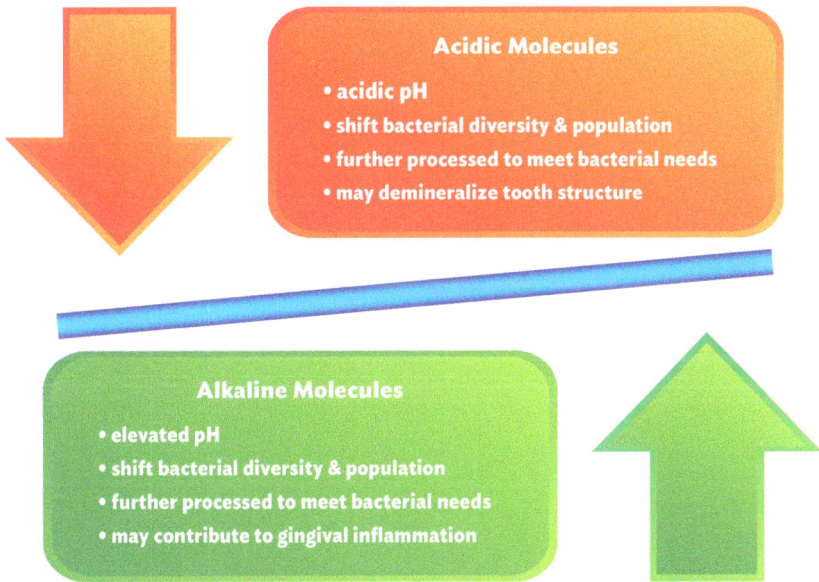

Acidic Molecules

• acidic pH
• shift bacterial diversity & population
• further processed to meet bacterial needs
• may demineralize tooth structure

Alkaline Molecules

• elevated pH
• shift bacterial diversity & population
• further processed to meet bacterial needs
• may contribute to gingival inflammation

Figure 2.4. Dynamic equilibrium arising from the neutralization of acidic and alkaline molecules produced by microbes residing in plaque. When in balance, a neutral pH is achieved and the risks of dental decay are significantly reduced.

Dental caries is of microbial origin, where acids produced within the local plaque environment permeate to the tooth surface and demineralize tooth structure. While bacteria may create these acids, what is the energy source? Answer: saccharides. This includes mono-saccharides (e.g., glucose), disaccharides (e.g., sucrose), oligosaccharides (e.g., kestose, which is a trisaccharide oligofructan) or polysaccharides (e.g., starch, cellulose, and long-chained fructans or glucans, such as levans or dextrans, respectively). **Figure 2.5** outlines the various saccharide sources, examples of saccharolytic bacterial that ferment saccharides, and the molecular output produced from the metabolic processes.

First, it is clear that there is more than one source of saccharides: in addition to dietary intake, saccharides are also sourced from the immediate plaque matrix, from storage within the walls of bacteria, and also from salivary glycoproteins like mucin. Dietary saccharides typically include sucrose (e.g., table sugar), some oligosaccharides (e.g., inulin or steviol glycoside (a trisaccharide and main compound in the *Stevia rebaudiana* leaves), and starches (e.g., potatoes). The extracelluar and intracellular polysaccharides are products from microbial species. Extracellular polysaccharides are a major contributor to

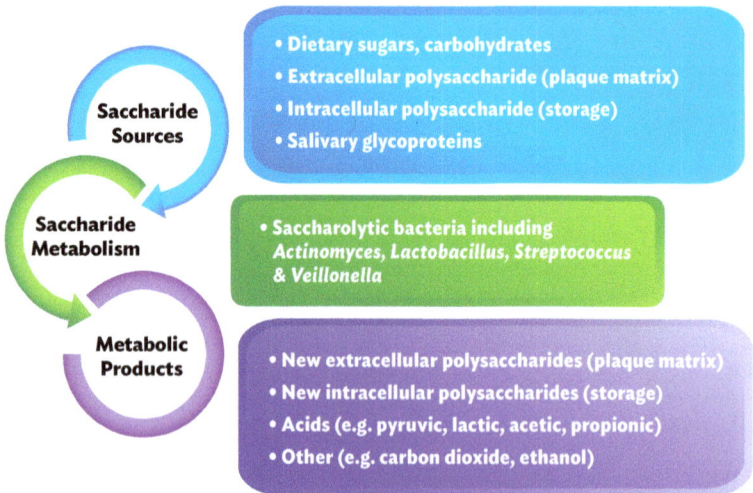

Saccharide Sources
- Dietary sugars, carbohydrates
- Extracellular polysaccharide (plaque matrix)
- Intracellular polysaccharide (storage)
- Salivary glycoproteins

Saccharide Metabolism
- Saccharolytic bacteria including *Actinomyces, Lactobacillus, Streptococcus & Veillonella*

Metabolic Products
- New extracellular polysaccharides (plaque matrix)
- New intracellular polysaccharides (storage)
- Acids (e.g. pyruvic, lactic, acetic, propionic)
- Other (e.g. carbon dioxide, ethanol)

Figure 2.5. Microbial consumption of saccharide sources and resultant metabolic products. This process pertains particularly to supragingival plaque.

plaque, serving as a substantive support and protective matrix for microbial colonization and growth, as well as promoting adhesion to the tooth surface [45,55–58]. Another fermentation product, intracellular polysaccharides are accumulated and stored within the microbial species, and utilized when there is a deficiency of available saccharides [45,58–61]. Finally, saliva naturally produces glycoproteins, such as mucins, that help coat the teeth with a protective film [62,63]; but, these glycoproteins can be catabolized (from both microbes and salivary enzymes), enabling glucose to be utilized for energetic processes [45].

Consistent with the nonspecific plaque hypothesis, the microbes largely involved in saccharolytic processes include species within the *Actinomyces, Lactobacillus, Streptococcus,* and *Veillonella* genera [45,64–67]. Microbes from these genera anaerobically ferment saccharides, generating new polysaccharides for storage (i.e., intracellular) and cohesive (i.e., extracellular) purposes, along with acidic molecules. Other molecules are also produced (particularly in the fermentation of glucose), such as carbon dioxide and ethanol.

Similarly but distinctively, other microbial species utilize proteins for energetic processes as summarized in **Figure 2.6**. In addition to dietary proteins, the mouth also provides dead tissue (e.g., microbes and cells), salivary constituents, gingival fluid, and desquamated tissue [40,45,54,66]. Enzymes such as protease and glycosidase found naturally in saliva and also produced from microbial species facilitate cleavage of proteins (e.g., glycoproteins, proline-rich proteins, etc.) into amino acids and peptides [45,68]. While peptidases can further process peptides, newly cleaved and existing host amino acids (e.g., glutamate or aspartate) are metabolized, forming acidic and alkaline molecules. For example, catabolism of cysteine by *Fusobacterium, Porphyromonas,* and *Prevotella* species produce molecules including pyruvate (which can further be processed) and ammonia, while *Streptococcus* and *Actinomyces* produce hydrogen sulfide [45]. The evolution of gingival pockets creates reservoirs of salivary nutrients while frustrating disruption of plaque formation: in turn, conditions favor microbial attachment, colonization, recruitment, and growth, with the nature of bacterial species propagating within these pockets correlating to the nature of acidic and alkaline molecules produced during the proteolytic processes.

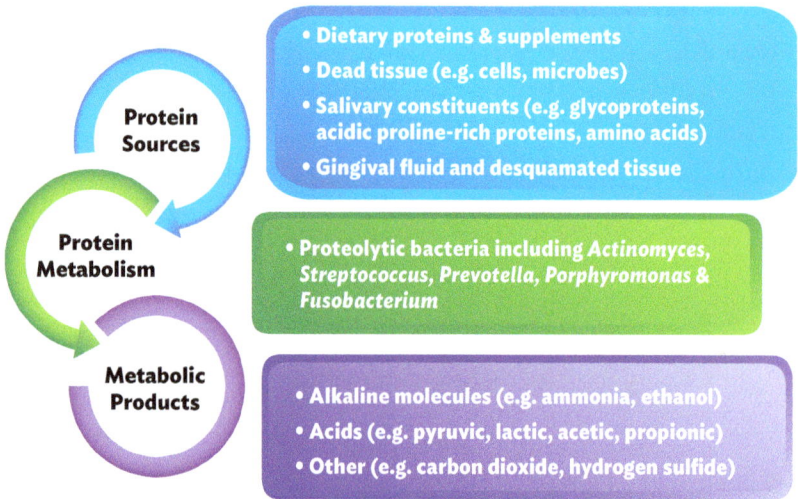

Protein Sources
- Dietary proteins & supplements
- Dead tissue (e.g. cells, microbes)
- Salivary constituents (e.g. glycoproteins, acidic proline-rich proteins, amino acids)
- Gingival fluid and desquamated tissue

Protein Metabolism
- Proteolytic bacteria including *Actinomyces, Streptococcus, Prevotella, Porphyromonas & Fusobacterium*

Metabolic Products
- Alkaline molecules (e.g. ammonia, ethanol)
- Acids (e.g. pyruvic, lactic, acetic, propionic)
- Other (e.g. carbon dioxide, hydrogen sulfide)

Figure 2.6. Microbial consumption of protein sources and resultant metabolic products. This process pertains particularly to subgingival plaque.

Following the plaque ecological hypothesis [45,51,67], when the plaque environment exhibits dynamic equilibrium, the production of acidic and alkaline molecules essentially neutralizes the pH and the risk for developing tooth decay is minimal; importantly, developments of any demineralization and/or irritations can be rectified with minimal intervention. However, when an acid-rich or alkaline-rich imbalance in the plaque ecology is created, this affects pH, therefore shifting microbial diversity and population as shown in **Figure 2.4**: imbalances in subgingival plaque are usually slightly alkaline, with the gingiva at risk for irritations and disease; in contrast, imbalances in supragingival plaque usually shift acidic, with the tooth structure especially susceptible to incipient enamel lesion formation, and perhaps progression to dentin caries ('acidogenic' and 'acidophilic' phases in **Figure 2.3**, respectively).

With respect to the oral environment, some principle acids produced during bacterial fermentation of saccharides and proteins are shown in **Figure 2.7**. Of particular interest, the differential between acetic and lactic acids is about one pK_a unit: this means lactic acid is about 10x as strong as acetic acid, and also demonstrates the nature of the acids produced during metabolic processes can vary considerably. While pyruvic is the strongest acid produced, it is readily consumed in further metabolic processes and thus does not appear to influence plaque pH as much as, for instance, lactic or acetic acid. And, some bacteria are heterofermentive, including *Veillonella*, which produces propionate, acetate, and succinate (along with carbon dioxide) via fermentation of glucose [69].

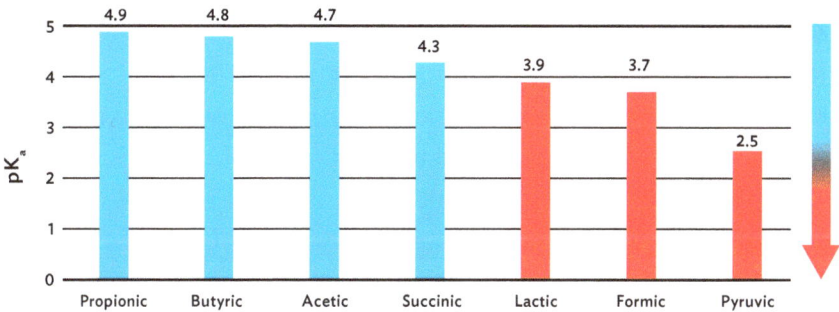

Figure 2.7. Principle acids produced during bacterial metabolism of saccharides and proteins. Some acids are further processed by certain families or species. By definition, lower pKa values reflect greater acid strength.

Importantly, expressed acidic products from metabolic processes can also be utilized as feedstock: for instance, *Veillonella* can convert lactate into formate, acetate, and propionate (e.g., for purposes of maintaining a less acidic pH environment), while some *Actinomyces* and *Lactobacillus* species can convert lactate into acetate [45,64,69].

Given that acids are readily produced, with some even used as further feedstock for certain metabolic processes, there continues to be interest in researching pH-raising, counter-balancing strategies, with a most popular approach emphasizing the production of ammonia. But is this approach effective? Here, I will pause briefly to present some outcomes of these efforts.

The production of ammonia via arginolytic activity to neutralize saccharide metabolism effects has been proposed [45,51,66]: several species within the *Actinomyces*, *Lactobacillus*, and *Streptococcus* families manifest the arginolytic mechanism [45], most notably *Streptococcus sanguinis* [70]. Although not clinically significant, supragingival plaque from children with lesion-free teeth (both primary and permanent) tended to have higher arginolytic activity compared to plaque from children with active enamel or dentin lesions [71]. But if arginolytic activity may be a possible biomarker for a potentially healthy mouth, can it be influenced? Or, might this be an example of where a correlation is mistakenly linked to causation?

One possibility of influencing arginolytic activity of microbial species may be through arginine supplementation [66]. However, clinical use of an 8% arginine dentifrice failed to significantly alter plaque diversity after eight weeks of use; at the same time, salivary diversity was altered to favor potentially pathogenic bacteria types *Prevotella* and *Veillonella* (the latter being significantly higher) [72]. But especially troubling was the effect on lactate production, which is a measure of saccharolytic activity: while lactate production was significantly inhibited during the eight weeks relative to baseline, the amount of lactate produced after cessation of the 8% arginine dentifrice increased significantly over the next two weeks when subjects returned to the baseline fluoridated control toothpaste. Based on this study, the shift toward possibly more pathogenic bacteria and the elevation in lactic acid production after discontinuance of arginine use does not stoke confidence for arginine supplementation.

Why did this study fail to promote a more promising microbial response? One can speculate that the significant increase in *Veillonella* species (and directional increase in *Prevotella*) may derive from the elevated ammonia levels produced during the eight weeks of 8% arginine use: perhaps *Prevotella* utilized a portion of the ammonia in amino acid synthesis for growth purposes [73], while *Veillonella* responded to the rise in pH with nonlactic acid fermentation products [45].

In a mixed microbial environment, and especially with respect to those most at risk for dental caries, the artful elevation of pH via ammonia-generating mechanisms might not present an effective approach for at least a couple of reasons.

Firstly, those manifesting dental caries (i.e., cavitation into the dentin) are likely hosting elevated levels of *Streptococcus mutans* [37,38]: though perhaps less likely involved in initial demineralization processes, *Streptococcus mutans* appears to be a major pathogen in caries progression [38,39,43,45,47]. Though some *Streptococcus mutans* found in animals may demonstrate arginolytic behavior, the serotype found in humans does not [44,66]. Furthermore, *Streptococcus mutans* is a bacterial beast: it metabolizes the widest variety of carbohydrates among all other Gram-positive bacteria; it readily ferments several acids (including lactic, formic, and acetic); it thrives in plaque environments while maintaining a near pH-neutral (7.5) intracellular environment; and, of particular interest, it utilizes ammonia as feedstock in its synthesis of glutamine, which is then utilized to power the biosynthesis of additional growth-related amino acids [74]. And even though agmatine may be metabolized by *Streptococcus mutans*, the metabolized levels of evolved ammonia are relatively low compared to those generated from the metabolism of arginine [75]. Thus, ironically and speculatively, for those demonstrating active dental caries, the ammonia produced from other bacteria, including that derived from arginolytic activity, may actually support *Streptococcus mutans* growth and activity, thereby frustrating neutralizing efforts and resulting in little to no therapeutic benefit.

Secondly, is the prospect of elevating plaque pH really new? And, if it isn't new, is it effective? The groundwork for studying saliva-induced ammonia had been realized since Pavlov's salivary gland-nitrogen

experiments in the late 1880s [76]. In 1934, two Chicago dentists published on their findings that *"ammonia content of the saliva appears to be the
immunizing factor in dental caries"* [77]. Shortly thereafter, patents were
filed and products were launched on the basis of generating ammonia to
elevate mouth pH and thereby depress dental decay risks (see Chapter
7 for additional detail) [78–80]. However, many independent studies
could not confirm the purported caries-fighting effects of ammonia,
including the following:

✓ Youngburg noted *"evidence tends strongly to show that caries is not
dependent on ammonia concentration in saliva"* [76]; and,

✓ Chernausek & Mitchell noted *"daily brushing of the molar teeth of
hamsters with a control and an ammoniated dentifrice resulted in significant reductions of caries experience of approximately the same magnitude"*
[81]; and,

✓ Davies & King published that *"under the conditions of the test, ammonium ion toothpowder failed to reduce the annual increment of dental
caries when its effect was compared with that of a controlled toothpowder."*
Furthermore, *"at the end of the study period there was no significant
difference between the Lactobacillus counts of the control and experimental
groups."* [82].

Thus, it seems pH elevation, as a means of inhibiting tooth decay
through the evolution of ammonia from metabolic processes, remains
elusive. And, despite ongoing research (now approaching almost 75
years with millions of invested dollars spent on research and development and experiments on rats, monkeys, and humans—all without a
consistent, suitable solution), the inability to effect a vaccine against
dental caries reflects the stubbornly dynamic, elastic nature of the
oral environment [83].

Altogether, these well-intentioned efforts underline the pitfalls in ascribing emphasis to either a single bacteria or even a group of bacteria that reside within the mixed, adaptive microniches (saliva, tongue, supragingival plaque, subgingival plaque, etc.) of the mouth.

Diversity of plaque acids in caries-free and caries-susceptible groups

In order to progress to the discussion of demineralization of the tooth, let's return to the commonly metabolized acid products shown in **Figure 2.7**. Among those listed, pyruvic, formic, and lactic acid are noted as the stronger of those potentially produced by microbial metabolism of saccharides and proteins. In particular, one pK_a unit corresponds to a factor of 10: this means lactic acid ($pK_a \sim 3.9$) is about 10x as strong as acetic acid ($pK_a \sim 4.7$), thus presenting a relatively greater threat to demineralization of tooth structure.

Given that bacteria possess machinery to metabolize the various **Figure 2.7** acids, are all of them found in abundance in the oral environment? And, can the type of fermented acid be influenced by external factors?

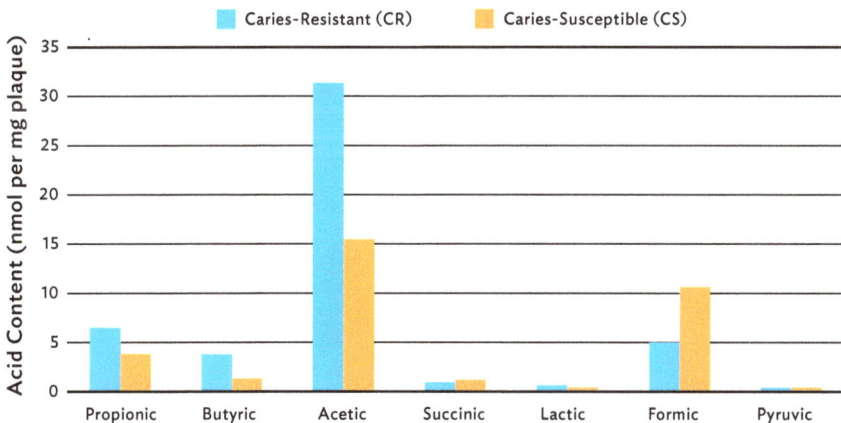

Figure 2.8. Mean amounts of acids naturally produced in plaque residing on the facial tooth surface of caries-resistant (CR) and caries-susceptible (CS) subjects, as collected by Vratsanos & Mandel [84]. The content of acid is expressed as nanomoles (nmol) acid per milligram (mg) of wet plaque samples obtained from tooth pairs 19 & 28.

While all of the **Figure 2.7** acids are present, not all are expressed equally: as an example, analyses of plaque samples from 'healthy' (i.e., 'caries-free') and 'risky' (i.e., 'caries-susceptible') subjects reveals striking plaque differences in acid diversity as shown in **Figures 2.8–2.10** [84]. In this study, the two cohorts refrained from oral hygiene activity for three days prior to plaque collection, which was collected at least three hours but not more than 12 hours after consuming food. **Figure 2.8** shows the various acids present in supragingival plaque, with acetic acid significantly higher compared to the caries-susceptible counter group. In addition to lower amounts of acetic acid, the plaque of caries-susceptible individuals also harbors higher levels of formic acid, which is 10x more aggressive than acetic acid. Notably, pyruvic acid, which is most likely to be further processed by microbial species, is found in negligible amounts in both study groups.

The histograms of **Figures 2.9** and **2.10** capture the acetic and lactic acid evolution from both cohorts when chewing sucrose gum over a 45-minute period: not only do caries-resistant subjects produce

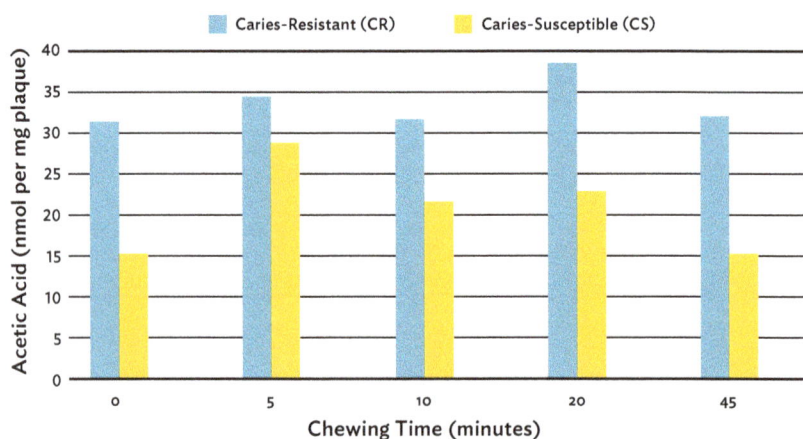

Figure 2.9. Mean amounts of acetic acid produced from 10 caries-resistant (CR) and 10 caries-susceptible (CS) subjects evolved by chewing a sucrose-sweetened chewing gum for up to 45 minutes [84]. The content of acid is expressed as nanomoles (nmol) acid per milligram (mg) of wet plaque sample. Plaque samples (3–4 mg) were collected from facial surfaces of tooth pairs at each time point (0 min: 19 & 28; 5 min: 5 & 15; 10 min: 20 & 30; 20 min: 2 & 12; 45 min: 18 & 29).

a higher amount of weaker acid (i.e., acetic acid) but they also produce lower amounts of stronger acids (i.e., lactic acid). To that end, in addition to producing greater formic acid [84], the caries-susceptible group experienced more than twice the lactic acid production relative to the caries-free group over the first 10 minutes of chewing, while only generating about one-third the acetic acid. Further discussion about acid attack on tooth structure, however, will be discussed shortly, where weaker and stronger acids can both play significant roles. But for purposes of the present discussion on fermented acids, the caries-susceptible group demonstrated higher total acid evolution (e.g., the sum of both acetic and lactic acids) relative to the caries-free group. These results are consistent with the relatively greater bacterial diversity also observed for those susceptible to caries activity.

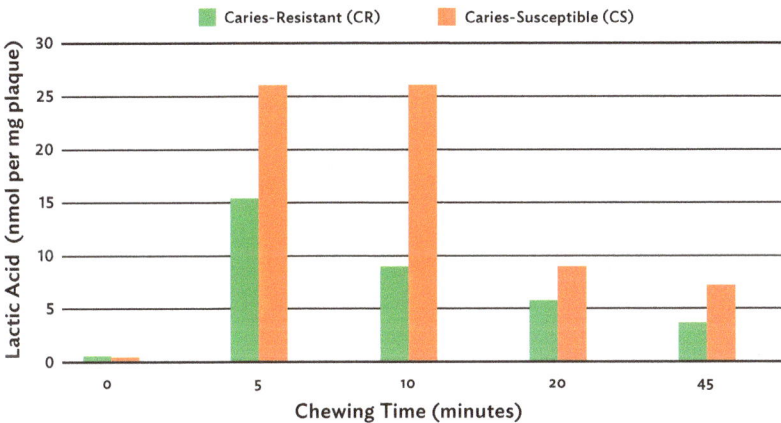

Figure 2.10. Mean amounts of lactic acid produced from 10 caries-resistant (CR) and 10 caries-susceptible (CS) subjects evolved by chewing a sucrose-sweetened chewing gum for up to 45 minutes [84]. The content of acid is expressed as nanomoles (nmol) acid per milligram (mg) of wet plaque sample. Plaque samples (3–4 mg) were collected from facial surfaces of tooth pairs at each time point (0 min: 19 & 28; 5 min: 5 & 15; 10 min: 20 & 30; 20 min: 2 & 12; 45 min: 18 & 29).

Plaque pH of caries-free and caries-susceptible groups

These results are consistent with independent plaque pH studies, including one study by Abelson & Mandel, who examined the buccal pH levels in two cohorts (10 caries-free, 10 caries-susceptible) as a function of salivary access in response to sucrose shocks as shown in **Figures 2.11–2.13** [85]. The protocol was similar to that used in the assessment of fermented acids as shown in **Figure 2.8–2.10**: the two cohorts refrained from oral hygiene activity for three days prior to plaque collection, which was collected at least three hours but not more than 12 hours after consuming food. The absence of saliva clearly inhibits pH recovery as shown in **Figure 2.11**. But in **Figures 2.11–2.13**, it is clear that caries-resistant individuals experience pH drops significantly different than their caries-susceptible peers, regardless of access to saliva or intake of sugary sources.

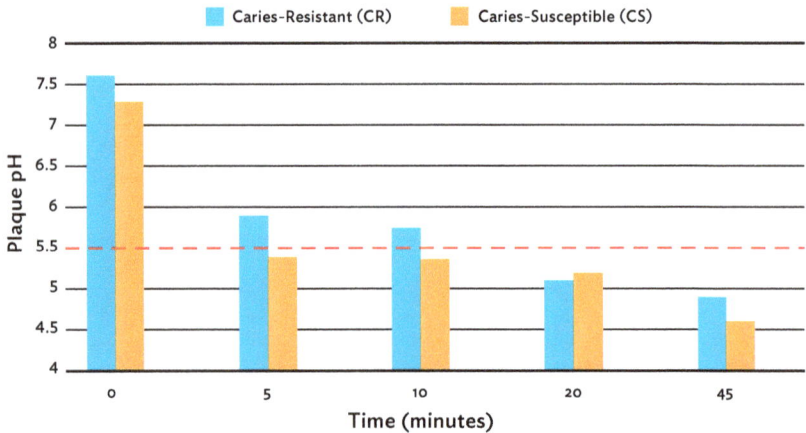

Figure 2.11. Mean plaque pH produced from 10 caries-resistant (CR) and 10 caries-susceptible (CS) subjects without access to saliva (i.e., staunched with cotton rolls). Initial pH was measured, then a 10% sucrose rinse was administered over a one minute period, followed by pH measurements on the cervical buccal surfaces of teeth 3, 6, & 8 at 5, 10, 20, and 45 minutes [85]. Note: the dashed red line at pH 5.5 approximates dissolution of enamel apatite.

Saliva

Perhaps not much appreciated until we experience dry-mouth conditions, saliva powers significant aspects of our lives: talking, eating (and associated digestive and alimentary processing), and even intimate interaction is much more feasible let alone enjoyable when the mouth

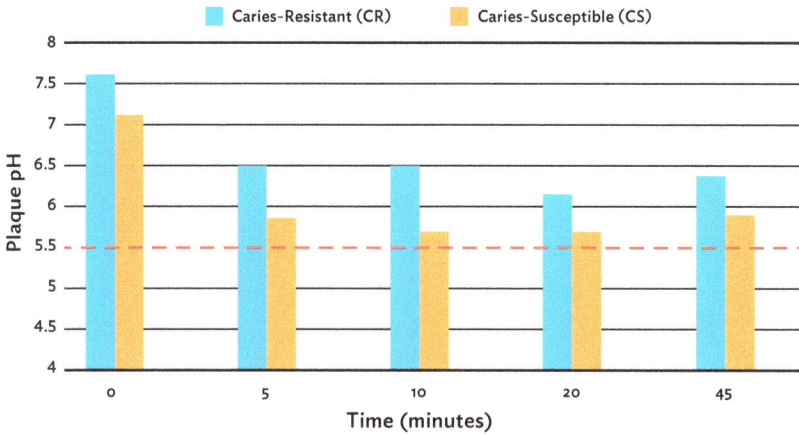

Figure 2.12. Mean plaque pH produced from 10 caries-resistant (CR) and 10 caries-susceptible (CS) subjects with uninhibited access to saliva. Initial pH was measured, then a 10% sucrose rinse was administered over a one minute period, followed by pH measurements on the cervical buccal surfaces of teeth 9, 11, & 14 at 5, 10, 20, and 45 minutes [85]. Note: the dashed red line at pH 5.5 approximates dissolution of enamel apatite.

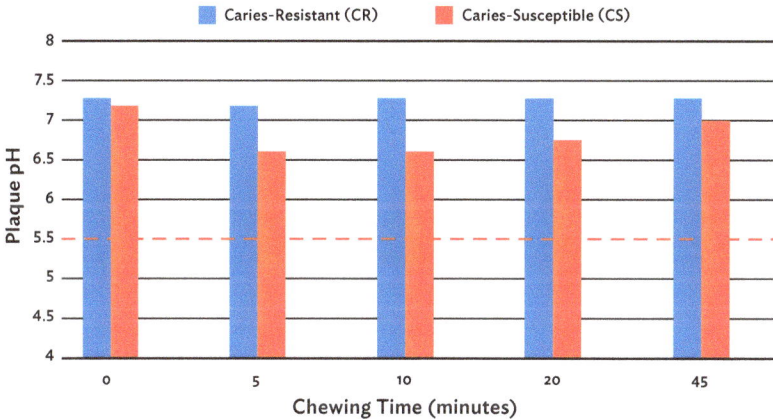

Figure 2.13. Mean plaque pH produced from 10 caries-resistant (CR) and 10 caries-susceptible (CS) subjects over the course of chewing a sucrose gum. Initial pH was measured prior to chewing the gum; then, pH measurements on the cervical buccal surfaces of teeth were measured at 5, 10, 20, and 45 minutes [85]. Note: the dashed red line at pH 5.5 approximates dissolution of enamel apatite.

has moisture. One must also appreciate the healing and protective effects of saliva, even in caries-susceptible persons, as it commands the health of the mouth: for instance, when the dentition (and the plaque on which it resides) is freely exposed to saliva as shown in **Figures 2.12** and **2.13**, the plaque pH did not dip below 5.5 (the pH near dissolution of tooth apatite [86]) over the 45-minute periods. But, saliva restriction overwhelmed the relatively healthier oral environment of caries-free persons by the 20-minute mark (**Figure 2.11**), where the pH dropped below 5.5.

Thus, while bacterial diversity and acid production obviously imparts effects in the mouth (for better or worse, which will be discussed in greater detail below), saliva provides a host of therapeutic and palliative effects in the maintenance of oral health, providing key functions such as [87–92]:

✓ Antimicrobial benefits (e.g. antibacterial, antifungal, antiviral)

✓ Cleansing, debridement, and carbohydrate clearance

✓ Water balance and pH regulation

✓ Source of mineralizing ions to counter demineralization processes

✓ Deposition of biofilms to limit bacterial adhesion and acid diffusion

✓ Initiation of digestive process

Secretions by several major (parotid, submandibular, sublingual) and minor glands, as well as the gingival fluid, give rise to the above properties [91]. Saliva pH varies but hovers around neutral, and is mostly comprised of water (~ 99.5%), with electrolytes, proteins, and antimicrobials comprising the remainder [91]. Salivary flow follows a circadian rhythm and increases during stimulation [91].

When saliva flow becomes restricted—for whatever reason—protective and healing effects are reduced, thus increasing the risk for tooth decay. For example, among several *Streptococcus* species evaluated in patients afflicted with head or neck cancer, *Streptococcus mutans* grew 10-fold (from 2.4% to 25.5%) three months after radiation therapy [93]. So in addition to the typical inhibition of salivary action resulting from radiotherapy, which is already problematic and serves as a major tooth decay risk [92,94], this pathogenic population increase underlines microbial sensitivity to saliva.

Other health situations also lead to conditions of hyposalivation, or dry-mouth, including those affected by oral or systemic diseases, including diabetes or Alzheimer's [92,94]. In addition to prescription therapeutics for management of chronic health problems, common medications such as aspirin, antihistamines, or even birth control pills can impart dry-mouth conditions, the severity of which, of course, depends on one's natural health and the medication dose [92,94]. Given this short list of examples, it is clear that a majority of the global population experiences at least some degree of dry-mouth sensation on a daily basis.

Notwithstanding the above-mentioned stresses, insufficient water intake, poor dietary choices, and dehydration stress the body's water requirements, and can result in dry-mouth conditions. Even improving one's body and overall health through exercise can lead to changes in saliva quantity and quality. As exercise is routinely recommended for a variety of reasons (e.g., mood, weight loss, overall health, and circulation), let's briefly consider some situations where exercise influences saliva.

In one scenario and in collaboration with the Wingate Institute for Physical Education and Sport [95], salivary impact was evaluated in participants engaged in one of two exercises: a single nine-minute submaximal aerobic exercise regimen, or a single 30-second Wingate anaerobic test. The submaximal test evaluated participants until near-maximum heart rate (~ 85% age-specific maximum heart rate) was reached through progressive workloads. The anaerobic test involved participants cycling at maximum speed at a set resistance. The study evaluated several metrics including saliva volume, sodium, potassium, calcium, magnesium, protein, lactate, and cortisol content generated both pre-exercise and within 10 minutes post-exercise; among these metrics and for purposes of discussion, saliva volume, lactate, and protein production are shown in **Figures 2.14** thru **2.16**, respectively [95].

Each participant served as their own control. For each metric, no significant differences were found between the two groups prior to each test. With respect to saliva volume, relative to pre-exercise salivary volumes, both exercise regimens produced significant drops, with the 30-second Wingate anaerobic exercise inhibiting the salivary rate the most. Lactate concentration in both exercise groups increased significantly relative to pre-exercise levels. The greatest concentration in lactate production occurred for the nine-minute submaximal exercise test, indicating the test produced a response closer to the anaerobic threshold. Also, in both exercise tests, protein concentration in saliva increased significantly, with the 30-second Wingate test yielding a higher post-exercise concentration. Elevations of protein concentration are consistent with other independent findings [96–98], and may account for the relative increase in viscosity.

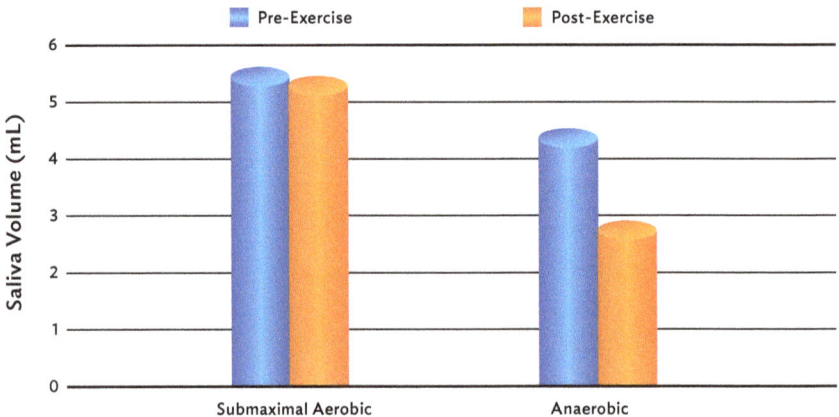

Figure 2.14. Mean saliva volume produced from 25 and 17 subjects participating in submaximal aerobic and anaerobic exercise, respectively [95]. Saliva was collected over a 10-minute period immediately following the exercise test.

Although some degree of dehydration may be expected during exercise, the relatively short exercise times in this study suggest elevations in protein concentration and viscosity may be attributed to increased secretions of certain proteins, such as MUC5B [97], which is a relatively large glycoprotein that readily adheres to the tooth surface as part of the protective salivary pellicle [96,97]. There were no significant changes in cortisol, sodium, or calcium content within each exercise group. The 30-second

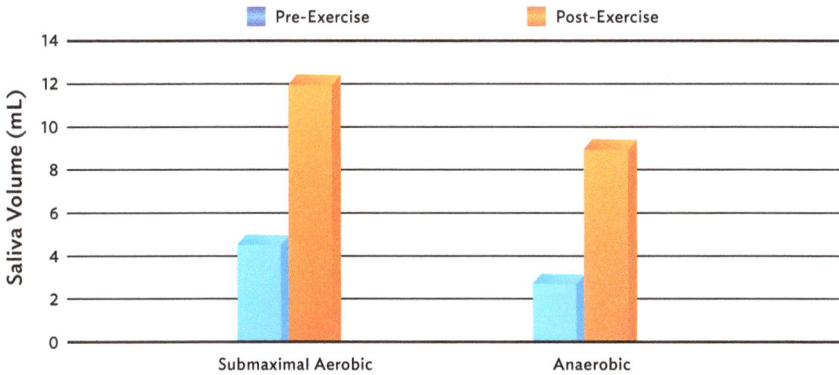

Figure 2.15. Mean lactate concentration produced from 24 and 8 subjects participating in submaximal aerobic and anaerobic exercise, respectively [95]. Saliva was collected over a 10-minute period immediately following the exercise test.

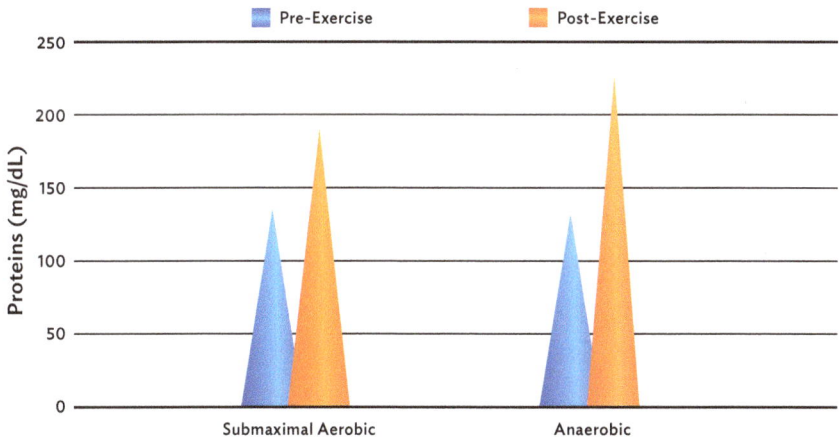

Figure 2.16. Mean protein concentration produced from 22 and 13 subjects participating in submaximal aerobic and anaerobic exercise, respectively [95]. Saliva was collected over a 10-minute period immediately following the exercise test.

anaerobic activity did produce significantly lower magnesium content while the nine-minute exercise had no effect. Also, potassium content significantly increased in both exercise tests, and, in conjunction with observed protein secretions, may reflect the body's sympathetic response to exercise.

Altogether, within 10 minutes of exercise cessation, the participants displayed increased viscosity (e.g., from lactate, protein, and potassium) and reduced saliva flow rates [95]. Similarly, saliva flow was greatly reduced in exercise-to-exhaustion tests at 80% and 55% maximum oxygen intake [98]. While these results are indicative of exercise performed near, at, or above the anaerobic threshold, low or moderate intensity exercises may not elicit the same salivary responses: for instance, saliva viscosity (due in part to increases in carbohydrate and glycoprotein mucin [MUC5B] concentrations and/or secretions) increased after 15 minutes of low-to-moderate intensity exercise, but saliva flow remained at pre-exercise levels [97]. In the course of rigorous exercise reliance on mouth-breathing is likely to occur [98]: in these instances, acute dehydration effects in the oral environment will occur, with the environment naturally recovering after exercise (especially with the aid of aqueous replenishment).

But for participants in more grueling regimens, additional concerns may also exist: observed in elite athletes, data reveals that repetitive, high-intensity exercise can lead to consistently low levels of mucosal proteins, including the salivary immunoglobulins IgA and IgM [99]. Although the reason for suppression is not yet fully known, reductions in these antibodies limit their ability to interfere with adherence of plaque-forming pathogens, and increases risk for respiratory illnesses [99].

So how might the oral environment be affected in an immuno-compromised situation? In head and neck cancer patients receiving radiotherapy, significant reduction in salivary proteins (including IgA, lysozyme, lactoferrin, etc.) occurs during treatment (e.g., 8 weeks) and persists (at least) three months post-therapy [100]. Concomitant with this decline is the increase in *Streptococcus mutans* [100], which suggests diminished efficacy of immunoglobulins and other protective proteins [92,94,99–101]. And, this study echoes a separate one discussed above on the ability of certain microbes to flourish in a saliva-poor environment [93].

I have opened the discussion on the importance of saliva from the perspective of its restriction and the effects on plaque pH and microbial diversity, which, in turn, are heavily influenced by, for example, moisture, antibodies, and proteins. But there is another key role of saliva, and this role was published by Dr. Head in 1912 [87]. So profound was this newly discussed role, that Dr. Brown of Milwaukee, Wisconsin, provided his commentary on Dr. Head's presentation: *"I believe that when Dr. Head has established the facts pertaining to saliva and enamel as he has presented them today . . . then saliva will have a significance that we have never before accorded it."* In conclusion to this presentation, Dr. Head commented, *"I cannot help feeling that the enamel is undergoing a series of changes, a sort of unseen action in itself, and that it is capable in its own molecular being of softening and hardening. . . ."* Of course, what Dr. Head is referring to is the ability of saliva to reharden (or, 'remineralize' [102]) softened enamel.

Dr. Head constructed perhaps the first (if not *the* first) microhardness apparatus designed for use by researchers in the life sciences. He used his invention to record measurements on enamel specimens exposed to acids from chemical reagents or fruits—sometimes diluted with water or saliva—as well as his own saliva. His measurements enabled observations that saliva restrains the softening power of acids yet also strengthens weakened enamel specimens, with the latter especially surprising to him (and his contemporaries) as the enamel component was thought to be "dead" or "inert," given its situs relative to dental pulp.

Some electrolytes secreted by salivary glands include calcium, phosphate, potassium, sodium, chloride, and iodide [103], with calcium and phosphate ions especially key in the dynamic remineralization and demineralization processes [104]. In fact, saliva is recognized as a key source of minerals driving formation of the hypercalcified layer associated with incipient lesions [102,105,106]. And, several decades after Dr. Head's pioneering work, by way of physical changes in the indentations from a diamond-shaped hardness indenter (i.e., Knoop), the quantitative demonstration of increased surface microhardness from synthetic calcium and phosphate solutions—with or without fluoride—confirmed the ability of softened enamel to be strengthened [86].

Realizing a healthy oral environment relies on access to saliva, in the event plaque is left undisturbed—for whatever reason, including poor hygiene practices, challenging medical situations, or otherwise—then salivary action will have reduced efficacy.

An excellent example is observed with patients wearing orthodontic brackets, where proper cleaning around the brackets typically remains elusive over the course of the intervention: the combination of bracket topography and poor lavaging reduces salivary accessibility (as well as any topical treatment), thus creating an environment favoring microbial adhesion and colonization [107–109]. This common iatrogenic situation leads to increased bacterial counts, plaque polysaccharides, and lower pH [107], where demineralization about the orthodontic fixtures ensues [108,109]. Long recognized clinically, incipient lesions can form within one month of bracket placement [108], and may affect, for instance, at least two-thirds of orthodontic patients [109].

Another problem area related to the reason many opt for orthodontic intervention is the relief of overcrowding and tight interproximal spaces. Again, limited salivary access (and minimal plaque disruption) can lead to tooth decay [1,11,110]; but, once relieved (even 10 years later!), little to no decay occurs [111,112].

Ergo, the aforementioned examples and discussion underline the multifunctionality of saliva. And, to ensure the benefits of saliva are realized, it is imperative that all oral surfaces have as much access to and contact by saliva. Of course, this is accomplished by disrupting plaque traps and dislodging foodstuff particulates, usually by brushing, flossing, and/or rinsing.

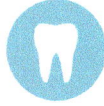

CHAPTER THREE

Ultrastructural Characteristics of Healthy (Sound) Enamel

IN THIS CHAPTER I PROVIDE SOME KEY DETAILS related to the microscopic assembly of enamel. Examining details of intra- and interprismatic enamel architecture can provide insight into demineralization and remineralization processes.

Microscopically, top and cross-sectional views of healthy enamel are shown in **Figures 3.1** [113] and **3.2** [114], respectively, and correspond generally to the enamel crowns shown in the column of images in **Figure 4.1** [115] in the next chapter. The top-view of enamel in **Figure 3.1** reveals scale-like topology, manifesting imperfect lobes aligned in parallel rows and finely resolved on three sides, but with the

Examining details of intra- and interprismatic enamel architecture can provide insight into demineralization and remineralization processes.

fourth side blending into a band-like region. These lobes are comprised of some 10,000 individually closely-packed crystallites collectively referred to as a 'prism body' or 'rod', and evolve from calcium-binding phosphoprotein secretions (i.e., amelogenin, ameloblastin, and enamelin) by a single ameloblast [116,117]. The negative image in **Figure 3.1** helps resolve three subregions of enamel (i.e., "head": H; "tail": T; interprismatic: IP), where the lobe "head" marks the growth front of the prism body and fades into the narrower "tail" region as the ameloblast becomes displaced and crystallite growth eventually ceases. This patterned arrangement of enamel can also be described as having keyhole-shaped prisms sheathed in a three-quarter arcade [118], and is addressed in greater detail below.

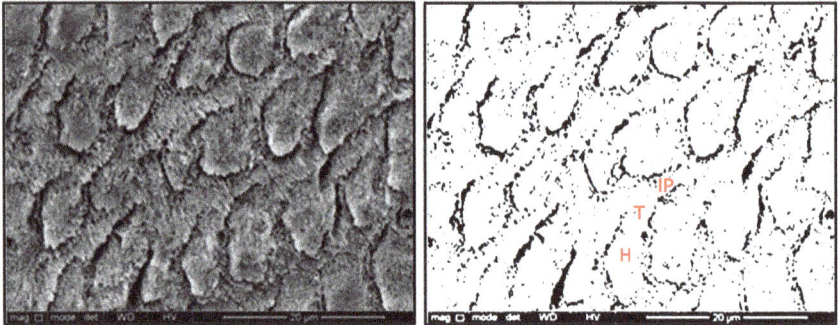

Figure 3.1. Top-view scanning electron micrographs of sound enamel at 5,000x magnification modified from [113]. The image on the right is a negative of the image on the left, and contains three sets of letters where H and T refer to the "head" and "tail" prism (or rod) components, respectively, while IP is the interprismatic region. Scale bars in the image footers correspond to 20 μm.

Both the "head" and "tail" regions are also referred to as the intraprismatic material [117]. The sizes of the 10,000 or so crystallites within the "head" of the prism vary according to the type and variation of the enamel [116,118–120]. As discussed previously and shown in **Figure 3.2**, transmission electron microscopy experiments reveal crystallite thickness on the order of about 26 nm and widths about 68 nm for permanent enamel, though the lengths vary considerably and can be quite long [27,29,31,33,118–121]. As observed with electron microscopy (e.g., **Figure 3.2**), the porosity within the "head" component is fairly tight, with nanosized channels or elongated pores (diameters between 1 and 10 nm) interspersed among the myriad crystalline laths [118,120–122]. And while the "head" crystallites exhibit preferred orientations within the prism plane as well as along the c axis, in contrast, "tail" crystallites appear to be aligned prominently along the c axis, especially with respect to the (002) plane [118]. Based on measured density measurements of enamel mineral content (about 87% by volume, v/v) [123], the "head" and "tail" regions of the keyhole-shaped prism bodies account for about 66% (by volume, v/v) of mature enamel (and, about 60% for primary enamel) [117].

Fueled by ameloblast activity during enamel formation, junctions naturally emerge at the growth edges of neighboring prism bodies, reflecting the imperfect meshing of mixed-crystallite orientations. These junctions comprise the interprismatic zone (e.g., IP in **Figure 3.1**). Three-quarter junctions formed about prism "heads" clearly reveal poor crystallite interlacing. As noted in the prism body demarcations in **Figure 3.1**, the fade of a prism body "tail" into the "head" of the subtended prism front appears relatively relaxed: here, crystallite spatial

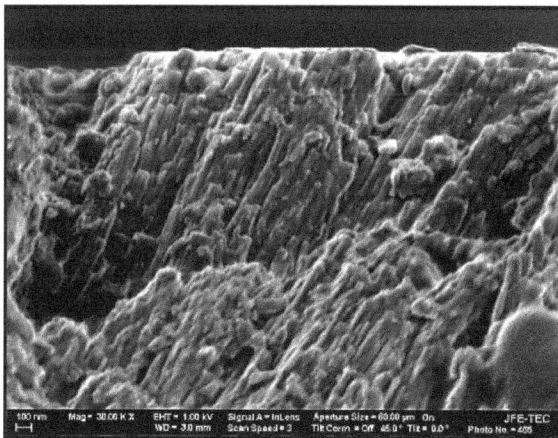

Figure 3.2. Scanning electron micrograph of a sound enamel cross-section at 30,000x magnification [114]. Scale bar in the image footer corresponds to 100 nm.

confinement and differences in growth kinetics are relieved, in part, through crystallite splay [118,120], with preferred crystallite orientations (which, as discussed above, are limited but prominent within the "tail" region) fanning up to an average of 40° from the prism axis [118,122]. The abutments about the intraprismatic material naturally produce increased porosity, with some pore diameters extending, for instance, up to about 60 nm [120,121,124,125]. Supported with the morphological details in **Figure 3.1**, this environment accounts for about one-quarter (~ 24%) of the volume of secondary enamel; for primary enamel, the fraction is even higher (~ 30%) [117,126].

As discussed above, the imperfect nature of crystallite growth and orientation leads to heterogeneous microporosity. Still, are there other factors involved? Adsorption experiments using different sorbates (e.g., krypton, water, methanol), along with thermal evaluations, point to the existence, confirmation, and importance of non-inorganic constituents in enamel: proteins and water.

Drying and ashing experiments reveal a relatively low protein-aceous weight fraction of enamel, which likely remains as residue from the original matrix proteins (e.g., ameloblast secretory proteins) [122] and may be as high as 1 wt. % [16,122,124,127,128]. Supporting the molecular sieve view of enamel [129], adsorbate experiments demonstrate an apparent constriction of pores due to organic matter [124,128,130,131,132]. Therefore, the existence of insoluble proteins [133] contributing to porosity ultimately bears on enamel permeability of various molecular species (e.g., undissociated and dissociated acids, minerals, and ions).

Similar studies probing water content reveal the presence of 'free' and 'bound' water, with variable measured water content (e.g., based on age, tooth, and site), but likely residing between 2% and 6% by volume [130,132,134,135]. Though 'bound' water (e.g., as hydroxyls in the crystallites, or that adsorbed by proteins) persists at low pressures [131], 'free' (i.e., labile) water also contributes significantly to the total water content [135]. Supported in part with data obtained from diffusion experiments, an approximate measure of microporosity may be related to labile water content [132].

The size and extent of enamel porosity is clearly affected by crystallite orientation and occupancy of proteins within pores. But these assessments critically depend on several factors, including the nature of the tooth and the experimental methodology used to probe porosity. Here is a glimpse into the studies elucidating pore characteristics, and will be followed by a short commentary on enamel microporosity.

Adsorption experiments reveal micropores smaller than 2 nm are especially adept at retaining water [131]. Further still, imbibition experiments utilizing a variety of refracting organic molecules (e.g., water, quinolone, alcohols) reveal molecular sieve-like action extends to pores having sizes less than 0.5 nm, with water demonstrating the greatest form birefringence in enamel (i.e., penetration) [129]. The existence of pores smaller than 10 nm has been associated with highly constricted pores within the organic matrix [130] and/or nanogaps residing within (e.g., dislocations, small angle boundaries, or atomic vacancies [26,27] or between (e.g., observed in **Figure 3.2** [114], and [118,120,121]) crystallites.

In further investigations, pore distributions probed with water have been obtained for canine teeth (0.7 nm and 1.3 nm), and incisors and molars (1 nm and 2.5 nm) [128]. When the water adsorption data are modeled to an elongated or cylindrical pore network, estimated surface areas (e.g., from about 4 to 9 m^2g^{-1} with water as the sorbate) appear to reflect crystallite characteristics within intraprismatic enamel [118,120–122]. Interestingly, these characteristics are similar to those obtained for modified forms of a popular carbon allotrope: bundles of alumina-hematite-seeded carbon nanotubes [136].

In contrast, for enamel exposed to a much larger sorbate (i.e., krypton), a low porosity (~ 0.1%) but broad distribution of pore radii (extending from 0.7 nm to around 30 nm, with the majority of the pore radii between 4 and 10 nm) were obtained. Calculated surface areas based on laminar porosity are an order of magnitude lower relative to experiments with water (i.e., ~ 0.4 m^2g^{-1} with krypton) [124]. When coupled with electron microscopy imaging where calculations estimate the mean prism junction surface area of permanent teeth (~ 0.23 m^2g^{-1} [117]), these data strongly suggest the relatively larger porosity (i.e., mesoporosity) fits the interprismatic junction profile [124,125].

Notwithstanding the microporosity data assembled to this point, there exists heterogeneous porosity in enamel that extends over three orders of magnitude and involves molecular sieve action (for sizes less than 0.5 nm), microporosity (for sizes less than 2 nm, which may also overlap the sieve region), and mesoporosity (for sizes between 2 and 60 nm). In consideration of this heterogeneity, contributing features to microporosity include the possibility of point defects in crystallites [26] and arranged rows of pores flanking the central lattice (Retzius) striation [122].

Within enamel, water and protein exist, though the nature of both remains of some debate (see for example [124,127–132] and the references therein). Further, variability in pore size assessments can frustrate those studying or reviewing this topic (including me!). But this review was necessary in order to better understand how the enamel framework may become degraded with acids. The intra- and interprismatic zones discussed here manifest unique characteristics that ultimately bear on enamel demineralization, which is discussed in the next chapter.

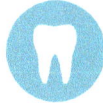

CHAPTER FOUR

Demineralization of Enamel Structure

IT IS CLEAR THAT MICROBIAL PLURALITY and oral ecosystem complexity underline the view that dental decay arises from a nonspecific pathogenic perspective (see, for example, [45]). In previous chapters I have addressed the production of fermented acids by bacterial species as well as the microscopic nature of enamel. In this chapter, I present the chemical underpinnings of the destruction of enamel due to acid attack. For further information, the interested reader is kindly directed to the references provided in this chapter.

The acids imparting enamel-dissolving damage include those produced from microbial influence and those that act directly on the tooth structure without the microbial 'middleman.'

The acids imparting enamel-dissolving damage include those produced from microbial influence (e.g., fermentation of carbohydrates) [84,137] and those that act directly on the tooth structure without the microbial 'middleman' (e.g., dietary or health/behavior-related acids)

[138]. Both of these demineralization processes (i.e., caries and erosion) will be discussed, along with dentinal hypersensitivity, which can develop from either caries or erosive damage. First, caries-based demineralization is presented.

Dental caries—clinical observations

Given that metabolism of carbohydrates produces acids (e.g., as shown previously in **Figures 2.8** thru **2.10** based on ref [84]) leading to tooth decay, clinically speaking, what do carious teeth look like? **Figure 4.1** reveals top (left column) and sagittal (right column) views of varying stages of tooth decay involving the enamel and dentin of molar teeth [115].

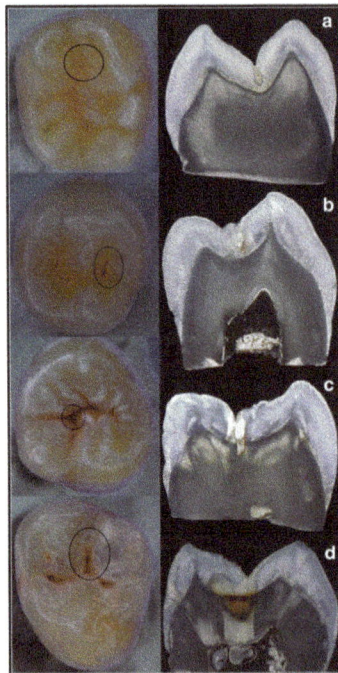

Figure 4.1. Photographic (left column) and histological (right column) images of molars with varying levels of decay (from [115]). The circles highlight the region of interest as shown in the corresponding histologic images. The four sets of images correspond to decay in outer (a) and inner (b) enamel, and then enamel plus outer (c) and inner (d) dentin.

An example where invasive intervention was required to repair a previously restored tooth is shown in **Figure 4.2**. In this case, the afflicted tooth exhibited cavitation extending from the enamel and into dentin. The original restoration, though functional for a time (in this case lasting more than 10 years), debonded from the tooth, thus requiring follow-on intervention.*

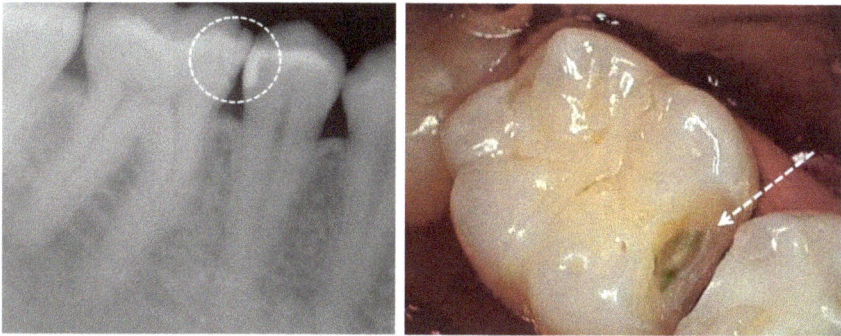

Figure 4.2. Clinical images (courtesy of Dr. Chris Hardin) of the author's mandibular molar with caries experience. The white dashed circle in the X-ray image (left) highlights the failure of the original restorative material. The clinical photograph (right) depicts the size and nature of the afflicted interproximal surface (white arrow). Phosphoric acid etch was used in lesion excavation, and necessarily extended into dentin.

*NOTE:

As explained in the caption, this failed restoration pertains to one of my teeth: so in addition to sharing my perspectives, I'm literally revealing a part of myself. And, yes, I was very surprised when the restoration failure happened, as it occurred during one of my routine flossing events and I didn't have prior experience with this. In fact, at first I didn't know if I had somehow chipped a tooth, or if it was a hardened food particle (e.g., popcorn kernel) lodged between teeth, or something else, but fortunately I was at home and was able to schedule an immediate appointment with my highly talented dentist—thank you again, Dr. Chris Hardin!

The examples above demonstrate stages of more advanced tooth decay but began with incipient enamel lesions. The initial stages of demineralization (or incipient lesion formation), though certainly unfavorable, can be arrested and even reversed under certain conditions (more on remineralization will be discussed in Chapters 8 and 9). Thus, enamel manifesting incipient lesions is routinely used to explore various aspects of tooth decay, including demineralization and remineralization processes, and is discussed in greater detail below.

Demineralization ensues when the remineralization-demineralization balance gets tipped unfavorably [34]. As shown in **Figure 4.1**, acid-induced demineralization begins in outer enamel, and if allowed to progress, extends through to the inner enamel, crosses the enamel-dentin junction, and then enters dentin. Clinically, the imbalance that initially produces net demineralization is marked by the evolution of chalky 'white spots' (i.e., incipient lesion formation), like those shown in the labial surfaces of the anterior teeth in **Figure 4.3** [139].

While incipient lesions in labial or buccal surfaces (e.g., like those in **Figure 4.3**) may be readily visible to the clinician, imaging techniques, such as soft X-ray imaging [140], fluorescence [141], and digital photography [115], are often necessary to explore more obscure sites (e.g., interproximal or occlusal regions).

Closer inspection of the incipient lesion reveals demineralization extends beyond the enamel surface and into the enamel subsurface.

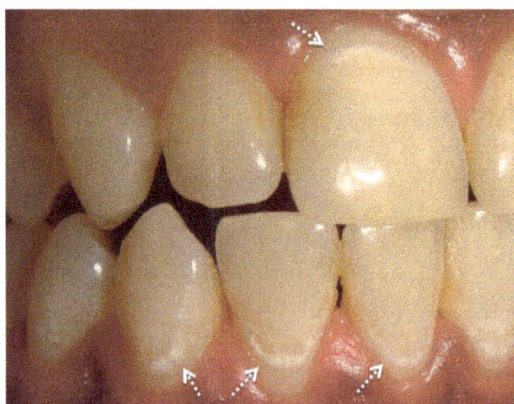

Figure 4.3. Clinical photograph of anterior teeth manifesting white-spot lesions near the gingival margin (as indicated with white arrows) [139].

Figure 4.4 (which shows a negative image of the right-half of the histological image **d** of **Figure 4.1**) allows one to easily reconcile bulk mineral loss (as indicated by the red arrow) that develops during lesion formation. Demineralization creates irregular-shaped regions largely devoid of mineral; however, microdensitometric measurements reveal islands of residual mineral within these largely mineral-free zones [142]. The thin layer of mineral capping the lesion is typically different than sound enamel [102,140], and is comprised of expanded prismatic material [30], or even aprismatic enamel [143].

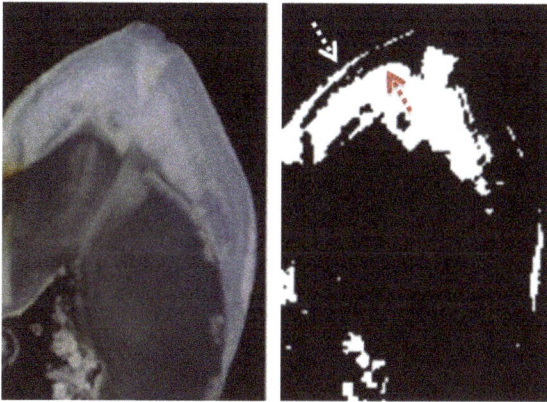

Figure 4.4. Original (left) and negative (right) histological images from the **Figure 4.1** [115] carious molar (d). Only the right-half of the crown is shown for purposes of discussion. The red dotted arrow indicates the dark lesion zone in the carious enamel crown. The white dotted arrow points to a thin layer of mineral formed during lesion formation, which is visible in the left-hand image and materially differs from sound enamel.

Dental caries—laboratory investigations

Synthetic approaches that successfully emulate natural lesions, while imperfect, allow for robust studies into caries formation, progression, arrestment, and reversal. One artful approach that I have used in much of my research involves a partially apatite-saturated blend of polyacrylic acid—which simulates the biofilm that adheres to (and protects) the tooth surface—and lactic acid—which is a predominant product among the several pathogenic acids produced by cariogenic bacteria as previously discussed [144]. This demineralization solution effects subsurface mineral loss *and* surface softening without surface erosion and/or affecting demineralization/remineralization processes [144,145]; in turn, this allows for facile, reproducible assessments at both the enamel surface and subsurface. These artificial lesions also demonstrate sensitivity to fluoride and remineralization, allowing for investigations into demineralization/remineralization phenomena [146–148]. Importantly, these simulated lesions are a staple of many of the global manufacturers who routinely research, develop, and evaluate topical fluoridated modalities in compliance with various regulatory bodies, including the United States Food & Drug Administration [149].

Because simulated white-spot lesions are routinely utilized for study and evaluation as surrogates for clinical incipient lesions, it is important to detail characteristics of these lesions. An example of the surface appearance of the simulated lesions is shown in **Figure 4.5**. In this example, the demineralized surface is smooth but bears modified three-quarter arcade (or, honeycomb-like) patterns reflective of sound enamel (e.g., **Figure 3.1**). Within this framework, the intraprismatic material appears especially susceptible to significant demineralization, resulting in bulk loss of mineral [125,126].

Some studies reveal that during acidic attack, central lesion cores (average diameters about 6 nm) develop orthogonal to the (100) plane, with subsequent demineralization following the longitudinal axis of the crystallite and spreading laterally to the equatorial faces (e.g., (100) and (120) planes) [33]; sometimes, the core destruction splits the crystallite into two halves [31]. While defects, missing atoms, or even the occupancy of easily dissolved components may reside within the crystallite cores [23,26,27,31,33,123], initial acidic insults along the facets and periphery are also observed [27], thus demonstrating demineralization is not necessarily site-specific.

Multiple length-scale images of sound and incipient enamel lesions are shown in **Figures 4.6** and **4.7**. The brightfield images reveal the

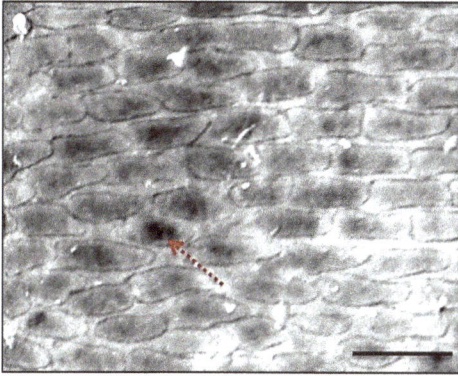

Figure 4.5. Scanning electron micrograph (top view) of an incipient enamel lesion at 3,500x magnification. The demineralization was performed by immersion in a lactic acid-polymer solution partially saturated with respect to hydroxyapatite (pH 5). Scale bar corresponds to 20 μm. The red dashed arrow indicates bulk loss of intraprismatic mineral.

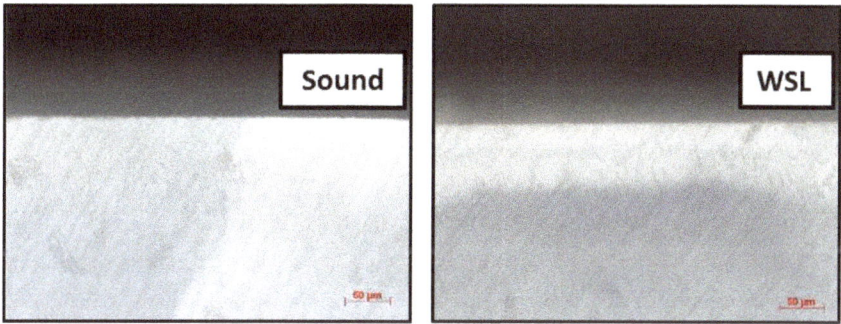

Figure 4.6. Brightfield reflected light images (200x magnification) of randomly selected enamel slice cross-sections for Sound and artificially demineralized (i.e., white-spot lesion, WSL) enamel (from [114]). The demineralization was performed by immersion in a lactic acid-polymer solution partially saturated with hydroxyapatite (pH 5). In each image a 50 μm scale bar is shown in red on the bottom right.

canted orientations of the crystallites, and also reveal the difference in optical density which extends to about 75 μm in the incipient lesion. At 2,000x magnification, the differences in density are even more clear, with sound enamel manifesting solid, nondescript crystallite packing, while the lesioned enamel bears crystallite ridges with overlaying texture; these differences are further resolved at 30,000x magnification, where lesioned enamel comprises shorter but wider crystalline fragments [27], while sound enamel manifests groupings of long and relatively tightly packed crystallites.

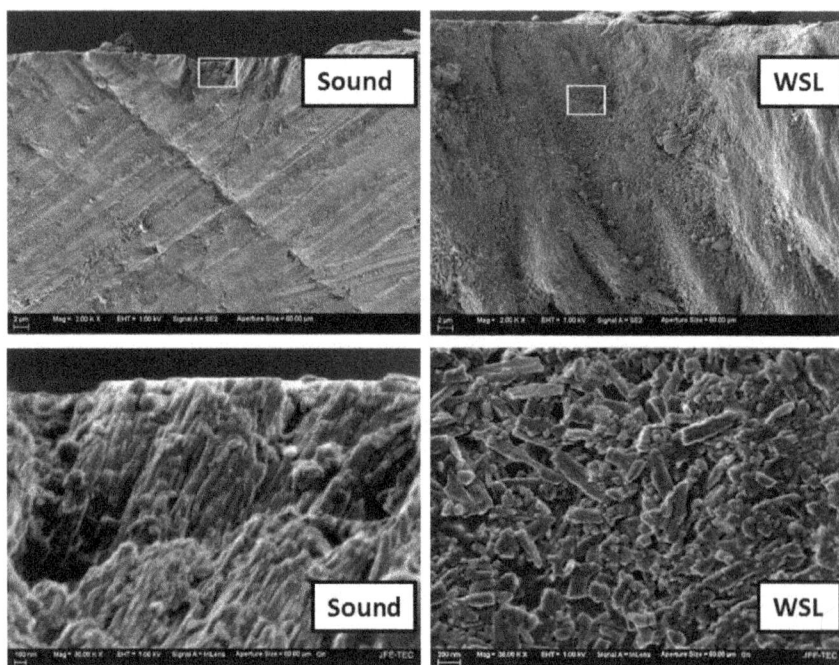

Figure 4.7. Scanning electron micrographs of Sound and white-spot lesion (WSL) enamel cross-sections at 2,000x (top row) and 30,000x (bottom row) magnification (from [114]). The demineralization was performed by immersion in a lactic acid-polymer solution partially saturated with hydroxyapatite (pH 5). In the top row, the scale bars correspond to 2 μm for both Sound and WSL. The 30,000x images (bottom row) correspond to the white box region shown in each 2,000x image (top row). In the bottom row, scale bars in the image footer correspond to 100 nm (Sound) and 200 nm (WSL).

Concomitant with the loss of crystallite density, size, and packing is the reduction in physical strength; as measured with a Knoop hardness indenter and shown in **Figure 4.8**, the microhardness of the simulated incipient enamel lesion is comparatively low (e.g., 10x lower near the enamel surface), down to depths approaching 80 μm. This lesion size is consistent with the brightfield image depicting lower optical density (**Figure 4.6**). Comparison between the WAXD and SAXS (wide-angle X-ray diffraction and small-angle X-ray scattering, respectively) patterns in the **Figure 4.8** inset reveals the loss of periodicity within the enamel lesion. The WAXD contribution of the finely resolved Debye ring (corresponding to the (100) equatorial reflection) reflects hydroxyapatite (HAP) crystallites [150–152]. The bright, sharply resolved but diminutive SAXS contribution suggests the presence of nonmineral material such as water, proteins, or even micopores manifest within intercrystallite spacings [151]. The SAXS signal appears more pronounced for lesioned enamel and likely indicates a profound shift in surface area due to evolution of voids (e.g., micro- and mesoporosity)

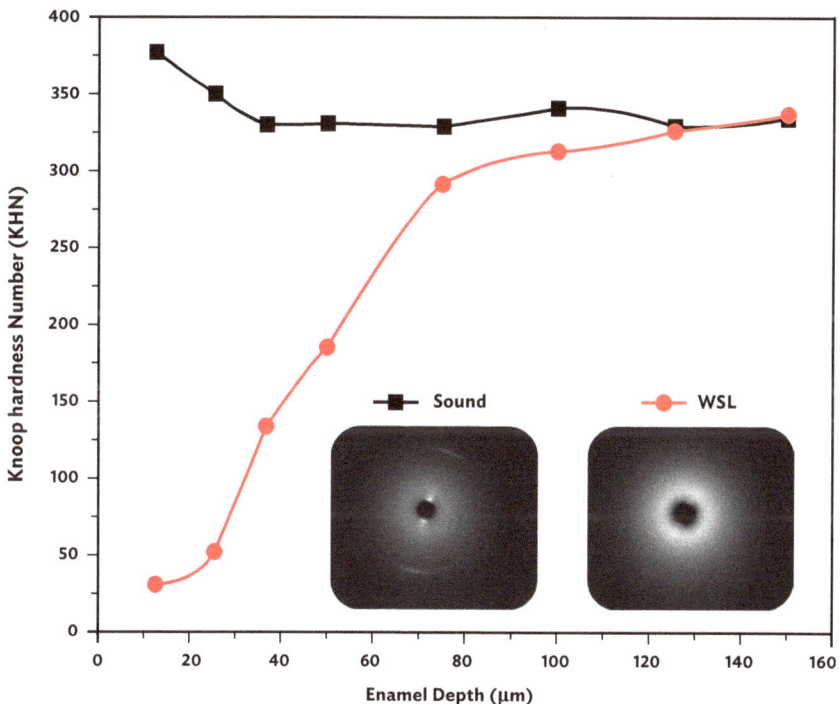

Figure 4.8. Cross-sectional microhardness line profiles for Sound and white-spot lesion (WSL) enamel (from [114]). Obtained in a separate experiment, the inset in the lower right depicts the simultaneous collection of WAXD and SAXS patterns within each enamel cross-section (about 30 µm from the enamel surface).

during lesion formation [27,151–155]; in this case, the relatively intense smear-like SAXS component suggests the lesion formation process produced substantial crystallite dissolution along all three crystal axes. While the relatively faint (100) reflection underlines loss of mineral, the morphology shown in the 30,000x electron micrograph points to wider [27], shorter and randomly-oriented crystallites. When coupled with the diminished microhardness measurements, the bulk mineral loss [156–157] and relaxed packing of shorter, mixed-orientation crystallites are characteristics of the incipient lesion.

As discussed above and shown in **Figure 4.9**, ultrastructural studies of carious lesion formation indicate dissolution of enamel may initiate within the (100) HAP plane where defects (e.g., edge dislocations, screw dislocations, small angle boundaries, atomic vacancies or rotations) in the imperfect enamel abound [23,26,27,31,33,123]. **Figure 4.9** supports these assessments, with significant reduction in the (100) periodicity of the white-spot lesion as shown in the WAXD profile (top graph) [114,151,152]. Also within the equatorial plane, the significant rise in SAXS signal, which peaks around 36 μm (bottom graph), suggests lesion formation effects a distribution of voids [114,151,152] ranging in size and shape that evolve from modifications in surfaces areas within intra- and interprismatic enamel; in essence, an overall increase in porosity is produced. Within the subsurface region it may also be expected that islands of mineral (varying in size and shape) may remain as part of the lesion formation process and, therefore, contribute to SAXS signal from crystallite surfaces [142]. The nearly concomitant recoveries of the WAXD and SAXS intensities around 100 μm in the WSL enamel are indicative of the nature of these shallow incipient lesions [114]; of course, these characteristics are not absolute for all lesions and, therefore, are expected to differ from other nonsimilar simulated lesions, including larger subsurface lesions [151].

The above discussion on incipient caries lesions emphasized lactic acid and the creation of subsurface lesions. Next, I present brief overviews

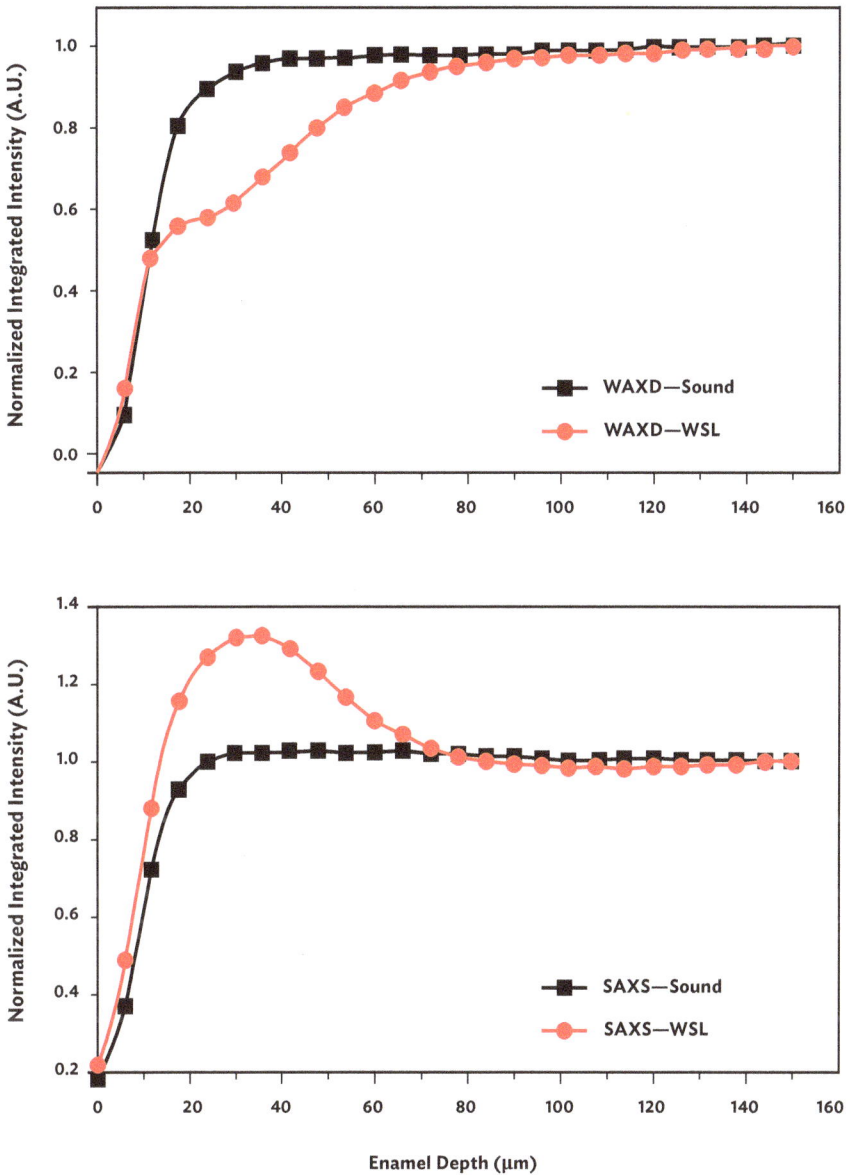

Figure 4.9. WAXD (top graph) and SAXS (bottom graph) profiles as a function of enamel depth (from the surface down to 150 μm) for Sound and white-spot lesion (WSL) enamel (from [114]). In each graph, the mean normalized integrated intensities are shown for the (100) reflection (WAXD, top graph) and small-angle equatorial scatter (SAXS, bottom graph).

of the effects of acids on dental erosion and dentinal hypersensitivity. As a number of excellent reviews abound in these specialized topics, I purposely limited my commentaries, and the reader is encouraged to explore the references used herein as desired. And as a teaser for Chapter 5, the chemical signatures of the acids leading to caries, erosion or hypersensitivity will be presented in greater detail.

Dental erosion and dentinal hypersensitivity

To begin, erosion is described as demineralization by acid attack on the tooth structure in the absence of plaque, producing surface roughening en route to significant mineral loss. Chronic erosive processes render the enamel weak, and can lead to tooth wear when subject to abrasive forces (e.g., by tongue, mastication, or even toothbrushing) [158]. An example of eroded enamel produced from a seven-day immersion in acetic acid (adjusted to pH 4) is shown in **Figure 4.10** [113].

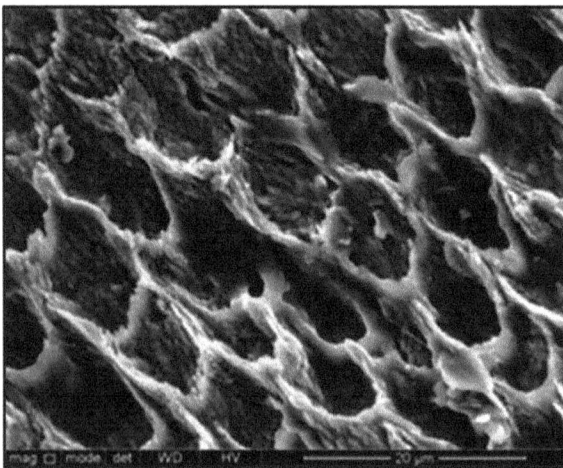

Figure 4.10. Top-view scanning electron micrograph of eroded enamel at 5,000x magnification (from [113]). Erosion was achieved through immersion in acetic acid (adjusted to pH 4) for seven days. Scale bar in the image footer corresponds to 20 μm.

Although **Figure 4.10** details surface morphological effects of erosion, the erosion process also extends to the enamel subsurface, although the subsurface characteristics are generally not as pronounced relative to caries lesions due to fundamental differences in the kinetics of formation; still, subsurface damage occurs at and below the enamel surface, the specifics of which are sensitive to various factors including pH and concentration of erosive acid [159–161]. And because erosion is not dependent on bacterial fermentation, erosive damage occurs over shorter timescales relative to carious lesions. As an example, laboratory studies demonstrate erosion from citrus fruit or beverages can occur in less than 15 minutes [162]; in contrast, incipient enamel lesions created in the laboratory usually require several days at minimum [144–147].

Just as habitual tooth grinding or uncorrected malocclusion may lead to attrition caries [163], unmanaged eroded enamel can lead to tooth wear [158]. Factors influencing the extent of tooth wear include repetitive intake of extrinsic acids (i.e., acidic beverages and foodstuffs) [158,164,165], as well as unhealthy behavior (e.g., bulimia) [166] or genetic disorders [167]. Additionally, aggressive exercise (including competitive swimming in gas-chlorinated pools [168]) can also impart erosive tooth wear [169]. Whatever its origin, the onset of erosion softens enamel, rending the tooth more susceptible to tooth wear, especially in regions where preexisting erosion has taken place [170]; due to the protective nature of the oral environment, erosive damage is largely based on chronic exposures to acid attack [158,161].

Unchecked demineralization dissolves enamel structure, progressing to cavitation and tooth wear, where the underlying coronal dentin, gingiva-protected tooth root, or in extreme situations, the dental pulp, become exposed (e.g., the clinical photographs of a patient exhibiting significant tooth-structure loss in reference [167] demonstrates the painful reality of rampant decay). In these instances, demineralization extends to both the hard *and* soft tissues, thus leading to dentinal sensitivity to otherwise common stimuli (e.g., temperature, sweetness, and air, fluid and tactile pressure).

Dentinal hypersensitivity is common worldwide [171,172], and espe-cially affects periodontal populations where root sensitivity is reported by nearly all categorical patients [173,174]. The etiology of dentinal hyper-sensitivity is largely but not perfectly understood. The thinning and loss of enamel, especially around the cervical margin, is certainly a dominant factor, while another is the gradual recession of gingiva [172–173,174]. With the loss of enamel from the crown surfaces, the underlying dentin, which is largely comprised of apatite-like mineral, Type I collagen, and water, becomes susceptible to demineralization [176,177]. Similarly, near the pulpal base, the cementum can become compromised as the gingiva recedes, leading to a breakdown in connective tissue [171,173–177].

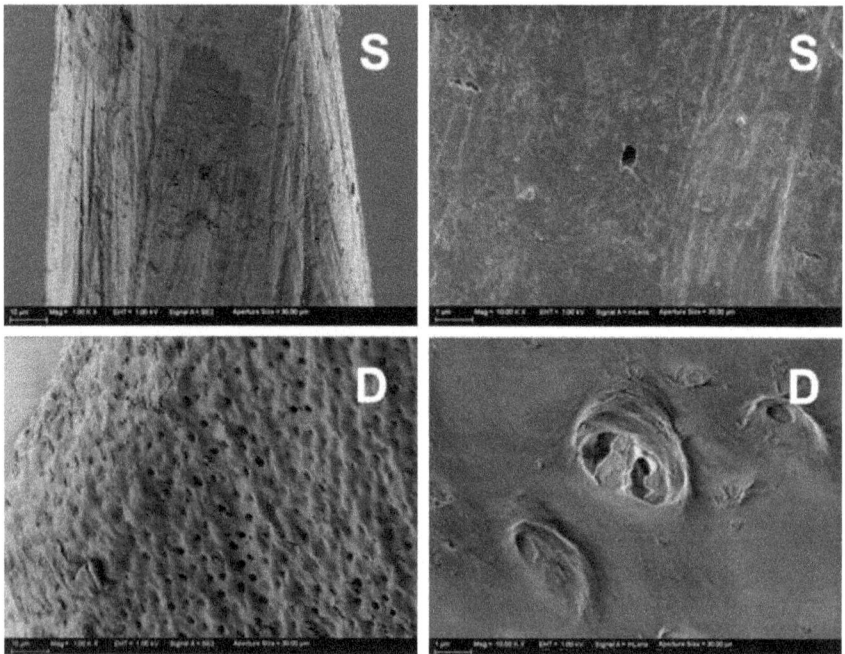

Figure 4.11. Scanning electron micrograph of sound (S, top row) and eroded (D, bottom row) dentin (20-minute immersion in 1% citric acid, pH 3.2) (from [181]). In each row the left and right images correspond to 1,000x (with 10 μm white scale bar on bottom left) and 10,000x (with 1 μm white scale bar on bottom left) magnification, respectively. Note the tubule diameters are heterogeneous in demineralized dentin (bottom row images), and are demonstrably larger compared to sound dentin (top row images).

As destructive processes (e.g., caries, abrasion, and erosion) progress, the integrity of the dentin mantle weakens, leading to, for instance, patency of tubules. The tubules are a complex structure, comprising fluid, minerals, and biological material, and manifest larger diameters near the pulp relative to the dentin-enamel junction [171–177]. When sufficiently demineralized, leakage and disruption of tubular fluid occurs, which in turn affects pulpal nerve receptors [171–176]. Permeability studies have helped identify patency of tubules as a major characteristic of dentinal hypersensitivity [174,178]. The most popular theoretical model supporting permeability studies is known as hydrodynamic theory [179], and has been invoked to support pursuits into desensitization of pulpal nerves and occlusion of dentin tubules [171–176,178–180].

Since dentinal sensitivity usually (but not only!) results from loss of mineral and exposure of dentin [172], it is sensible to explore some characteristics of demineralized dentin. Indications of dentinal caries include discolorations, obvious cavitations or missing tooth structure, and the general unhealthy appearance of the tooth as shown in **Figure 4.1**. Separately, erosion is also associated with dentinal decay but differs in its characteristics (including appearance) with respect to caries, thus warranting further discussion. The following discussion details some key characteristics differentiating sound and eroded dentin substrates.

Morphological images of sound and eroded dentin specimens from extracted bicuspids are shown in **Figure 4.11** [181]. In the figure, the erosion of dentin was achieved in a static solution of 1% citric acid (pH 3.2) for 20 minutes. Like well-worn leather, the intertubular region of eroded dentin appears stressed and contrasts with the relatively 'fresh' appearance of intact dentin. But even more distinctive is the stark comparison with respect to tubule openings: eroded dentin comprises gaping tubule openings, expanding to diameters at least twice as large compared to healthy dentin. These images underline the deleterious effects erosion has on soft dental tissues, depleting the tubular, peritubular, and intertubular regions of mineral [183,184].

From a compositional perspective, the tubular and peritubular dentin regions are rich in calcium and phosphate, but also harbor an appreciable magnesium content [183,184]; therefore, similar to demineralization of enamel apatite where Mg^{2+} is especially susceptible to fermented acids [123], these may also serve as weak points for erosive insults as well [183].

Further insight into the morphology of dentin substrates bearing tubular structures includes noninvasive assessments as shown in the submicron X-ray tomography renderings in **Figures 4.12** and **4.13** [181].

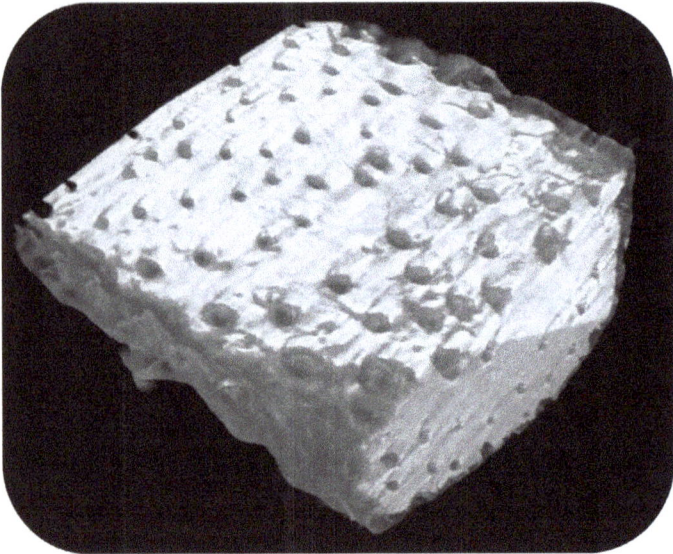

Figure 4.12. 3-D reconstruction of a section of demineralized dentin noninvasively probed using submicron X-ray tomography [181]. In this screenshot, tubule openings are visible on the surface. For the full animation that includes passage through one of the tubules, see [182].

For a unique perspective into a dentin tubule, the reader is encouraged to watch the animation from which the screenshots were obtained from reference [182]. Though the image in **Figure 4.13** indicates a largely parallel alignment of tubules, the reality is that significant variations exist among the teeth and within a tooth [185]; and when coupled with the unique situation of a given person, it is reasonable to eschew a 'one-size-fits-all' approach in assessing and treating one experiencing dental erosion and/or dentinal hypersensitivity. In fact, it may be these inherent variations, which can be extremely difficult clinically to noninvasively probe let alone correct, contribute to different assessment methods and subsequent treatment recommendations of dentinal hypersensitivity [171].

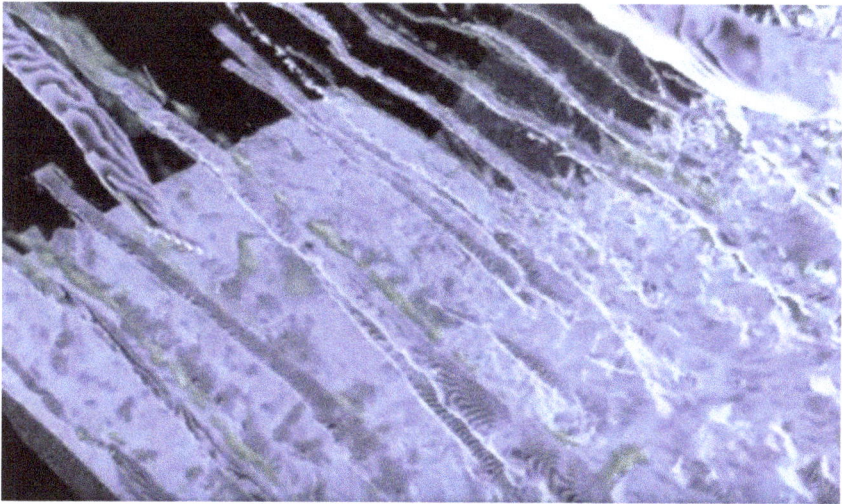

Figure 4.13. 3-D reconstruction of tubule structure within a dentin substrate non-invasively probed using submicron X-ray tomography [181]. In this screenshot, a cross-sectional view from within the dentin in **Figure 4.12** reveals the arrangement and heterogeneity of the dentin tubules. For the full animation, see [182].

Using submicron X-ray tomography, non-destructive depth-dependent assessments of the apatite mineral profiles of sound and eroded dentin can be made, such as shown in **Figure 4.14** [181]. The data trends in the figure reveal clear differences not only between sound and eroded dentin but also between tubular and intertubular dentin within the sound or eroded dentin substrates. For sound intertubular dentin, mean (standard deviation) mineral concentrations of ~ 1.16 (0.05) g·cm^{-3} were obtained across the measurement depth of ~ 4.95 μm; in contrast, sound tubular mineral concentrations diminished almost linearly (R^2

~ 0.97 ± 0.04) from ~ 1.22 (0.15) g·cm^{-3} at the tubule opening down to ~ 0.6 (0.18) g·cm^{-3} at the ~ 4.95 μm depth, and are similar to other tomography experiments (~ 1.4 g·cm^{-3}) [186,187]. This gradual decrease in mineral concentration indicates sound dentin tubules are comprised of multiple constituents and phases, supporting, for instance, ions, water-based fluids, and biologically active agents (including odonto-blasts) [175,176,188]. Such compositional milieu then bears on dentin permeability and biological signaling [173–176,178,188].

Consistent with the morphological differences observed in **Figure 4.11**, the short-term exposure to citric acid produced relatively consistent mean (standard deviation) apatite mineral concentrations within the tubules of ~ 0.15 (0.18) g·cm^{-3} over the same dentin depth (~ 4.95 μm). This rela-tively flat mineral content differs markedly from the tubular mineral profile obtained for sound dentin and indicates the erosive challenge was sufficient in expelling tubular constituents (at least down to ~ 4.95 μm). Relative to the tubular region, the intertubular region remained more resilient to the erosive challenge: here, the mean (standard deviation) mineral concentration increased linearly (R^2 ~ 0.98 ± 0.00) from ~ 1.02 (0.05) g·cm^{-3} to ~ 1.15 (0.06) g·cm^{-3} (at a depth near ~ 1 μm). Despite the differences in the nature of demineralization dentin along with experi-mental differences, these mineral values are similar to that obtained on carious dentin (i.e., between ~ 0.30 and 0.43 g·cm^{-3}) [186,187]. The approximate order of magnitude difference in apatite mineral content between tubular and intertubular regions demonstrates the compositional sensitivity of tubules and underlines the critical importance of the col-lagen framework to dentin durability [173–177,184].

The purpose of this chapter was to explore the sensitivity of the hard and soft components of the tooth to acid attack. Importantly, extrinsic factors, including diet, behavior, or preexisting history of decay were not addressed in order to focus attention solely on the properties of the demineralized tooth. Acknowledging the inherent variation (including anomalies and imperfections) that may exist for a given person or a

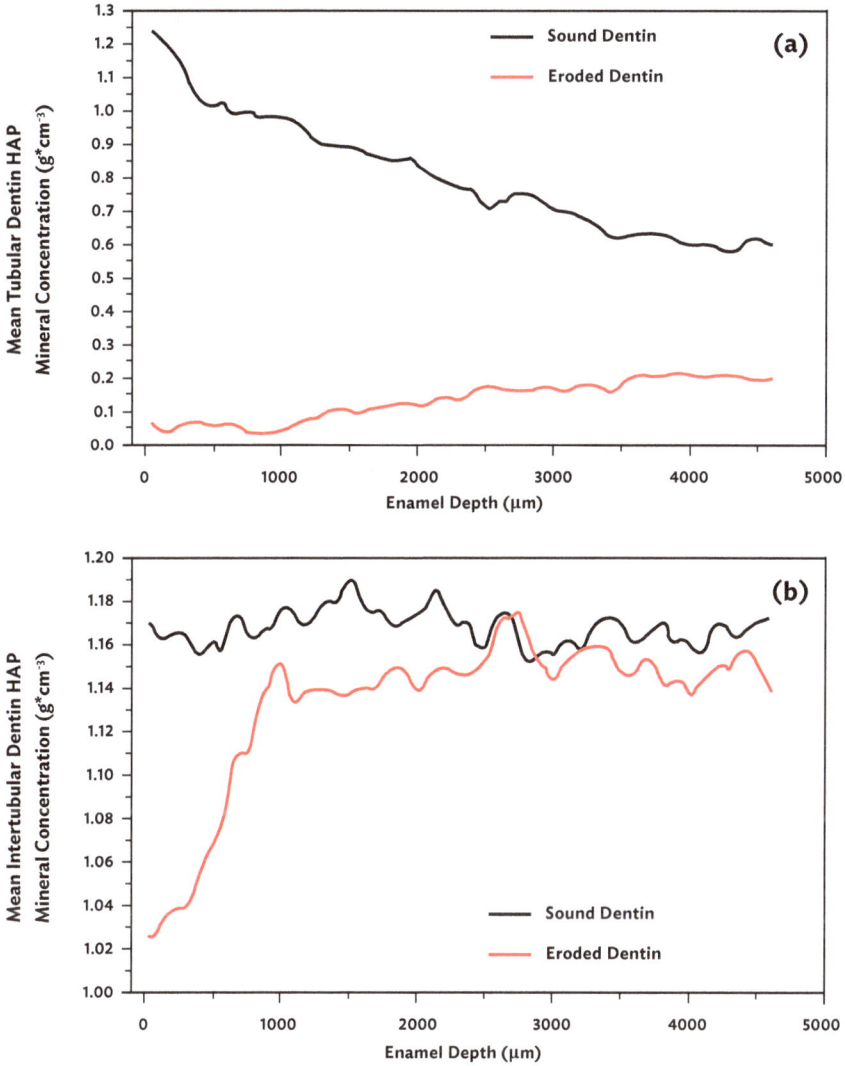

Figure 4.14. Mean mineral (hydroxyapatite, HAP) concentrations for tubular (a) and intertubular (b) regions as a function of depth for sound and eroded dentin from the dentin surface down to 4.95 μm (see [181] for further details).

specific tooth, demineralization of tooth structure generally appears as described in this chapter. Although specific examples were described in some detail, it is important to stress the intrinsic heterogeneity of the structure and properties of the tooth will naturally affect demineralization, such as:

✓ The natural birefringence of enamel [102,122,129,140,189];

✓ Differences in porosity, and subsequently diffusion, from tooth-to-tooth [124,128,130–132,190];

✓ The size, shape, and intermeshing network of tubules within dentin [185];

✓ Range in crystal sizes throughout enamel, including that arising from the repetitive demineralization/remineralization processes that lead to relatively larger crystals within the outermost enamel surfaces contacting the oral environment [27–29,31–33,191–194];

✓ Variability in strength and acid-resistance of enamel due to, for example, defects, composition (e.g., magnesium and carbonate), and low levels of ameloblast activity [26,27,116,123,195,196].

As shown in **Figures 4.5** and **4.10** an important feature shared by both white-spot formation and enamel erosion is the apparent resiliency of the interprismatic junction material [113,162,197]. Though the material within this region is also subject to demineralization, it appears more resistant to demineralization compared to the interprismatic material, and, therefore, commands further perspective. In closing out this chapter, in my view there are three principle factors leading to the relative 'acid-resistance' of the junction, each of which will be followed by a short commentary:

1. The relatively lower specific surface areas of the interprismatic junction pores compared to intraprismatic pores; and,

2. The presence of residual proteinaceous content within the inter-prismatic zones; and,

3. Irregular and discontinuous crystallite interlacing within the interprimastic regions that contrasts with the relative continuity of closely-packed crystallites.

First, while junctions facilitate flow of acids (including dissociated and undissociated constituents) within enamel [125], the intraprismatic material manifests reactive surfaces that essentially serve as the 'targets' for acid attack. As discussed previously, the specific surface areas within the intraprismatic region are more than 10x as large as the junction density pores, and this translates into greater susceptibility to wetting and subsequent demineralization. Perhaps a useful model is that of a shooting target, where the diminishing concentric circles terminate with the bull's eye: with respect to enamel, the large outer circles represent the junction material and its meso- and microporosity [124,128,130,131], while the bull's eye corresponds to the more com-pact intraprismatic material along with the attendant micron-level and submicron-level porosity [118,120,132,135]. These latter characteristics would help explain why acid attack seems to initiate within the intra-prismatic regions [31,33,121].

Second, although relatively low in content, the nature of the protein component may impart significant effects by inhibiting dif-fusion through pores via constriction [128,132,190]; importantly, this may also help protect against demineralization, much like salivary mucins adhere to enamel and provide anti-demineralization protection [63,198,199]. With respect to the latter, the proteins may influence fluid transport of molecular and ionic species (including acids) within the enamel regions [128,130–133,190]. Since much of the organic content appears to be trapped within interprismatic regions (which, therefore, includes the junction material) [117,122,128,130,133,190], the passage of fluid to regions bearing less organic content (i.e., within the intraprismatic regions [31,33,117,121]) will be more susceptible to both demineralization and remineralization processes.

Third and final, closely-packed crystallites manifesting high surface areas help propel the wetting action of water and acidic molecules (whole or dissociated) along the continuous laths. In contrast, the poorly intersecting laths in the interprismatic regions—as well as the "tail" component of the intraprismatic zone—are inherently discontinuous, presenting relatively higher energetic barriers to acid adhesion and subsequent dissolution. Still, fluid readily penetrates throughout the interprismatic region, effecting geometric (e.g., elongations and/or pore widening) and chemical (e.g., formation of non-enamel-like mineral) distortions [110,121,125,143].

Altogether, these three inherent properties of enamel (i.e., surface area, protein content, and crystallite packing) help explain the contrast as to why, during an acid attack, the interprismatic junctions survive attack despite bulk intraprismatic mineral loss. There are likely other factors also in play, to be sure, but it is clear that enamel structure influences the nature of dissolution by acids.

The next chapter takes a closer look at the acids involved in demineralization.

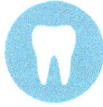

CHAPTER FIVE

On the Nature of Demineralizing Acids

One feature of a dynamic ecosystem is the response to a stimulus. So, the oral environment responds to, for example, foodstuffs, oral hygienic activities, effects from systemic medications, and medical procedures. Although saliva naturally imparts healthy balancing effects by, for instance, offsetting acidic assaults [34,91], often the pace of remineralization, which involves progressions of mineral phases to apatite [200,201], cannot compete with demineralization, and dissolution of enamel mineral ensues. This dynamic balance is critically based on extrinsic and intrinsic variables such as diet, oral hygiene regimen, as well as the quality and quantity of saliva, which can be impaired due to certain medications (e.g., antihistamines) or medical procedures (e.g., chemotherapy treatment) [88,90–94].

Whether demineralization is caries-like or erosive-like, if allowed to progress, acid attack results in bulk mineral loss from enamel, exposed root structure, or dentin (e.g., **Figures 4.1** and **4.2**). Some of the most acid-susceptible targets within tooth mineral include magnesium and carbonate species, missing species, and physical defects [23,26,27,31,

33,116,123,195,196]. But acids differ in more than just name, so what makes some acids more damaging to tooth structure than others?

While I previously touched on the diversity of fermented acids in Chapter 2, in this chapter I explore why and how some acids are more damaging to the teeth than others based on a variety of characteristics including acid strength, diffusion and size of undissociated and dissociated acids, and stability with calcium complexes. The purpose of this important chapter is to establish the chemical basis for the acid-susceptibility of tooth structure. The information presented here helps introduce the nature of acids found in foods or those produced by microbes, and will be discussed in greater detail in Chapter 6. The content discussed herein is imbued with many enlightening references and the reader is encouraged to refer to these as needed.

Whether demineralization is caries-like or erosive-like, if allowed to progress, acid attack results in bulk mineral loss from enamel, exposed root structure, or dentin

The initiation, extent, and rate of enamel dissolution collectively involve many factors including pH, buffer strength, acid type and concentration, and presence of mineralizing ions (e.g., calcium, phosphate, fluoride, magnesium, etc.) [34,144,145,202–207]. Additionally, plaque pH, salivary clearance, and microbial metabolism bear on the availability of acidic species to penetrate into enamel, where microporosity (which is influenced by geometric arrangement, as well as the nature of water, proteins, and crystallite packing as noted previously) and ultrastructure impact acid diffusion (i.e., both dissociated and undissociated) and, therefore, the extent of demineralization [121,124,125,127–132,189–195,202–208]. Nevertheless, in the demineralization equation, acids remain the outsize variable whether enamel dissolution involves microbes [11] or not [209].

Two compilations of acids commonly found in either tooth decay or in foods/beverages are shown in **Figure 5.1** and **Table 5.1**. **Figure 5.1** is arranged according to increasing pK_{a1} (or, decreasing acid strength) for eight acids, while the equilibrium details corresponding to each dissociation are established in **Table 5.1**. Although more acids are involved for sure, I chose those routinely found in at least one of these major areas: microbial fermentation (i.e., lactic, acetic, propionic); laboratory and clinical models involving acids and tooth structure (i.e., lactic, acetic, propionic); and, those commonly found in foods or beverages (i.e., phosphoric, citric, malic, ascorbic, benzoic, acetic).

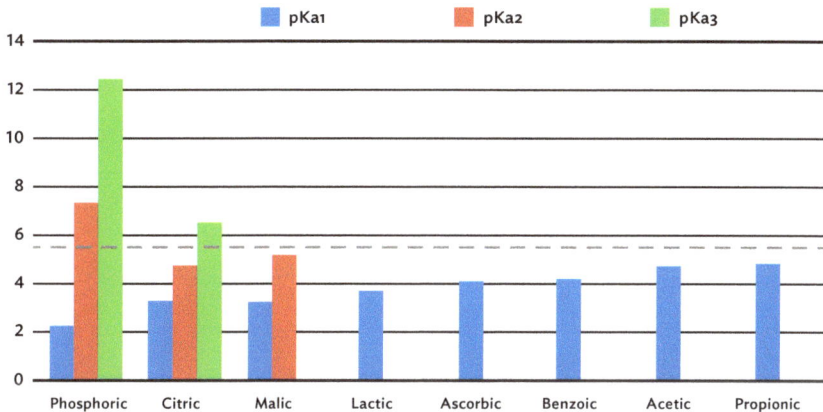

Figure 5.1. Equilibrium dissociation constants for several inorganic and organic acids [210]. The acids are arranged according to increasing pK_{a1} values (i.e., decreasing acid strength). The gray, dashed line approximates a pH threshold for initial demineralization. The equilibrium constituents of these acids are listed in **Table 5.1**.

A comment before pressing further: I have purposely excluded carbonic acid because at pH < 8 (which falls within the range of virtually all comestibles and drinks fit for consumption [210]) this acid (and its dissociated counterparts) is not found in large amounts relative to dissolved carbon dioxide gas, CO_2. The reaction between CO_2 and water to form carbonic acid is kinetically slow, so dissolved CO_2 survives in abundance [211]. Naturally, depressurized (i.e., opened or uncapped) beverages infused with CO_2 will soon 'go flat' (i.e., lose carbonation) once exposed

NOMENCLATURE	SPECIES	EQUILIBRIUM REACTION	DISSOCIATION CONSTANT, pK_a
Phosphoric Acid	H_3PO_4		
Phosphate$^-$	$H_2PO_4^-$	$H_3PO_4 \leftrightarrow H_2PO_4^- + H^+$	$pK_{a1} = 2.16$
Phosphate^{2-}	HPO_4^{2-}	$H_2PO_4^- \leftrightarrow HPO_4^{2-} + H^+$	$pK_{a2} = 7.21$
Phosphate^{3-}	PO_4^{3-}	$HPO_4^{2-} \leftrightarrow PO_4^{3-} + H^+$	$pK_{a3} = 12.32$
Citric Acid	$C_6H_8O_7$		
Citrate$^-$	$C_6H_7O_7^-$	$C_6H8O_7 \leftrightarrow C_6H_7O_7^- + H^+$	$pK_{a1} = 3.13$
Citrate^{2-}	$C_6H_6O_7^{2-}$	$C_6H_7O_7^- \leftrightarrow C_6H_6O_7^{2-} + H^+$	$pK_{a2} = 4.76$
Citrate^{3-}	$C_6H_5O_7^{3-}$	$C_6H_6O_7^{2-} \leftrightarrow C_6H_5O_7^{3-} + H^+$	$pK_{a3} = 6.40$
Malic Acid	$C_4H_6O_5$		
Malate$^-$	$C_4H_5O_5^-$	$C_4H_6O_5 \leftrightarrow C_4H_5O_5^- + H^+$	$pK_{a1} = 3.40$
Malate^{2-}	$C_4H_4O_5^{2-}$	$C_4H_5O_5^- \leftrightarrow C_4H_4O_5^{2-} + H^+$	$pK_{a2} = 5.11$
Lactic Acid	$C_3H_6O_3$		
Lactate$^-$	$C_3H_5O_3^-$	$C_3H_6O_3 \leftrightarrow C_3H_5O_3^- + H^+$	$pK_a = 3.86$
Ascorbic Acid	$C_6H_8O_6$		
Ascorbate$^-$	$C_6H_7O_6^-$	$C_6H_8O_6 \leftrightarrow C_6H_7O_6^- + H^+$	$pK_a = 4.04$
Benzoic Acid	$C_7H_6O_2$		
Benzoate$^-$	$C_7H_5O_2^-$	$C_7H_6O_2 \leftrightarrow C_7H_5O_2^- + H^+$	$pK_a = 4.20$
Acetic Acid	$C_2H_4O_2$		
Acetate$^-$	$C_2H_3O_2^-$	$C2H_4O_2 \leftrightarrow C_2H_3O_2^- + H^+$	$pK_a = 4.76$
Propionic Acid	$C_3H_6O_2$		
Propionate$^-$	$C_3H_5O_2^-$	$C_3H_6O_2 \leftrightarrow C_3H_5O_2^- + H^+$	$pK_a = 4.87$

Table 5.1. Summary of nomenclature for acid constituents, along with the corresponding equilibrium reactions and pK_a values for the acids listed in **Figure 5.1** [210]. Information is grouped according to each acid (e.g., phosphoric, citric, etc.), and are arranged in order of decreasing acid strength.

to normal atmospheric conditions. Everyday evidence of the slow reaction between CO_2 and water is borne out by the relatively long shelf-lives of sealed carbonated beverages (both cans and bottles), which provided they remain unopened, will still 'pop' at the press of a tab or twist of a cap.

Among the acids in **Figure 5.1** and **Table 5.1**, some display relatively stronger association to calcium than others: as an example, **Figure 5.2** illustrates the response of several acids to the addition to a $CaCl_2$ solution (pH 5.6), where lactic, malic, and citric produced the greatest pH depressions (1.28, 0.2, and 0.15, respectively). Notably, the diminishing trend in pH depressions (shown in green) mirrors the acid strength trend according to **Figure 5.1** and **Table 5.1** (i.e., citric > malic > lactic > ascorbic > benzoic > acetic), and demonstrates that stronger acids (which tend to dissociate in solution) favor interaction with calcium; in doing so, complexation of the acid anion with calcium ions lowers the acid anion concentration, thereby lowering the pH.

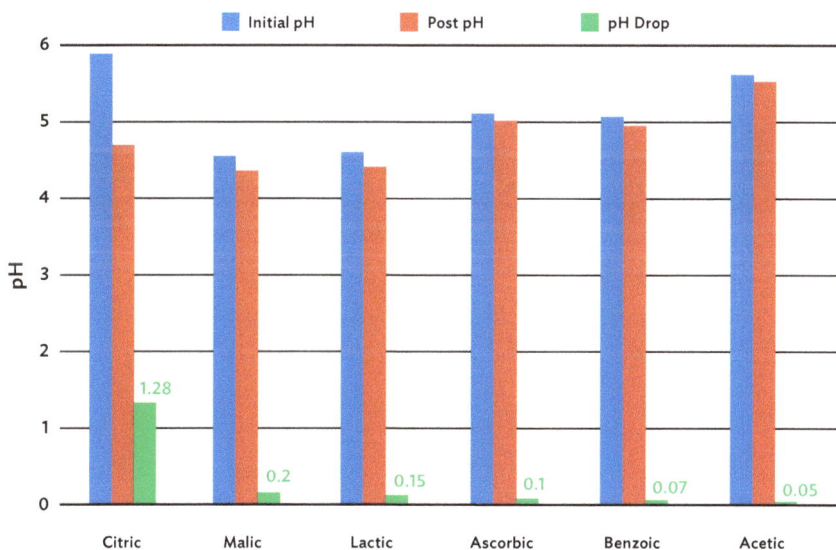

Figure 5.2. Impact on pH of addition of 0.1 N $CaCl_2$ (pH 5.6) to solutions of 0.1 N organic acid solutions [212]. The data are arranged according to increases in pH drops as noted with the data labels in green.

The interest in calcium-acid complexation is clear since this bears on susceptibility of tooth structure to acid-induced demineralization. To further this important characteristic, carboxylate-Ca^{2+} stability constants are given in **Figure 5.3**. These data are arranged according to increasing carboxylate-Ca^{2+} stability, which subsequently reflects the risks for enamel demineralization. The trend clearly shows complexation stability increases with carboxylate valency, with malate^{2-}, phosphate^{2-}, citrate^{2-}, tartrate^{2-}, and citrate^{3-} exhibiting the greatest stability among the acid constituents in **Figure 5.3**. For perspective, the ethylene tetraacetic acid (EDTA)-Ca^{2+} stability constant (i.e., log K_{Ca}) is about 11, and is more than twice the stability of citrate^{3-}-Ca^{2+} (which is ~ 4.7). Lactate$^-$, phosphate$^-$ and citrate$^-$ have relatively less damaging potential but still appear more aggressive compared to

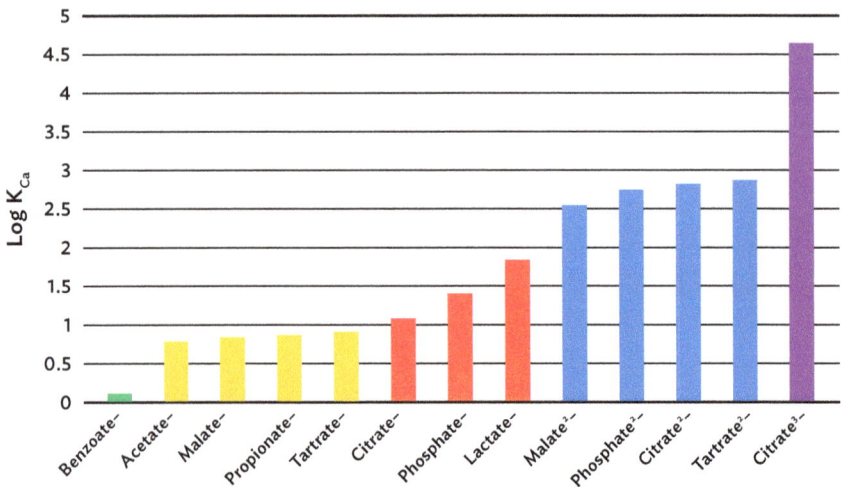

Figure 5.3. Stability constants (log K_{Ca}) of acid anion-Ca^{2+} complexes [213–216]. Risks for enamel demineralization (via acid anion-Ca^{2+} complexation) increase with anion valency. For additional perspective, ethylene tetraacetic acid (EDTA), which is commonly used to isolate metal ions in solution, imparts strong, stable, and ring-like chelation with calcium: the pK of EDTA-Ca^{2+} complexation is more than twice as high relative to the trivalent citrate-Ca^{2+} shown above (i.e., log K_{Ca} ~ 11) [217]. From a generalized perspective, risk for dental caries would involve monovalent ions, while risks for dental erosion involve higher-order valency ions.

benzoate⁻, acetate⁻, malate⁻, propionate⁻, and tartrate⁻, which are among the least damaging from a Ca^{2+}-complexation perspective. Importantly, the trending in **Figure 5.3** largely mirrors that for acid strength (**Figure 5.1** and **Table 5.1**).

In addition to acid dissociation and calcium-complexation, diffusion coefficients and hydrated radii of the acids and their respective constituents provide further differentiation. This is especially important since experiments reveal caries lesion formation and progression may be sensitive to acid ionization, where undissociated acidic molecules (e.g., acetic acid) diffuse into and react (via release of the acidic proton, H^+) with a susceptible mineral site [204,206]; in fact, acetic acid is known to penetrate into enamel [208], along with other weaker acids including propionic, butyric, and even succinic acid [207].

Additionally, three principle acids readily produced in the plaque during fermentation of sugar have been identified *in vivo*: lactic acid, acetic acid, and propionic acid [218], where acetic acid is abundant prior to the cariogenic event, but after the event lactic acid is found in higher amounts [218]. Earlier in Chapter 2 regarding plaque acids, a separate study was described that found a group of caries-resistant individuals who naturally expressed significantly higher acetic acid content and generated much less lactic acid during a cariogenic event relative to those susceptible to caries [84]. Thus, these acids bear tremendous importance in the caries process and deserve further scrutiny.

Among diffusion coefficients of at least 10 x 10^{-10} m^2s^{-1} as listed in **Figure 5.4**, undissociated acetic acid and its dissociated acetate constituent exhibit the greatest diffusion in water, followed by propionic acid, lactate, benzoic acid, and lactic acid. While acetic, benzoic, and propionic acid are relatively weak, lactic acid (and its lactate counterpart) has the distinction of bearing strong acid properties (e.g., pK_a and log K_{Ca}) with similar diffusivity, thus helping to define its potency in demineralization of tooth structure. But while these monovalent acids manifest relatively high diffusion rates compared to the other acids (e.g., monovalent and higher-order valency acids, as well as the corresponding constituents), these still pale in comparison to H^+ and OH^-, which are 93.1×10^{-10} m^2s^{-1} and 52.7×10^{-10} m^2s^{-1}, respectively; additionally, the high diffusivity of H^+, which travels more than four times as fast as F^- in solution, underlines its potentiality in destabilizing tooth structure, since the process of mineral dissolution appears to be diffusion controlled [205].

To that end, it has been proposed that undissociated acetic acid, and perhaps other weaker acids (e.g., propionic, butyric, etc.), may penetrate deeper into enamel by virtue of "pump-like" action [208], whereby dissociation by lactic acid (which works in concert with acetic acid *in vivo*) leads to production of H^+ that then associates with available acetate ions; in turn, the newly associated species (i.e., acetic acid) is proposed to penetrate into and subsequently react with enamel to produce demineralization [208]. But while undissociated acids may contribute at least some H^+ en route to demineralization (e.g., sourced from undissociated acetic acid [205,207]), is the extent of demineralization critically linked to undissociated acids? And, what is the role of acetic acid in demineralization processes?

To answer these questions, let's first consider the interrelationship between undissocated acids and pH. If a goal is set to achieve a desired fraction of undissociated acid, then efforts to do so (namely, depressing the pH) will naturally increase H^+ as the pH is lowered: for example, the pK_a of acetic acid is about 4.8, which corresponds to ~ 50% acetic acid [220], while at pH 4.4 the relative acetic acid fraction is ~ 70% [220]; although the difference in undissociated acetic acid contents may be ~ 20%, there is 2.5x more H^+ at pH 4.4 compared to pH 4.8, which is an amount sufficient to accommodate robust association with reactive anions and yet still have H^+ available for acidic purposes (e.g., attacking mineral structure).

It also helps to explore the transport and size (e.g., hydrated radii) properties of diffusing species and this is shown in **Figure 5.5**. Among

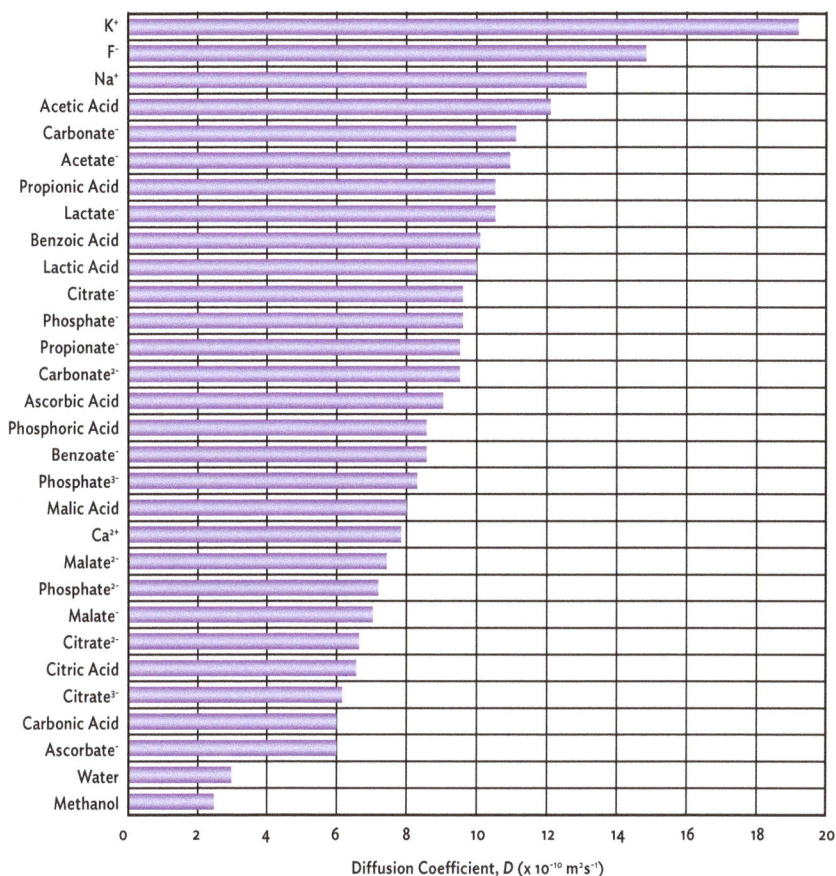

Figure 5.4. Experimental diffusion coefficients in water (corresponding to 20°–25°C) for acid constituents listed in **Table 5.1,** along with K^+, Na^+, Ca^{2+}, F^-, water (H_2O) and methanol (CH_3OH) [132, 219–234]. For reference, diffusion coefficients (also in units of 10^{-10} m^2s^{-1}) for H^+ and OH^- are 93.1 and 52.7, respectively [219].

the four smallest species, acetic acid stands out as an exception among the ions. About 20% larger than acetic acid and ranging between 2 Å and 2.5 Å are acetate, lactate, and lactic acid, which are presented according to diminishing diffusion coefficients (which, on average, are also about 20% smaller than that for acetic acid). Diffusion coefficients of the remaining ions tend to further diminish with increasing hydration size. I also included water (the diffusivity of which may be impacted by repulsive and attractive hydrogen-bonding effects and becomes significant when water adsorbs and occupies micropores [243]) and methanol (which enamel imbibes quite extensively [129]) for reference purposes. While having an effective hydrated radius of about 2.8 Å [240], the diffusivity of H^+ overwhelms other molecular and ionic species (e.g., its diffusivity is more than 6x, 7x, and 8x greater than fluoride, potassium ion, and acetic acid, respectively), and would seem to be *the* factor in the diffusion-controlled carious lesion formation and

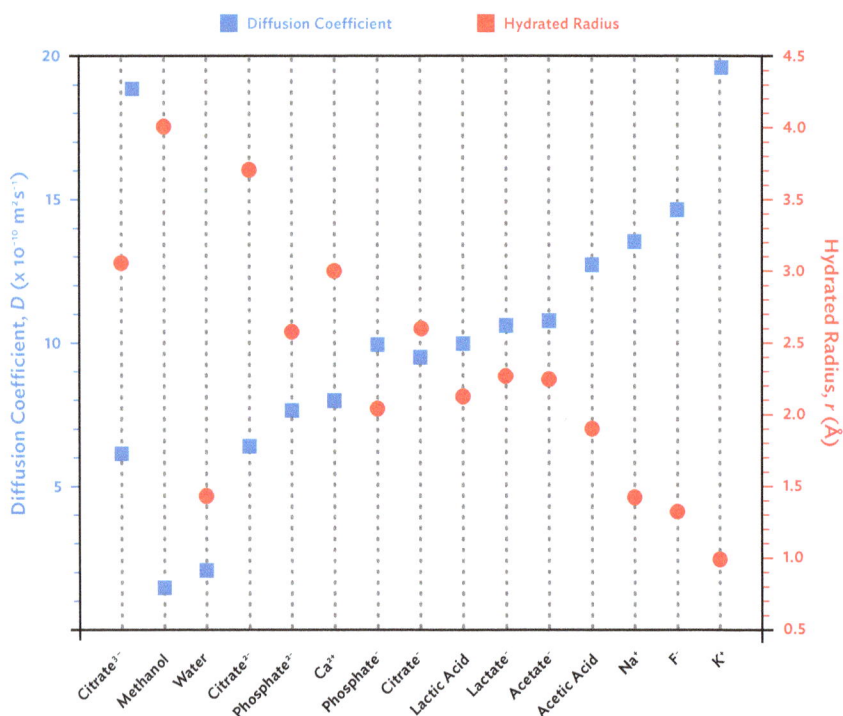

Figure 5.5. Experimental diffusion coefficients in water (corresponding to 20°- 25°C) and approximate hydrated radii for acid constituents listed in **Table 5.1,** along with K^+, Na^+, Ca^{2+}, F^-, water (H_2O) and methanol (CH_3OH) [132,220,221,231,235–242]. For reference, the diffusion coefficients (also in units of 10^{-10} m^2s^{-1}) and hydrated radii (also in units of Å) for H^+ and OH^- are 93.1 and 52.7 [219], respectively, and the hydrated radii (also in units of Å) are 2.8 Å and 3.0 Å, respectively [240]. Note the middle (~ **citrate⁻**) of this 'X' plot marks the separation in the nature of demineralization to either more erosive (on the left-half) or more caries-like (on the right-half).

progression processes [204]. Based on diffusive properties alone, it is clear H^+ exerts a powerful influence on the stability of tooth structure, especially at or below the apatite-sensitive pH 5.5.

Additionally, H^+ profoundly affects key sensory regions that may bear on enamel penetration and reactivity: sourness and astringency [244,245]. These two sensations (the former a primary response, and the latter a tactile one) appear to be critically dependent upon pH. Using a constant-acid concentration technique to evaluate several variables (pH, acid concentration and anionic species), only sourness was influenced by acid concentration and anionic species [245]. Importantly, at a given pH (between 2.8 and 4), changes in each acid concentration (i.e., lactic, malic, tartaric, and citric) did not register significant differences in astringency; however, for each acid, small adjustments in pH (from 4 down to 2.8) brought about significant differences in astringency (e.g., 3x the astringency from pH 4 to pH 2.8 for lactic acid) experienced by the panel of participants [245]. Thus, maintaining a given acid concentration but lowering the pH brought about substantial differences in astringency.

But what does this mean for enamel and the caries process? Astringency is the sensory response to a substance that results in the puckering, shrinking, or drawing of epithelia [245]. Importantly, while sourness diminishes at dilute acid concentrations, astringency becomes noticeably heightened. As previously discussed, enamel comprises fragments of stroma that become embedded or pinched during enamel formation, contributing to an inkwell-like pore constriction that may exist at the junctions and interprismatic regions [122,128,130,246].

These trapped proteins, which comprise amino acid residues such as proline [133] and salivary proteins (again, including proline) [88,91,92] are sensitive to astringents (e.g., tannins [247]) and may, therefore, impart afferent-like characteristics in the transport of H^+, especially within constricted regions that open into a relatively larger volume (i.e., at the neck region of the inkwell pore system [130]).

Heretofore, the possibility of pH effecting astringent-like responses (e.g., puckering or drawing forth action) originating from trapped protein residues within the interprismatic region has not been contemplated. The afferent-like nature of these proteins may, therefore, contribute to the permeation of acids within interprismatic enamel [117,125,190]. As discussed previously, permeation of acidic species within the junction region then facilitates mineral loss, which occurs within the intraprismatic region [110,117,121,125]. Since diffusion of acids appears to be an activated process [130,204], astringent action by H^+ on protein fragments would seem to lower this barrier while helping to explain the resiliency of the junction material that survives during, for example, erosive events [113,159,162,197].

Now let's turn to acetic acid: is there something special about this weak acid that distinguishes it from other acids? To answer this question, the results from three independent studies are considered.

First, in a study previously discussed (see **Figures 2.8** thru **2.10**), caries-resistant volunteers naturally produced significantly higher baseline plaque levels of acetic acid compared to the caries-susceptible group. To account for this observation, the researchers suggested the relatively higher acetic acid content results from the catabolism of lactate by the *Veillonella* species (which were found in larger concentrations for the caries-resistant group) which, in addition to some *Actinomyces* and *Lactobacillus* species [45,64,69]), may contribute protective acetate buffering benefits [84]. Therefore, this study points to a possible microbiological origin in the naturally high amount of acetic acid expressed in some individuals' oral flora.

Second, Geddes observed baseline acetic acid plaque levels were significantly higher in patients prior to a cariogenic challenge as shown in **Figure 5.6**. In this study, the explanations for the prompt and marked acetic acid reduction have been attributed either to salivary clearance or metabolic processing [218].

Finally, a separate laboratory study involving a binary acid system comprising acetic and lactic acids was performed to further assess the

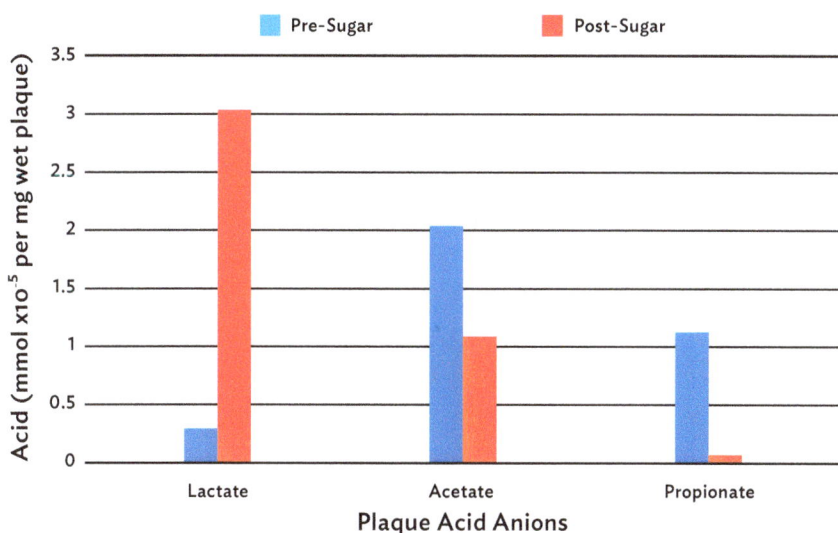

Figure 5.6. Plaque acids and corresponding contents recovered from the dentition of four participants before (Pre-Sugar) and after (Post-Sugar) a 5-minute exposure to one lump of sugar [218].

reduction in acetic acid described above. Here, the authors observed that acetate preferentially entered an enamel slab immersed in an acid system lacking any microbes: about 48% of the acetate was absorbed into the slab over the 65-hour event (at 37°C), along with a concomitant loss of H^+ resulting in pH elevation from 2.57 to 4.64 [208]; notably, despite small differences in diffusion coefficients and hydrated sizes, essentially none of the lactate absorbed into enamel. The authors proposed a "pump-like" mechanism was in play (as noted earlier), where dissociation by lactic acid (which would work in concert with acetic acid *in vivo*) encourages acetic acid association, which, in turn, helps diffuse into and subsequently demineralizes enamel [208]. If so, one might expect acid-enamel complexation to produce some kind of mineral deposits either on the slab or in solution, but the authors were silent on this matter.

In my view of these well-designed, well-conducted studies, the following can be concluded:

1. The relative acid ratio of acetic-to-lactic is higher in resting plaque but alters during cariogenic events [84,218];

2. Especially observed in caries-resistant people, acetic acid is found in abundance during resting, noncariogenic periods [84];

3. While acetic acid may be produced by action on lactate for patho-genic purposes, it may also be produced by commensal microbes (e.g., some *Veillonella* species) for benign purposes, including pro-tective buffering effects [84]; and,

4. Relative to lactic acid, acetic acid potentiates preferential absorption into enamel (including at pH where both acids would be found in undissociated form) [208].

Given the modest transport (e.g., diffusion, size) differences between acetic and lactic acids, perhaps the natural biological presence and production of acetic acid is intelligently designed for another purpose.

Published in 1898, Dr. Kahlenberg wrote on the unexpected astrin-gent notes exhibited by dilute concentrations of acetic acid; in fact, though only 6% dissociated, acetic acid stimulated astringent sensations (and even produced sour notes as well!) [244]. For comparison, Dr. Kahlenberg notes that Dr. Richards witnessed this unique observation in independent tests involving the strong inorganic acid, hydrochloric acid (HCl): though acetic acid solution exhibited astringency about 33% as strong as HCl, only 0.07% of acetic acid was dissociated. While strong and/or dilute acids are expected to exhibit astringency, this response is not usually observed for weak acids.

Thus, a sensational though unexplained property of acetic acid is its inherent astringency, particularly in undissociated form.

Given that the organic content of enamel has a significant impact on enamel despite its low content, the astringency of acetic acid would be clear: by drawing forth the requisite proteins (e.g., proline) [133], which already bear considerable water-binding characteristics [127–132], the already constricted pore openings become further pinched, rendering resistance to absorption and penetration [117,125,130,204], and, therefore, reduced risk of intraprismatic demineralization by stronger acids (e.g., lactic, citric, etc.).

Keeping in mind lactic acid is readily produced in high amounts during a cariogenic event but does not always lead to cariogenic results (e.g., as observed in caries-resistant people in **Figure 2.10**), the possibility of acetic acid functioning as a putative astringent within the interprismatic region enamel needs to be considered. And, consistent with Dr. Kahlenberg's research more than 100 years ago, astringency becomes particularly sensitive to dilute concentrations of acetic acid, and would be commensurate with, for example, the relatively low amounts produced by plaque microorganisms (e.g., *Veillonella*).

In order to explain why acetic acid may be dominant in resting plaque as well as present in caries-free individuals, I surmise that the natural microbial production of acetic acid facilitates penetration into enamel presumably via its unique astringent properties (which become magnified at dilute concentrations), and acts principally on the organic matter confined within the intraprismatic enamel regions. That acetic acid may be beneficial in this way is supported with clinical and laboratory observations (as discussed here), and may also be an example of commensal bacteria working to counter pathogenic processes.

But if protection created by acetic acid was surmounted and penetration (and subsequent demineralization) into enamel was to occur, this would be an activated process [130,204], requiring the following:

✓ Low pH (likely less than 4);

✓ High concentration of undissociated acids (e.g., acetic acid, lactic acid) for penetration into enamel;

✓ Higher flux of H⁺ or anions (e.g., lactate, acetate); and,

✓ Extended transport/demineralization times.

Concomitant with a drop in pH due to extrinsic or intrinsic acids, a nonsmall fraction of H⁺ may diffuse into enamel via demineralization processes, as well as via astringency. Whatever is the source of the pH drop, the dynamic balance (e.g., **Figure 2.4**) becomes disrupted when remineralization processes cannot meet the rate or extent of demineralization.

It follows that many of the above conditions could simply be achieved by the extrinsic introduction of large amounts of fermentable carbohydrates over a considerable amount of time (e.g., 20 minutes of potato chip munching, or sucking on a sticky or sour candy). It also follows that extrinsic introduction of foods and drinks comprising acetic acid may also jeopardize tooth structure.

Returning to **Figure 5.5**, the middle (~ **citrate⁻**) of this 'X' plot appears to mark the separation in the nature of demineralization to either more erosive (on the left-half) or more caries-like (on the right-half). In particular, it seems that the smaller and more diffusive acids (and their dissociated constituents) are typically involved in caries-like lesions, while the larger and slower diffusive species are involved in erosion. Furthermore, it seems the strength of the acid increases in moving from right to left, with acetic acid and citric acid being among the weakest and strongest acids listed, respectively. Based on the diffusion data shown, one can then identify additional acids (and corresponding constituents) listed in **Figure 5.4**.

Importantly, the pH of the acidic incursion directs demineralization toward caries-like or erosive, with additives, acid type, and concentration, and other factors imparting further demineralization characteristics. As discussed in Chapter 4, caries-like lesions are usually macroscopically smooth, while eroded enamel exhibits significant pitting and jaggedness [113,197]. Erosive lesions are readily produced in straight solutions of acid buffers [113,159,162,197], while artificial caries-like lesions are formed without surface erosion or pitting through use of protective membranes, fluoride, or a combination of these [144,145,196,206,207,248].

While acetic and lactic acids are used routinely to emulate caries-like lesions [144,145,196,206,207,248], dental erosion like that shown in **Figure 4.10** generally encompasses a larger range of acids; in fact, erosion of enamel results from inorganic and organic acids, and includes, for example, phosphoric, hydrochloric, citric, and lactic acids [145,203,249–256], some of which are routinely used in conservative, cosmetic, and restorative procedures [251–263], such as the tooth shown previously in **Figure 4.2**.

With respect to more invasive procedures involving the root, the options adjust to include acids with strong chelation effects and those effective at neutral pH [264–267]. Common in endodontic procedures, the root canal is typically irrigated with a ~ 17% EDTA solution at neutral or slightly basic pH to prep the tooth for obturation [267]. EDTA, a large polydentate ligand comprising four anion (i.e., oxygen) and two neutral (i.e., nitrogen) ligand sites, forms very stable calcium complexes (e.g., this is why it is used in sequestering calcium, magnesium, and lead from drinking water [211]) and is, therefore, used in smear layer removal, along with any undesired calcification within the canal. That EDTA (log K_{Ca} ~ 11) elicits rapid, stable calcium complexation and subsequent mineral demineralization even under neutral pH, demonstrates the power of its chelation effect [211,264–267] and its ability to interact directly on the tooth structure instead of relying on pH to generate soluble ions (e.g., Ca^{2+}) for complexation. These pronounced effects are not exhibited by citric acid under neutral pH conditions: presumably, because there are no soluble ions (e.g., Ca^{2+}) available to couple with citric acid, no decalcification of root mineral occurs [264]. As such, fully dissociated citrate^{3-} (log K_{Ca} ~ 4.5, per **Figure 5.3**) still remains subject to the generation of solution ions (e.g., Ca^{2+}) by pH (e.g., pH 7 versus pH 1), while more potent chelators (e.g., especially polydentate ligands like ETDA and others [217]) achieve decalcification via relatively pH-insensitive chelation [264–267]. Still, decalcification is accomplished using low-pH citric acid solutions, and is on par with neutral solutions of EDTA: for instance, EDTA (15%, pH 7) and citric acid (15%, pH 1.6) produced similar decalcification, although EDTA achieved this more quickly [266,267]. But perhaps limited by repre-cipitation of calcium phosphate minerals or interactions with collagen, little decalcification differences exist for increased concentrations of citric acid solution at low pH: for example, similar decalcification was observed from citric acid solutions comprising 10% (pH 1.5) or 20% (pH 1.2) [267]. With respect to phosphoric acid, different concentra-tions (i.e., 5% or 37% phosphoric acid, with both having pH ~ 1) do not decalcify as well as citric acid or EDTA [265,266]; like citric acid, perhaps these limitations are due to a combination of reprecipitation of dissolved mineral phases and a relatively weak chelation effect.

Though of some debate, aggressive whitening with concentrated peroxides (e.g., 35% hydrogen or carbamide peroxide) can also lead to bulk enamel loss and/or roughening [268–270]. Peroxides are strong oxidizing agents and their bidentate nature imparts chelation effects that can lead to enamel erosion. Like EDTA solutions, peroxides readily chelate with calcium around neutral pH. Similar to synthetic solutions used to create subsurface caries-like lesions, many whitening formulations now contain polymers, fluoride, and other additives in order to mitigate potential surface damage. Though effective, whitening systems affect individuals differently, so caution should be exercised to minimize enamel damage en route to a whiter smile.

Separately, conditioning the tooth surface to accept a treatment necessarily involves erosive-like demineralization. Examples include microabrasion of superficial enamel defects [255,256], resin-infiltration of incipient lesions [257–260], or placement of sealants as a preventive measure [261–263]. The relatively poor chelating ability of phosphoric acid helps to limit the action of phosphoric acid on the tooth structure (unless extended etch times are used), thus giving more control to the clinician. While phosphoric acid solutions are favored in cosmetic and minimal intervention strategies [252,254,256,266], ultimately the etch quality and quantity depends on the skill of the clinician and the characteristics of the patient and dental environment; for these reasons, sometimes self-etch systems (which usually include phosphoric acid derivatives, carboxylic acids, or acidic monomers) are preferred [251,271,272].

Whether intrinsic or extrinsic, acids clearly have an impact on dental structure. Recognizing that in an oral environment where natural salivary pellicles freely form on the tooth surface, numerous experimental observations (many of which are referenced in this chapter) support my submission of a generalized perspective regarding tooth demineralization by acids:

1. at pH favoring demineralization of tooth structure (pH ~ 5.5), dental caries generally arises from modest complexation of monovalent acids (e.g., lactic, acetic), while higher-order valency (e.g., citric, phosphoric, malic) drives dental erosion;

2. weak monovalent acids remaining undissociated (e.g., acetic acid, propionic acid, etc.) may exhibit greater diffusion (i.e., penetration) into enamel relative to dissociated species (e.g., acetate⁻, propionate⁻, etc.), and when in excess (e.g., via extrinsic sources), tend to effect subsurface lesions;

3. strong acids, especially those with higher valency (e.g., citric, phosphoric, malic) as well as strong calcium-chelators (e.g., EDTA), exhibit greater stability (relative to weak acids) when complexed to Ca^{2+} and tend to effect dental erosion;

4. caries-like lesion formation by strong or weak acids is pH-dependent;

5. excluding strong chelators of calcium (e.g., EDTA), effects of acids become attenuated at normal salivary pH (e.g., citric acid at pH ~ 7);

6. astringency correlates with pH, and bears on penetration of acids and demineralization of tooth structure;

7. intrinsic undissociated weak acids (e.g., acetic acid) may provide some protection against demineralization; and,

8. a continuum of demineralization exists and is not restricted to acids fermented by microbes nor is it limited to erosive episodes; instead, a combination of factors (which are critically dependent on local pH and acid type) ultimately produce net dental demineralization when exceeding remineralization processes.

In this chapter I have presented some important properties of acids affecting our teeth. The above view supports a dynamic situation that may reflect actual (i.e., clinically observed) demineralization. Of course, as an exception, excessive behaviors or conditions will naturally tip the nature of demineralization (i.e., caries-like or erosive-like): for instance, if one avoids citrus foods altogether, then risk for dental erosion is lowered; alternately, if one regularly engages in sticky, sugary foodstuffs, dental caries risk becomes elevated. These examples provide a glimpse into how acids in the comestibles we consume present risks and are explored in detail in the next chapter.

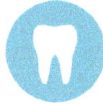

CHAPTER SIX

Acids and pH: Demineralization Risks of Foods, Drinks, and Other Comestibles

THE PURPOSE OF THIS CHAPTER IS TO EDUCATE the reader on certain aspects of foods and beverages, especially the pH and small organic/inorganic acid composition of many different foods and drinks. Of course, this presentation is not inclusive of all foods due to the multitude of global possibilities and variations.

Notably, data regarding sugar content (or, carbohydrates) of foods is not presented because sugars, while an important (and albeit casual) factor in tooth decay, impact individuals differently for various reasons. For example, because sugars must be digested by microorganisms in order to exert a detrimental force, such catabolism depends on, for instance, an individual's ecology and biochemistry. To that end, the evolution of acids and/or plaque by sugar fermentation (requisite in caries-related decay) can be managed by the use of topical fluorides, sugar-free (or, sugar alternative) comestibles (including gums, lozenges, and mints), and physical disruption of plaque (e.g., toothbrushing, flossing). Still further, for those individuals inherently resistant to caries activity, discussions on avoidance (or limitation) of sugar (or, carbohydrates) from an oral health perspective may not be constructive.

In contrast, pH and small organic/inorganic acids (e.g., phosphoric, citric, malic, lactic, etc.) directly impact an individual's dentition through chemical dissolution whether the demineralization is erosive or caries-based. It follows that pH and acid characteristics of foods and drinks may impart causative factors in the weakening of tooth structure.

While this exposition identifies certain foods or beverages that may carry increased risks for demineralization, the purpose is to educate the reader on the pH and/or acid composition, and not to demonize the food or drink: thus, one may still partake in the food or drink in question, but can do so from an informed perspective. In doing so, this chapter is unique in that it distinguishes itself from other information/educational sources advocating or protesting certain foods, drinks, or behaviors. Of course, sugar-free and acid-free foods will present less risk to your oral environment, but it is unreasonable to expect high compliance from restrictions or eliminations of certain foods, drinks, or other comestibles. In short, quality-of-life* factors play a major part of habit. So from a dental demineralization perspective, foods and drinks are presented to help facilitate discussions and decision-making.

> ***NOTE:**
>
> If one wants to avoid sugars, that is fine, but realizing that life can be fairly long, full of activity (for better or worse), and ever-evolving, I find it unrealistic to subsist solely on pH-neutral and/or low-sugar/low-carbohydrate foods and drinks. This view is consistent with clinical studies demonstrating diets low in carbs exude similar benefits relative to those higher in carbs (i.e., low-fat diets). Perhaps you'll agree with me. So don't shy from that celebratory toast or moment of indulgence when the occasion arises. But do understand the risks involved to your teeth. Then, mitigate those risks with the various options and tools discussed here and elsewhere.

About sugars and carbohydrates

It is no secret that the foods and drinks we consume can affect our oral health. Standard advice from a dental professional will usually include the cautionary exhortation to limit (maybe even avoid!) sugary foods, and of course, this is based on the casual correlation of sugar and tooth decay [273–276]. In fact, with respect to foods, there are many recommendations including perhaps at least one of the following (e.g., [277]):

It is no secret that the foods and drinks we consume can affect our oral health.

✓ Avoid (or limit) sugary foods, snacks, and drinks;

✓ Do not prolong meals, especially if they are carbohydrate-rich;

✓ Limit the number of meals and/or snacking throughout the day;

✓ Eat sliced nuts instead of whole, or consume sliced fruit instead of whole (e.g., an apple) to reduce the risk of compromising tooth, restorative, orthodontic, and prosthodontic structures;

✓ Aspirate acidic beverages via a straw, careful to direct the fluids toward the back of the mouth to limit contact with the teeth;

✓ Avoid brushing teeth immediately after consumption of an acidic beverage or food;

✓ Partake in a sugar-free gum, lozenge, mint, etc. after a meal.

While the above have merits, these recommendations (and others) often fail because they are too unrealistic, challenging, restrictive, or demeaning.

Firstly, human life is fundamentally and naturally centered on food, with meals numbering at least three times a day on a conservative basis (e.g., breakfast, lunch, and dinner). These meals become augmented and snacks are introduced depending on one's cultural immersion and activities (e.g., on average, there are about eight eating events in the United Kingdom [278]). For instance, one who exercises infrequently, regularly, or seriously, will add at least one more consumptive event to their daily schedule, whether it is to build strength or simply to rehydrate.

Often the economics and dynamics of one's life cannot regularly allow for 'tooth-friendly', balanced meals. This includes aspects of the home, family, work, school, sport, and social environment, along with age-related sensitivities (e.g., children, adolescents, and adults) [279,280]. And, social and/or special events typically involve various types of foods and drinks (e.g., weddings, anniversaries, birthday parties, graduations, promotions, formal dining events, etc.): it can be challenging (and possibly regarded as impolite) to not only restrict oneself to certain foods but also to consume the meal quickly, especially as others maintain a pace commensurate with the dining experience and conversation. Imbibing wine is another example: these events are not limited to five minutes but can last for hours. Separately, it is inconvenient, messy, or even un-fun to slice an apple (assuming a knife or other implement is handy or even appropriate) or aspirate an appealing beverage through a straw all the while ensuring it is aimed at the back of the tongue or the throat, thus missing the 'target' sensory taste buds of the tongue altogether; and, be careful: biting or chewing the straw can exacerbate erosive effects [281,282].

And as carbohydrates constitute the bulk of human macronutrition (i.e., our cells fundamentally need energy replenishment after all!), sugars (yes, even natural sugars such as that found in fruits) are necessary for our daily function (as those with hypoglycemia can readily attest) as dictated by the Krebs Cycle [69]. Sugars (e.g., intrinsic/natural, added, artificial and substitutes) help render a food or drink more palatable and/or enjoyable, and may be necessary for active individuals (especially those engaged in routine and/or demanding physical activity including sports and manual labor), as well as those struggling to meet daily nutritional needs due to a certain medical condition. From an ingredient perspective, sugar also provides key substantive and preservative properties to foods and drinks, thus rendering limitations to the view that sugar can 'simply' be removed or replaced from a product without affecting taste, mouthfeel, or shelf-life.

Like most activities on Earth (e.g., sunbathing, exercising, working, socializing, eating, drinking, medicating, etc.) moderation and education is key. There is debatable question, and even derision, regarding 'added sugars'. Naturally, the risk for abuse of any consumable is manifestly present (including carbohydrate-rich foods) but this is where *education* and, if desired, *therapy* (e.g., mental, emotional, physical, behavioral, as well as holistic approaches) can play big roles in the overall health of an individual [283].

With respect to 'added sugar' (including sugar added to drink and foods; honeys and syrups; fruit juices and concentrates), the World Health Organization suggests children should strive for less than 10% of total energy intake to reduce risk of caries [284]. While this may be an excellent guideline, few consumers (including those stressed-out, time-crunched, and/or exhausted parents) understand recommended daily caloric intake [285], always look at the nutritional fact panel (e.g., 11%) [286], or have time to digest the information [287]. Among those giving the nutritional fact panel more than a passing glance, most consider total caloric value and/or fat content rather than sugar content [286]. As a testament to the confusion surrounding nutrition, consumers are even less likely to readily distinguish sugars from calories and do not wish to allocate time to do so: for example, as noted in [287], study participants expressed that *"There must be a high calorie value in whatever is replacing the salt and sugar to make it nearly the same.*" or "*. . . when you're shopping you don't have time to think about it!*" Therefore, the identification and understanding of 'added sugars' from 'sugars' approaches a level of detail that winnows implementation on a routine basis to only those well-versed (including professionals) in the subject of nutrition—in short, resolving tree-level detail from the forest of nutrition is often too confusing and unrealistic. And in a note of caution, simplifying the presentation of nutritional content for a given foodstuff may not be enough, as consumers with relatively poor nutrition knowledge appear strongly motivated to make an unhealthy nutritional purchase [288].

Given the extant complexities in analyzing and understanding the quantity of macro- and micronutrients one needs for 'proper' nutrition (let alone the sources and types of proteins, carbohydrates, and fats), it may seem appealing (and at least less confusing or time-intensive!) to swear off sugars (or, carbohydrates) altogether. But forgoing sugar (or carbohydrates for that matter) is essentially a diet plan, and a sobering reason diets fail is due to the struggle to maintain quality of life changes or constraints [289]. While health benefits may be experienced from low-carbohydrate (i.e., high-fat and/or high-protein) diets, such benefits are at least as good as high-carbohydrate (i.e., low-fat) diets [283,289], so attaining long-term, superior benefits by avoiding carbohydrates (or sugars) may not be realistic. In fact, consistent with the need for sugars/carbohydrates in the body, there are significant health-based reasons for which exclusion of sugars/carbohydrates may not be preferable: for example, low-carbohydrate diets may elicit undesirable effects including skeletal muscle degeneration (as observed in amyotrophic lateral sclerosis (ALS) mice) [290] or gastrointestinal disorders (observed in humans) [291]. Plus, while sugar is a casual causative factor in tooth decay, not all sugars exert the same influence within or among individuals: for example, sugar clearance from the oral environment is linked to an individual's saliva flow and age, along with the nature of the sugar-containing format (e.g., biscuit, tablet, liquids) [292,293].

And, in an admittedly rare and certainly eyebrow-raising instance, some have purported the virtues of sugar [294].

While this chapter emphasizes pH and small acid characteristics of various foods and drinks, it is prudent to address how the fermentation of sugar/carbohydrate affects the oral environment. As recognized in the opening paragraphs of this chapter, the consumption of sugar and carbohydrates bears directly on the oral flora, with the evolution of polysaccharide matrices (i.e., plaque) and small organic acids (e.g., lactic acid), along with changes in pH and microbial ecology.

Examples of the change in pH and generation of lactic acid that may result from consumption of several foodstuffs are shown in **Figures 6.1** and **6.2** [137]. In this instance, plaque was sampled from the lingual surfaces of the maxillary premolar teeth before and after consumption of the foodstuff or rinsing (i.e., with the 20% glucose solution). The rinsing of the glucose solution helps establish a baseline (at least for sugary liquids) for pH-recovery in the lingual plaque. The inability to recover pH upon consumption of the fig cookie demonstrates the

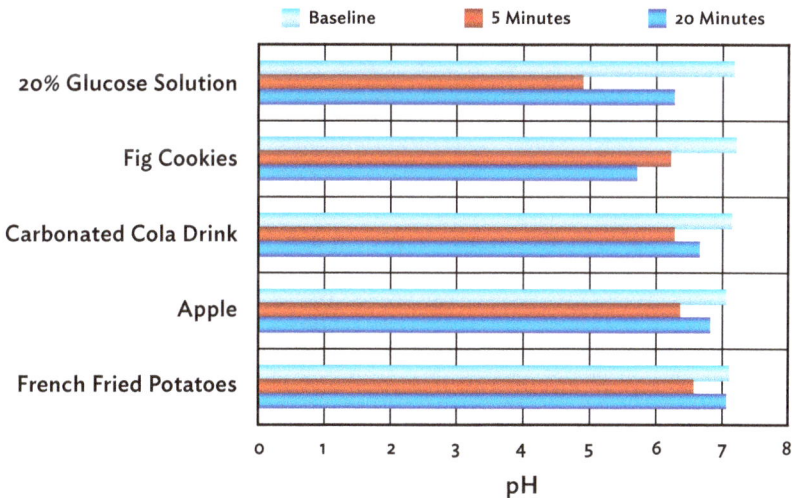

Figure 6.1. pH plaque measurements at baseline and at the 5-minute and 20-minute marks for several foodstuffs and a control 20% glucose solution rinse. pH measurements were made from lingual plaque collected from maxillary premolars from five volunteers [137].

influence of a sticky foodstuff. In fact, this was also observed in the lactic acid measurements made from the plaque samples as well, as shown in **Figure 6.2**. Relative to baseline, all foodstuffs produced significantly higher lactic acid even at the 5-minute mark, but the clearance of the nonsticky foods, which also included the acidic foodstuffs (i.e., carbonated cola, orange juice, and apples), at the 20-minute mark reflects the innate ability of the oral environment to reestablish equilibrium [137].

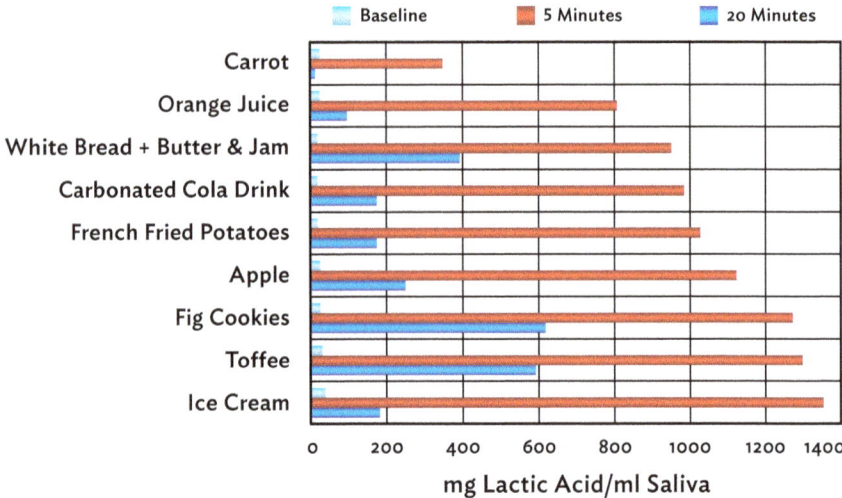

Figure 6.2. Lactic acid measurements at baseline and at the 5-minute and 20-minute marks for several foodstuffs. Lactic acid measurements were made from lingual plaque collected from maxillary premolars from five volunteers [137].

In contrast to the at-risk volunteers pertaining to **Figure 6.3**, ten healthy volunteers with low caries incidence were monitored for pH changes induced from a variety of foodstuffs [295]. **Figure 6.4** details the changes in approximal microsite (upper and lower jaw in the premolar regions) and pooled plaque (from at least 20 tooth sites). In general, the pooled plaque exhibited higher pH readings relative to only the approximal regions, thus underlining the heterogeneous nature of plaque [42]. Based on the 10% sucrose solution, a less dramatic drop

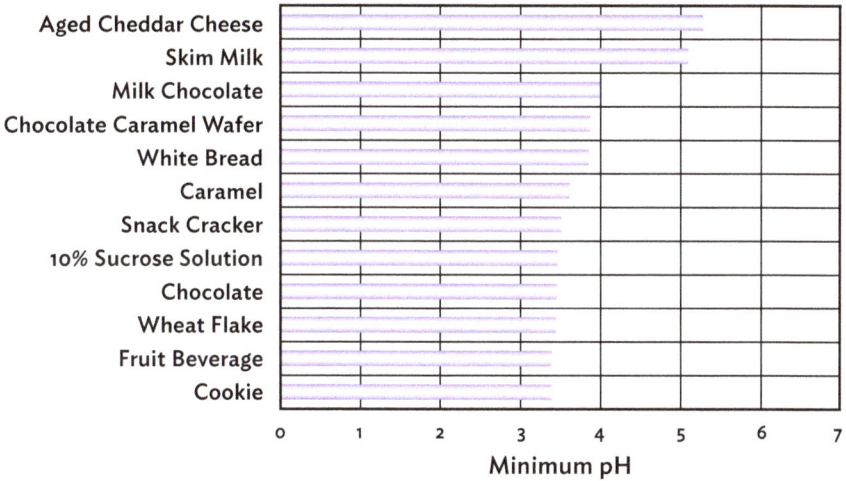

Figure 6.3. Minimum plaque pH measurements after consumption of several foodstuffs and a control 10% sucrose-solution rinse. pH telemetry measurements from a microelectrode were made from interproximal molar and/or prostheses plaque from five volunteers exhibiting a history of caries and acidogenic flora [273].

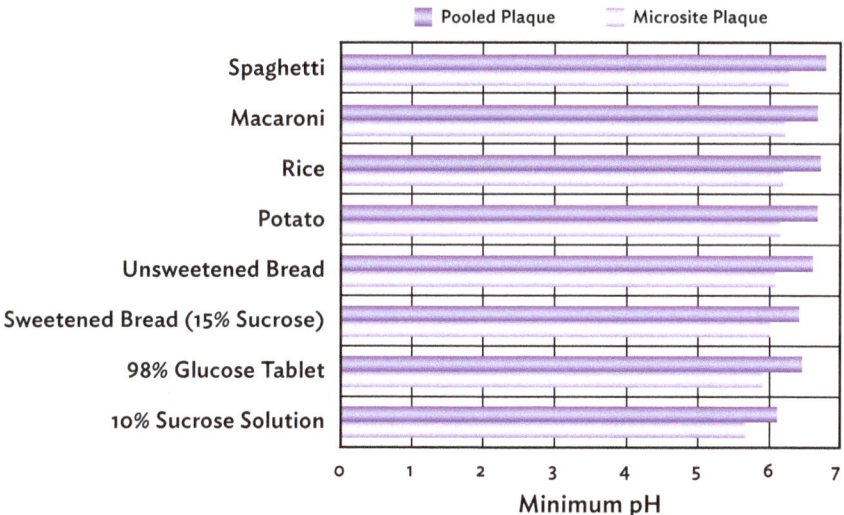

Figure 6.4. Minimum plaque pH measurements after consumption of several foodstuffs and a control 10% sucrose-solution rinse. pH measurements were made from pooled plaque (from at least 20 sites) and approximal-only molar sites from 10 volunteers with low caries experience [295].

in pH was observed relative to that in **Figure 6.3**, indicating the volunteers' plaque was much less acidogenic (i.e., the lowest pH was above 5.5 compared to around 4 in **Figure 6.3**), and is consistent with the relative lack in caries experience. Still, the presence of glucose or sucrose led to lower pH values relative to more complex and/or processed carbohydrates, such as the potato, rice, macaroni, and spaghetti.

The results from the low caries incidence described in **Figure 6.4** echoes the pH measured in food-saliva mixtures, with a few notable exceptions: candies having cherry, grape, or lemon flavor (all of which had initial pH < 4) led to very low candy-saliva pH (between 3 and 4) relative to cinnamon- or mint-flavored candies (which had initial pH > 6), as well as many flour-containing and/or sugar-containing foodstuffs (where the food-saliva final pH was usually above 5) [296].

Finally, the effect of sugary foodstuffs on microbial composition was evaluated over a 5-day period [278]. In this study, participants supplemented their existing (and uncontrolled) diets with four foodstuffs: lemonade (250 ml 5x per day), biscuit (5x per day), toffee (1 piece 5x per day), or sugar lumps (1 lump 5x per day). At the end of the 5-day period, plaque was collected from fissure (**Figure 6.5**) and smooth (**Figure 6.6**) surfaces from two permanent molar teeth in each of the

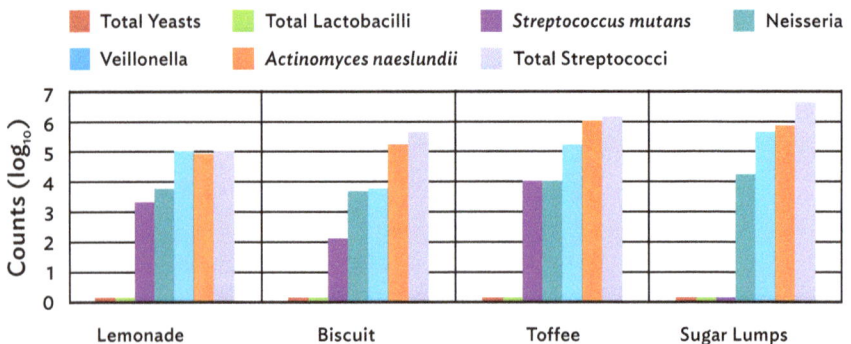

Figure 6.5. Microbial populations recovered from fissure surfaces of participants supplementing their existing uncontrolled diets with lemonade (250 ml 5x per day), biscuit (5x per day), toffee (1 piece 5x per day), or sugar lumps (1 lump 5x per day) for a total of five days [278].

20 participants. The data in **Figures 6.5** and **6.6** reveal the relative dearth of yeast and *Lactobacillus* microorganisms relative to the other evaluated microbes (i.e., *S. mutans*, *Neisseria* species, *Veillonella* species, *A. naeslundii*, and total *Streptococci*). Additionally, between fissure and smooth surface types, the latter surfaces generally harbor higher populations of microbial species.

Among the four foodstuffs, the toffee and sugar lumps (which were largely comprised of sucrose) yielded slightly more counts relative to lemonade and biscuits. While the foodstuffs did not generally alter microbial make-up, there were two exceptions: lemonade facilitated higher smooth surface counts of *Lactobacillus*, while sugar lumps resulted in near negligible levels of *S. mutans* within fissure surfaces. With respect to *S. mutans*, it seems that 'sticky' formats (i.e., toffee) may be of greater importance relative to nonsticky items (i.e., lemonade, biscuit, or sugar lumps) and this holds true for both fissure and smooth surfaces. Notably, the data show *S. mutans* is not critically dependent on sugar content, since lemonade and the biscuit each had less sugar (5.8% and 22%, respectively) relative to either toffee or the sugar lumps (both of which constituted more than 90% sugar). While *Veillonella* and *Neisseria* species also did not appear sensitive to sugar, *A. naeslundii* and other *Streptococci* species did.

While some general increases in microbial populations were observed, these did not appear to be as strongly dependent on sugar content relative to the sugar-containing format (e.g., toffee versus lemonade, biscuit, or sugar lumps). In fact, a highlight of this work is that the stickiness of the sugar-containing format may be a significant risk factor, and is consistent with other results (e.g., see [137] and **Figures 6.1** and **6.2**), whereby foodstuffs with retentive characteristics can help promote functional attachment and/or intracellular polysaccharide storage.

Still, the greatest population increases (on average and especially for fissure surfaces) were observed for nonmutans *Streptococcus*, which necessarily includes both commensal and pathogenic species. Additionally,

A. naeslundii counts also increased, consistent with expectations since plaque derived from saccharolytic activity is typically rich in *Actinomyces*, along with nonmutans *Streptococcus* and *Veillonella* (commensal and pathogenic species) [45,64–67].

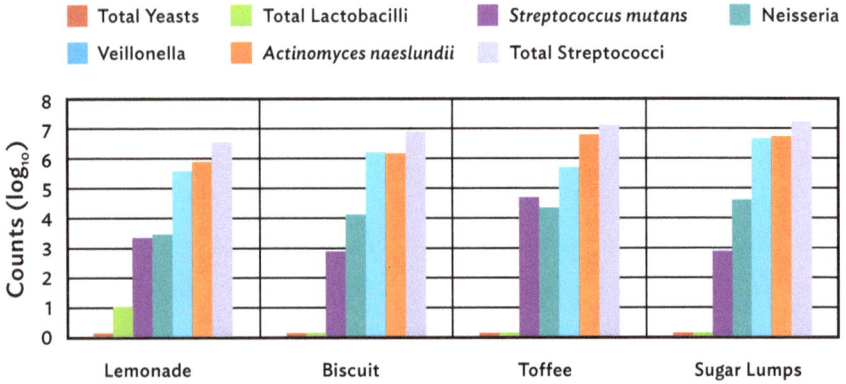

Figure 6.6. Microbial populations recovered from smooth surfaces of participants supplementing their existing uncontrolled diets with lemonade (250 ml 5x per day), biscuit (5x per day), toffee (1 piece 5x per day), or sugar lumps (1 lump 5x per day) for a total of five days [278].

As discussed earlier in this chapter, broad recommendations to avoid sugars (i.e., 'free', 'added', or otherwise) are not realistic or sustainable. In the event of active caries, the oral environment is likely abundant in acidogenic plaque, and interventions (including invasive, if applicable) are recommended. But caries or not, without physical disruption of pathogenic biofilms, avoidance of sugars and other carbohydrates will have limited effects.

So while the evolution of sugar-derived plaque is a critical and necessary step in the formation of incipient enamel lesions, the variability in microbial species (including the varying levels of commensal versus pathogenic species) among individuals [37–43] suggests a more sustainable way of managing plaque is to ensure adequate plaque removal, which is a tenet of minimally invasive dentistry and will be discussed in Chapter 10 [297].

If I were pressed to propose one restriction/recommendation for sugar-based foods given the information presented at this stage, it would be this: among sugary comestibles, those that are stubbornly sticky (i.e., those requiring increased effort in removing due to the ready attachment to tooth structure) confer the most negative effects, including:

✓ a sustained low-pH environment;

✓ ample production of tooth-destructive acids (e.g., lactic acid); and,

✓ proliferation of pathogenic flora.

Though 'sticky' could apply to many foods, this does not include syrups and honeys per se but would include taffy, toffee, and other sugary foods that present friability frustrations; sticky candies and suckers; certain sticky popcorns; and, generally other comestibles that would require intervention beyond swilling with water or quick finger-sweeping for dislodgement. (Note: use of a fingernail would apply as requiring above-normal intervention, as would toothpicks, toothbrushes, floss, or whatever else that is used to remove the obstruction.) Of course, these findings and recommendations are not new: even Aristotle proposed the decay-inducing effects of the tasty fig fruit was due to its sticky intercalation within dental interstices between teeth, as well as within gingival and periodontal pockets [298].

Besides the many foods that may have the potential to elicit caries-based (i.e., plaque-based) decay, which includes those rich in cereal grains (e.g., wheat, rice, corn), monosaccharides (e.g., sugar) and polysaccharides (e.g., starches), there exist others that present different demineralization risks: namely, dental erosion. While some of these erosive foodstuffs and beverages may comprise sugar, others may not. Even further, behavior (including purposeful and otherwise) drives much of the resultant damage to tooth structure. The causative factors in these instances include pH and small organic/inorganic acids, and unlike plaque-based decay, do not require the microbial middleman to destroy the dentition.

Erosion of tooth structure via pH and small organic/inorganic acids of foods and drinks

Without the microbial middleman, these factors act directly on the tooth structure, thereby reducing the timescale for demineralization while promoting the loss of mineral through chemical (i.e., erosion) and physical (i.e., abrasion and attrition) processes [138,165]. With respect to physical removal of mineral, abrasion involves instruments, including toothbrush action and/or abrasive particles, while attrition describes tooth wear due to, for instance, teeth-grinding; usually dental erosion involves chemical and at least one of these physical forms of mineral loss [165]. Importantly, concomitant with the loss of mineral, habitats may emerge that encourage biofilm formation (i.e., plaque), thus presenting another risk factor (i.e., caries) that may accelerate and/ or compound demineralization of the tooth.

But, like the variability in an individual's risk for developing dental caries, dental erosion also appears to be individual-dependent [299,300]. Still, while all tooth surfaces are inherently at risk for erosion, the upper labial tooth surfaces are particularly susceptible due in part to a lack of nearby salivary glands that could otherwise expedite acid clearance: for instance, healthy volunteers rinsing with a 2% citric acid solution (pH 2.1) exhibited relatively poor salivary clearance within this region; in fact, over the nearly two-minute waiting period, the retention of citric acid was about 20x and 3x higher compared to citric acid concentrations at the sublingual site and lower labial tooth surfaces, respectfully [299]. Or simply put, the most visible teeth of one's smile are especially susceptible to dental erosion. This example demonstrates how foods and drinks can affect dentition differently, and also reveals the ability of small organic acids to reside in the oral environment, even in a healthy population with unencumbered saliva flow.

When salivary flow is minimal, which is a frequent situation (e.g., at rest and during sleep; due to dehydration from exercise, medicine use, or inadequate hydration; or, due to genetic factors), or otherwise compromised (e.g., such as those with inadequate buffer capacity due to health or medical reasons; or, those experiencing acidic plaque environments due to poor oral hygiene and/or active decay), the insulting food or drink will impact the dentition more aggressively, sometimes having an outsize effect (e.g., protracted wine-drinking behavior in social or private situations).

Other factors besides pH and acid type certainly contribute to the overall risk of a foodstuff or drink, such as the total free H^+ content (which is also known as titratable or neutralizing acidity, and has been regarded as even more important than pH [301]), degree of saturation, viscosity, surface tension, salivary stimulus, etc. Irrespective of acid type, a low (i.e., acidic) pH is required to effect dental softening or demineralization (and pertains to both caries and erosive processes), and thus serves as a requisite primary indicator. And, unlike other factors, pH and acid type are parameters that can be readily determined or identified; toward this end, an association between dietary acidic intake (including food and drink source and corresponding acids) and dental erosion has been observed [302].

Since dental erosion develops with chronic chemical etching, our daily nutritional needs are innately intertwined with this risk. By exploring these aspects of foods and drinks (i.e., pH and acid type), perhaps the continuous consumption of foods and drinks (including snacks, meals, rehydration events, and so on) can be designed to help protect the integrity of the teeth.

pH and small organic/inorganic acids

Understanding pH and acid type of foods and drinks helps assess possible demineralization risks, especially for those opting for certain high (or, low) macronutrient diets (e.g., high-protein, high-carbohydrate, high-fat) and/or diets based on philosophies (e.g., raw food diets, vegetarian diets, etc.) [301,303–305]. Obviously, there are other components of foodstuffs that bear on the overall demineralization risk, including the nature of the macro- (e.g., proteins, carbohydrates, and fats) and micronutrients (e.g., calcium, phosphate, zinc, iron, etc.). But as a critical reminder from the last chapter, although acids are important in assessing possible demineralization risks, pH remains a primary factor, with small acid effects imparting additional risk factors.

I now present an extensive series of figures that highlight the pH and/or small acid composition of many foods (including fruits, vegetables, and plant-derived foods) and beverages (freshly prepared or ready-to-drink). While fairly comprehensive, these lists cannot be expected to be all-encompassing due to the myriad foodstuffs available throughout the world, let alone those subjected to analyses. Still, these lists are presented to help provide insight into some important foodstuff properties. Perhaps this information can facilitate healthier choices for foods and/or drinks when several options are available (e.g., one type of root beer might comprise phosphoric acid, while another might not), while also bringing awareness to perhaps unhealthy behavior (e.g., swilling or puffing the mouth with a swig of a low-pH sports drink).

For reference and discussion purposes, the pH at which dental enamel begins to demineralize ranges between 5 and 5.5 [306]. Importantly, while the pH values listed in this chapter refer to foods and drinks, it is the *saliva* and *plaque* pH, and not the food or drink per se, that modulates the demineralization-remineralization balance; however, since foods and fluids can be retained in biofilms (e.g., pellicle and plaque), food and drink pH remain causative factors in dental demineralization.

pH of common foods

A continuum of food pH ranging from highly acidic (lemons, pH ~ 2.3) to slightly basic (egg white, pH ~ 8) is presented in **Figure 6.7**. Please note that beverage pH is not included in this figure but is reserved for in-depth presentation later in this chapter. This food-pH relationship was compiled from data collected by the US Food & Drug Administration

[307] and provides a glimpse into the library of food pH; although not comprehensive, this is a good place to start in order to familiarize oneself with expected pH values and the reader is encouraged to access the reference ([307]) if further information is desired.

Based on **Figure 6.7**, one can readily see that diets high in pork, poultry, fish, and dairy are likely to confer tooth-friendly benefits (i.e., those having pH values > 5, which is the low end of the minimum threshold for enamel demineralization [306]). Wheat-based products (e.g., flour, biscuit and bread) and some vegetables (e.g., potatoes and corn) also have relatively benign pH values, so if any demineralization develops, this is due to action from the microbial middleman (as discussed previously). Importantly, corn syrup and sugar are not low-pH foodstuffs (i.e., the pH is around 5), so again, the action of the microbial middleman will drive potential demineralization. Butter and cocoa, which are commonly used in baked goods (often with sugar), also manifest pH values that appear tooth-friendly (pH values > 6), so these do not present inherent erosive properties; however, alteration of these ingredients in a baked good to produce a more acidic—and perhaps a more appealing—flavor profile may override potential tooth-neutral (or, tooth-friendly) benefits. At the low-to-mid-pH end of the spectrum, fruits (e.g., figs, apples, blueberries, pomegranates, and lemons), jams and honey, buttermilk, and some vegetables or leafy greens (e.g., sorrel and string beans) represent greater risks for erosive (i.e., immediate) demineralization; among these, sticky foods (such as figs and dates) likely present greater risks to demineralization relative to nonsticky foodstuffs.

Segue to small organic/inorganic acid and/or sugar content and/or pH considerations of certain foods

The **Figure 6.7** pH table provides a broad range of foods with the aim of becoming generally familiar to potential tooth demineralization risks. But another factor is small organic (and/or inorganic) acids. But which foodstuffs will or will not be presented, and why?

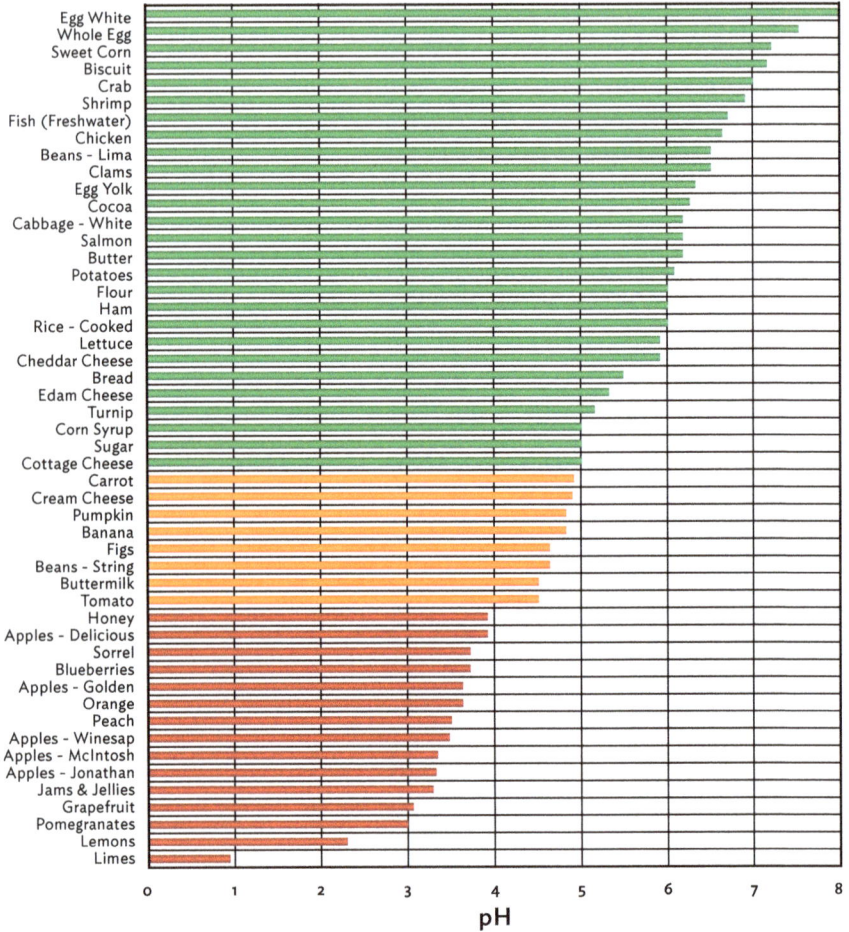

Figure 6.7. pH values of some common food items as determined by the US Food & Drug Administration [307]. Colors are shown to help approximate pH regions that may present relatively high (pH < 4), moderate (4 < pH < 5), or low (pH > 5) risks for dental erosion.

Packaged or baked goods (like crackers, cookies, breads) generally do not comprise a large amount of native or added organic acids: while organic acids such as lactic, acetic, or propionic acids that may be present during fermentation, these are typically evolved during baking processes [308,309]; but acids introduced as additives, such as citric, malic, and tartaric, are often incorporated for taste, flavor, and/or preservation purposes [310]. Solid, prepared foodstuffs, which are usually higher in carbohydrate content, would usually give rise to caries-based decay through fermentative processes; as such, given the pH ranges presented above, along with the fairly nonaqueous state in which they are presented (e.g., packaged goods are commonly low-moisture products), the relative risk of demineralization arising from erosive processes is comparatively low.

Lactic acid is usually present in meats (including beef, poultry, and fish) [309]; generally, the meat category manifests pH values higher than 5, and thus present reduced risks for tooth demineralization. Therefore, meats will not be discussed in this section.

Nuts, seeds, and grains, while contributing to a healthy diet, providing benefits against diabetes, cardiovascular and inflammatory diseases, and prostate and colorectal cancers [311,312], do not comprise an abundance of small organic acids. Rather, these contain an abundance of phytic and phenolic acids [309,313–317] as part of the phytochemical composition [313], but these are not involved in tooth demineralization processes; as such, these will not be discussed here, although the milks of some of these will be presented later in this chapter. [Note: intact nuts, seeds, or gains, however, can pose risks for attrition caries and/or structural weakening of either the natural, restored, or otherwise modified tooth; thus, care should be taken when eating these foods. As a guideline, for instance, sliced options are preferable over whole.]

So where does this leave us? Over the next immediate sections, fresh fruit and vegetables are assessed since these manifest an abundance of small organic acids; importantly, they also serve as familiar components of healthy eating, and in 2011, vegetables and fruits ranked second and fourth among food categories in US households not participating in the Supplemental Nutrition Assistance Program (SNAP) [318]: out of the approximate $31.5 billion US dollars in expenditures by these households, these categories contributed $2.8 and $2.3 billion US dollars, respectively. Though healthful, diets rich in vegetables and fruits also present elevated risks for dental erosion [301,303–305]; in fact, the relatively poor tooth health of the *inhabitants of the West-India islands and of other southern climates* due to *acid liquor and fruits* was well known by 1769 [319]. (This observation may be considered a bit ironic, given that general dental health in Europe at this time wasn't particularly pristine.) In presenting the acid content, a basic risk assessment for the 'as is' food, along with the myriad recipes and preparations that may exist, can be achieved. Note that all acid (and sugar, where applicable) content presented should not be regarded as absolute due to inherent variability that arises among analytical techniques and research laboratories; instead, these data should be considered from a relative perspective. Again, these assessments are not meant to be inclusive of all foods found throughout the world; however, one should be able to readily gain familiarity so that a general understanding can be used to identify potential demineralization risks.

Small organic acids in common edible plants (Mediterranean)

Leafy vegetables, commonly consumed fresh or cooked and in various cuisines, have long been utilized in Mediterranean cuisine and medical practice. Fifteen species of wild edible plants common to the Mediterranean region (e.g., Italy, Spain, Greece, and Portugal) were collected from central Spain and analyzed for acid content [320]. Three of the five acids identified are shown in **Figure 6.8**: ascorbic, malic, and citric acid; the other two, oxalic and fumaric acid, were most and least abundant relative to the other three acids, respectively. Relevant to those favoring diets with low oxalic acid content (as this reduces potential calcium absorption and possible urinary calculi formation), dandelion, wild leek, skeleton weed, black bryony, chicory, and hops exhibited low oxalic acid content (i.e., less than 68 mg per 100 g sample). But of particular interest from a dental demineralization perspective, the greatest variation was observed among the ascorbic, malic, and citric acids.

The leafy vegetables listed in **Figure 6.8** are ranked in order of decreasing ascorbic acid content. While the milk thistle provided the least acids overall (and next to least ascorbic acid content), this plant was the most hydrated among the 15 evaluated, so the very little dry matter remaining (i.e., less than 7%) clearly reflects water-solubility sensitivity of the acids. Among the 15, only dandelion and sorrel are predominantly consumed raw (e.g., as salads), while the rest are usually stewed. Given that sorrel has a pH around 3.5 (from **Figure 6.7**), it appears this derives in large part from its relatively high ascorbic acid content (i.e., it ranks fourth in the list). Notably, black bryony is highest in both ascorbic and citric acids, the latter of which comprised 90% of the total acid content; additionally, the content of ascorbic acid in this vegetable complements the daily recommended intake (RDI) for adults [321], and provides a baseline of sorts for comparison with the other leafy vegetables. Practically always stewed prior to consumption (a practice dating back to antiquity), the broth of the black bryony can be expected to be high in citric and ascorbic acids, and, therefore, may naturally present elevated risks for

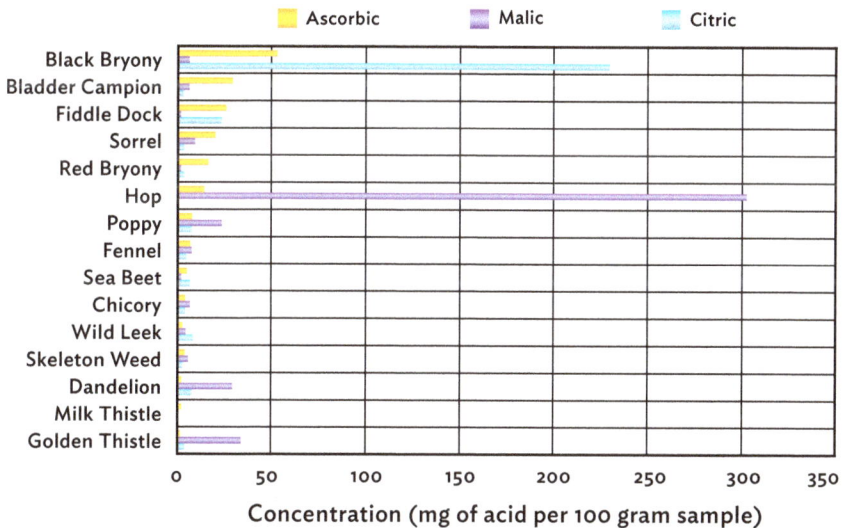

Figure 6.8. Small acid content (mg of acid per 100 grams of dry plant material) of 15 common edible Mediterranean plant species [320].

dental erosion. Hops, the young shoots of which are typically incorporated into omelets, have an abundance of malic acid, which is relatively less destructive compared to citric acid (e.g., **Figures 5.1–5.3** and **Table 5.1**); additionally, hops contain about 40% of the adult RDI for ascorbic acid which, although less than black bryony, remains at a level above many foodstuffs consumed in an average diet.

Small organic acids in some common vegetables

The ascorbic, citric, and malic acid contents of common vegetables especially familiar in western diets are summarized in **Figure 6.9**. Arranged in diminishing citric acid content, potatoes, tomatoes, wheat germ, broccoli, and cauliflower have the highest citric acid content. Notably, although these vegetables generally manifest higher levels of acids than the leafy ones previously discussed, the pH of these vegetables is relatively higher (e.g., **Figure 6.7** [307]): thus, the constitution of these vegetables demonstrates that though acids may be present (and in relatively abundant concentrations), the pH may be such that demineralization risk is minimal. As discussed in Chapter 5, pH drives demineralization, as realized, for instance, in the evaluation of two citric acid solutions at either pH 1 or pH 7.4: between these two solutions, the neutral one (i.e., pH 7.4) did not impart any demineralization when applied to dental enamel [264].

Let's consider potatoes as an example: potatoes (plain or non-sweetened) have a general pH near 6 (except for sweet potatoes, which have a pH 5.3 [307]) but also have relatively high citric acid content. Due to a relatively tooth-neutral pH, dental erosion risks are likely minimal. Still, modest drops in salivary pH upon consumption were observed (e.g., **Figures 6.1** and **6.4**), so plaque trap sites—between teeth, within occlusal crevices, around orthodontic brackets, etc.— present cariogenic risks.

Returning to **Figure 6.9**, while malic acid content is generally low, many of the vegetables have ascorbic content that meets the RDI and is important in iron absorption. Among the least acidic vegetables are pumpkins, eggplants, cabbage, turnips, and beetroot greens. While turnips and cabbage constitute relatively little acid and also relatively modest pH (~ 5.2 and 6.2, respectively from **Figure 6.7** and [307]), pumpkins have a lower pH (~ 4.8). In contrast to the potato, which has relatively high pH and high acid content, the constitution of the pumpkin has low pH and low acid content, and, therefore, presents relatively greater demineralization risks. Such risks can be neutralized through strategies such as incorporation of higher-pH foods at mealtime (e.g., milks, cheese, eggs, fish, other higher-pH vegetables, or even tea or coffee), or postmeal saliva stimulation with sugarless gums or mints to expedite pH recovery.

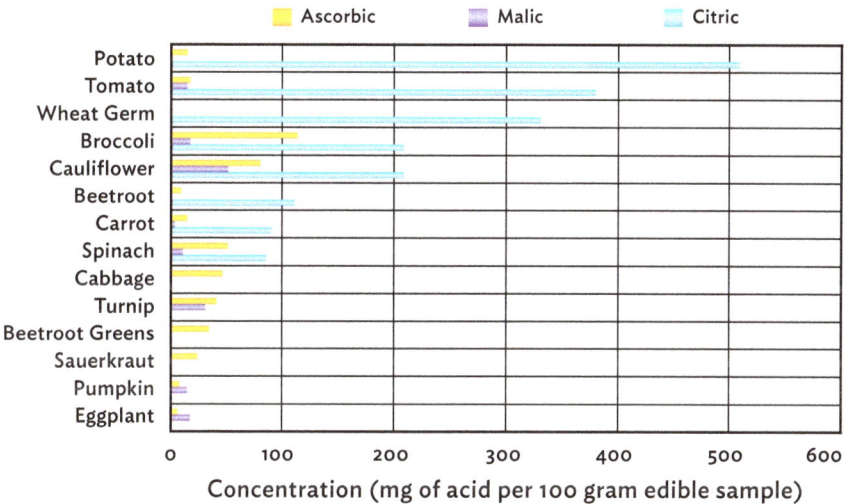

Figure 6.9. Small acid content (mg of acid per 100 gram edible sample) of 14 common vegetables [322].

The malic and citric acid contents of some other vegetables, in the order of diminishing citric acid content, are shown in **Figure 6.10** [309]. Among these vegetables, there are many with relatively high malic acid content, especially the root vegetable horseradish, along with mushroom, onion, and cucumber, all of which lack abundant citric acid content. Parsnip and artichoke have modest levels of citric and malic acids, while Brussels sprouts, green peppers, and beetroot are rich in citric acid. Still, despite the citric and malic acid concentrations, most of the vegetables in **Figure 6.10** have pH higher than 5 [307], so risk for tooth demineralization is relatively low.

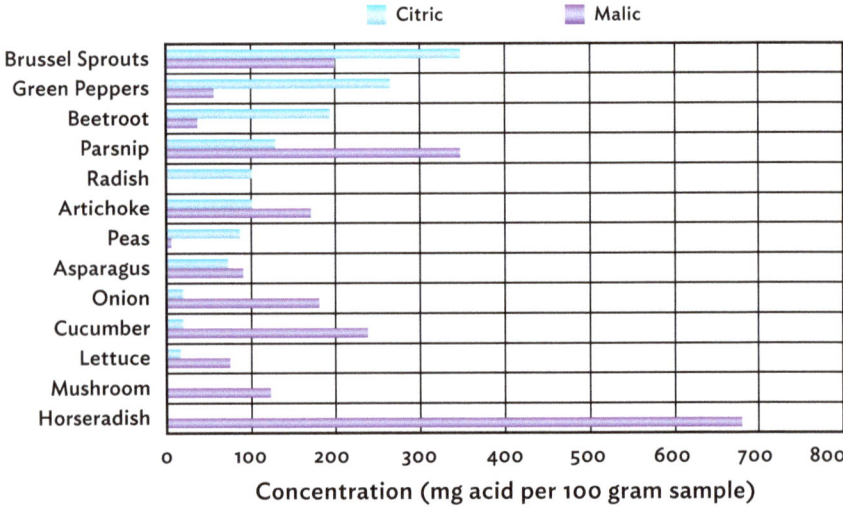

Figure 6.10. Small acid content (mg of acid per 100 grams of edible vegetable sample) of some other common vegetables [309].

Small organic acids in some common (and perhaps less common) fruits

The ascorbic, citric, and malic acid contents, along with the sucrose, glucose, and fructose contents of five common fruits (banana, peach, apple, kiwi, and strawberry, all sourced in Spain) are summarized in **Figure 6.11** [323]. Based on the figure, the dominant component in each food is sugar and the fruits are arranged in diminishing sucrose content. Strawberries have the least sucrose, but a fair amount of glucose and fructose, while bananas have the highest sucrose content, along with an abundance of glucose and fructose. Peaches have high sucrose and fructose contents, while apples are dominant in fructose and kiwis are glucose-rich. All fruits are relatively low in ascorbic acid, with none detected for bananas, peaches, or apples. Malic acid is most prominent in apples, followed by bananas and peaches, while kiwis and strawberries are rich in citric acid.

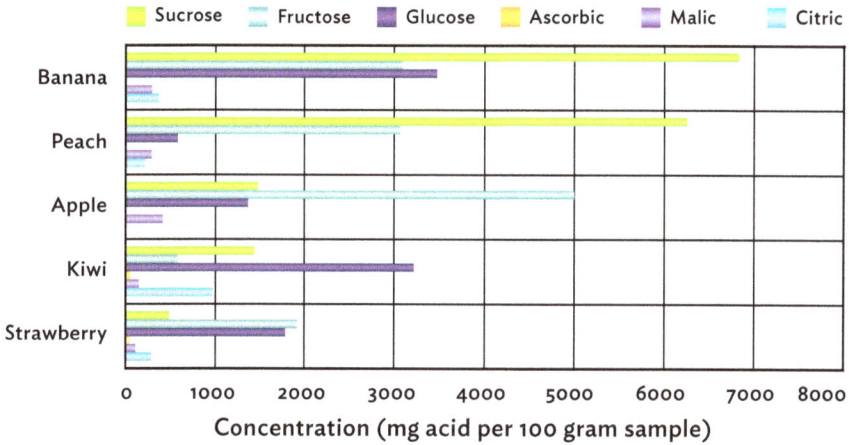

Figure 6.11. Small acid and sugar content (mg of acid or sugar per 100 gram sample) of five common fruits: strawberry, peach, apple, kiwi, and banana [323].

With respect to citrus fruits, the contents of ascorbic, citric, malic, and lactic acid of 10 fruits (sourced in Romania) are compared in **Figure 6.12** [324], with the top-to-bottom order ranked according to diminishing citric acid content. Among the four acids shown for these fruits, the ones presenting the greatest potential for demineralization are citric and lactic acids (e.g., **Figures 5.1–5.3** and **Table 5.1**), and these fruits have, on average (with some having more or less), about 88% and 4% of each of these, respectively. Supporting the 'citrus' moniker, these fruits also exhibit higher citric acid content than the vegetables in **Figures 6.8** and **6.9**. Malic and ascorbic acid content is, on average, about 6% and 2%, respectively. The most robust citric acid content belongs to lemons and limes, both of which exhibit the most acidic pH (e.g., **Figure 6.7** and [307]), and helps explain the mouth-puckering effect produced when consumed 'as is'. The range in citric acid content spanning oroblanco and clementine fruits is comparable to that of kiwis (**Figure 6.11**). Limes, which exhibit an even lower pH relative to lemons, also constitute the highest malic acid content among the citrus fruits: its malic acid is comparable to that of apples (**Figure 6.11**), although lime pH is more acidic (**Figure 6.7**).

Supporting the association of citrus fruits with vitamin C, these fruits exhibit relatively high levels of ascorbic acid compared to leafy vegetables (e.g., **Figures 6.8**), and are comparable to many of the vegetables listed in **Figure 6.9**. Additionally, lactic acid, which is a dominant acid involved in dental caries, was found in relatively higher concentrations in lemons (~ 2%), minneola [~ 9%; minneolas (also known as 'tangelos') are a cross between tangerines and grapefruits], sweet and mandarin oranges (~ 10% and ~ 8%, respectively), and oroblanco [~ 24%; oroblancos are seedless hybrids developed from pomelo (also known as 'shaddock') and grapefruit, and are also known as 'sweeties'].

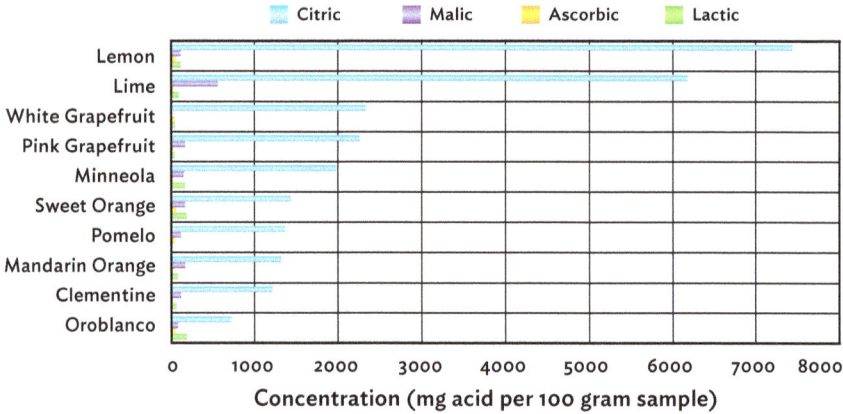

Figure 6.12. Small acid content (mg of acid per 100 gram sample) of various citrus fruits [324].

Acid and sugar content, as well as pH, of 11 berries (sourced from Finland) are presented in **Figures 6.13** and **6.14**, respectively. Among the berries, the currants (red, white, and black), red raspberry, and lingonberry yield about 5x more citric acid than malic acid; strawberry and bilberry have about 2x more citric acid; gooseberry and cranberry have nearly the same acid content; and, black crowberry and cloudberry are dominant in malic acid (about 2x more relative to citric acid). The currants (red, white, and black) exhibit citric acid content comparable to grapefruit, while cranberry, lingonberry, red raspberry, and gooseberry contents are comparable to that of oranges (**Figure 6.12**). Strawberry, cloudberry, and black crowberry have the least citric acid (and, overall acid content) and are among the least acidic berries (e.g., **Figure 6.13**). All 11 berries exhibit greater acid content relative to the banana, apple, peach, kiwi, and strawberry, although the kiwi citric acid content rivals that of the gooseberry. Differences in total acid content between the two strawberry groups (one from Finland and the other from Spain) are observed, and while the relative ratios are similar (about 2 and 3 times more citric acid than malic acid for Finnish and Spanish strawberries, respectively), clearly geography (and, therefore, climate, agricultural methods, etc.) can impart compositional differences.

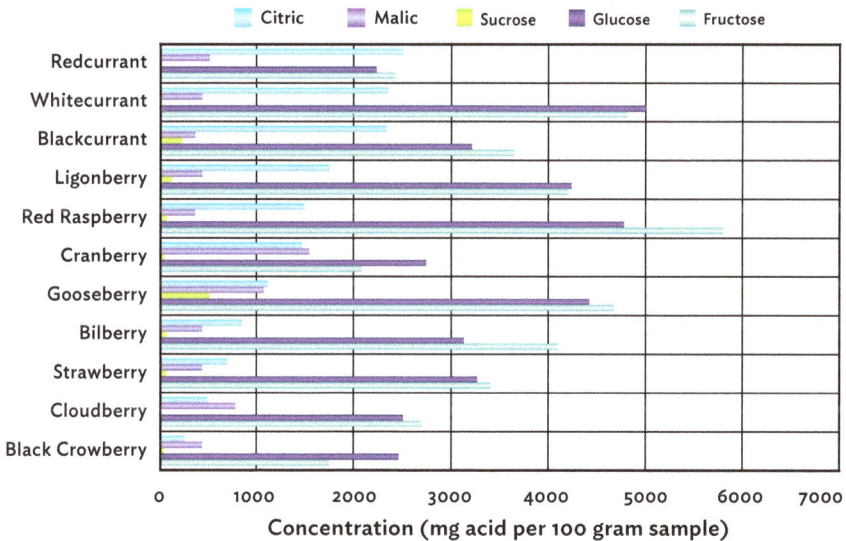

Figure 6.13. Small acid and sugar content (mg of acid or sugar per 100 gram sample) of various berry fruits [325].

The sugar composition of the berries is also pronounced, especially with respect to glucose and fructose. While bananas and peaches have higher sucrose content (**Figure 6.11**), all 11 berries have higher fructose and/or glucose content relative to sucrose, indicating the berries produce sweet notes in addition to sour character. Among the currants (all of which are fairly sour), the whitecurrant and redcurrant appear to be the most and least sweet, respectively. Among those most sweet, red raspberry leads, followed by whitecurrant, gooseberry, lingonberry, and bilberry. Strawberry and blackcurrant also have high sugar content, although the pH and acid content differ markedly. Similarly, the disparity in acid content and pH is also observed among the least sugary berries: cloudberry, black crowberry, redcurrant, and cranberry.

Though imperfect, the pH (**Figure 6.14**) correlates well with the total acid content (i.e., citric plus malic acid), indicating the acids contribute significantly to overall pH. While not the most sour or sweet, cranberry is most acidic (pH ~ 2.4), having comparable pH to the highly acidic (**Figure 6.12**) lemon (pH ~ 2.3) (**Figure 6.7**).

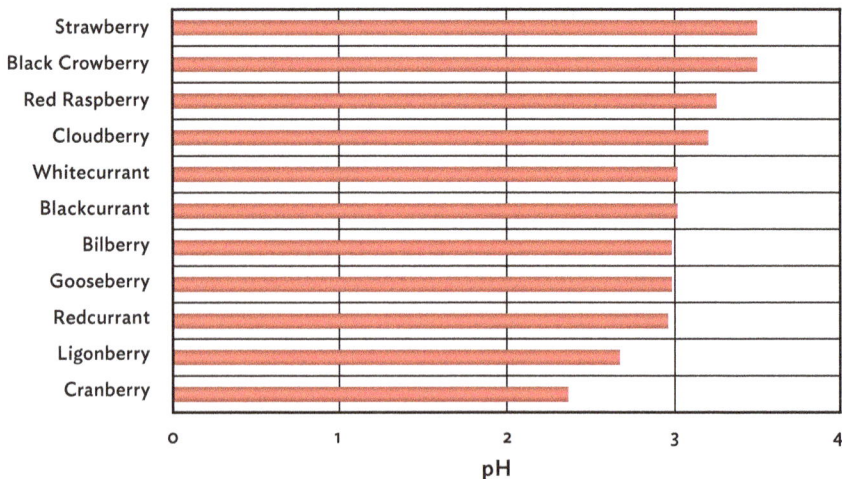

Figure 6.14. pH of various berry fruits (corresponding with **Figure 6.13**) [325].

Finally, the malic and citric acid content for other common fruits are shown in **Figure 6.15** [309], this time according to diminishing malic acid content. These fruits generally have pH < 5 [307], consistent with the other fruits in this section. Relative to the citric acid contents of lemon and lime (> 6,000 mg citric acid per 100 gram sample), and the grapefruit and currants (> 2,000 mg citric acid per 100 gram sample), rose hip, morello (i.e., sour) cherry, date, and plum exhibit the highest malic acid content (> 1,000 mg malic acid per 100 gram sample) among all fruits, with apricot, sweet cherry, and quince exhibiting comparable malic acid content relative to cranberry and gooseberry.

Altogether, these fruit data demonstrate that, like vegetables, the two most prevalent acids among all fruits are citric and malic acids, knowledge that has been known since the mid-18th century [326]. While pomme (i.e., apple-like, such as apples, pears, and grapes) and drupe (i.e., those manifesting a large central seed within the flesh, such as apricot, cherry, plum, and peach) fruits typically manifesting higher malic acid content, all other fruits, such as citrus (e.g., lemons, limes, and oranges), tropical (e.g., banana, mango, and pineapple), and berries, generally have high citric acid content. Consideration of both pH and acid content can help determine relative risk for tooth demineralization: for instance, the pH of dates and plums are about

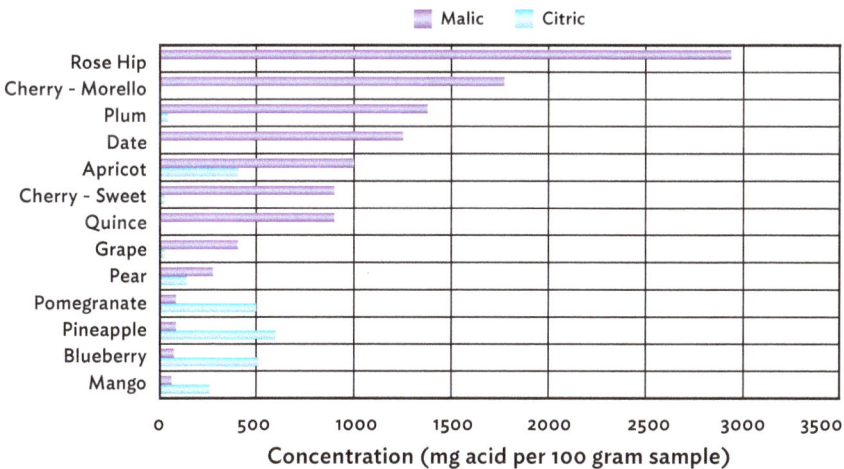

Figure 6.15. Small acid content (mg of acid per 100 gram sample) of some other common fruits [309].

6 and 4, respectively, despite both fruits having higher acid content than bananas, which have a pH approaching 5 [307].

Mitigating potential demineralization risks arising from high-acid or low-pH fruits and vegetables

In many instances, salivary flow and buffer capacity will likely dictate the extent of demineralization risk for a given individual; so, when salivary action may be limited (due to medicines, fatigue, dehydration, periods of rest, etc.), the risks for demineralization will naturally be elevated. When coupled with the pH values of several of the fruits, which are all less than 5, (e.g., **Figure 6.7** and [307]), it appears each presents increased risks for tooth demineralization relative to vegetables from both dental caries and dental erosion perspectives. As such, while these fruits certainly bear nutritional benefits, one should be aware of possible erosive risks, especially if consumed frequently or for long durations. Behavior such as sucking the lobes of lemons or oranges may increase the chance for demineralization and should be cautioned against. Fruit and vegetable fibers, seeds, or particles lodged in or between the teeth, around orthodontic brackets, or about restorations present pathways for acids to flow and bacteria to aggregate, and thus should be removed as soon as possible. Importantly, due to the acidic nature of these foodstuffs (i.e., pH < 5), one should avoid immediate toothbrushing in order to reduce compounding the risks for dental erosion and/or attrition [165,172,277].

With respect to countering pH, higher-pH foodstuffs and beverages may provide some protection when consumed after the acidic food or drink. Sialagogues such as hard cheese, salted nuts, sugar-free gums, mints, and other similar comestibles, can also help stimulate saliva to encourage remineralization. Fluoridated water and even some teas (which will be discussed later in this chapter) may also help promote nonacidic plaque environments while accelerating remineralization due to low levels of fluoride.

Segue to beverages

The discussion up to this point has focused primarily on pH and acid content of foods. Now, an extensive presentation of beverage pH and acid content will be presented, and includes waters, teas, coffees, juices, sports drinks, carbonated drinks (i.e., colas or sodas), alcoholic beverages, creamers, and milks. Again, this list is not meant to be inclusive of all beverages consumed throughout the world; however, the library of drink types amassed certainly allows for analog comparisons. But how does this relate to dental decay? Just as high-fructose corn syrup poses more damaging systemic risks than sugar (e.g., from sugarcane or beets) [327–329], beverages are implicated as a prime factor in the amount and extent of tooth decay, especially among lower socioeconomic populations [330–332], and mostly notably and sadly, in children [330,331]. Although not discussed here in great detail, sugary beverages (including carbonated beverages, fruit, energy and sport drinks, etc.) may present links to certain systemic diseases [333]. Therefore, in order to better address oral health risks, more detailed information needs to be known about the products we're imbibing. Even further, such information may bear on relationships linking dietary choices and systemic health.

pH and organic/inorganic acids of carbonated beverages (i.e., sodas or colas)

Recently reported expenditures compiled from 2011 grocery expenditure data reveal sweetened beverages rank second and fifth in Supplemental Nutrition Assistance Program (SNAP) and non-SNAP households, respectively [318]. This accounts for over $3 billion and does not include bottled water, coffee, tea, milks, or juices. Needless to say, sweetened beverages comprise a major fraction of the US diet, ranking behind the meat, poultry and seafood group for SNAP households, along with the vegetable, high fat dairy/cheese, and fruit categories for non-SNAP households.

With each person in the US estimated to imbibe about 40 gallons in 2016 [334], carbonated soda remains a familiar and tasty beverage. In fact, one study purports up to 50% of college students imbibe at least one soft drink daily [335]. And, because carbonated beverages are complicit in dental erosion risks [336,337], it is of particular interest to consider the pH (**Figure 6.16**, based on [338]) and acid type (**Figures 6.17** thru **6.19**) of various carbonated beverages from various manufacturers.

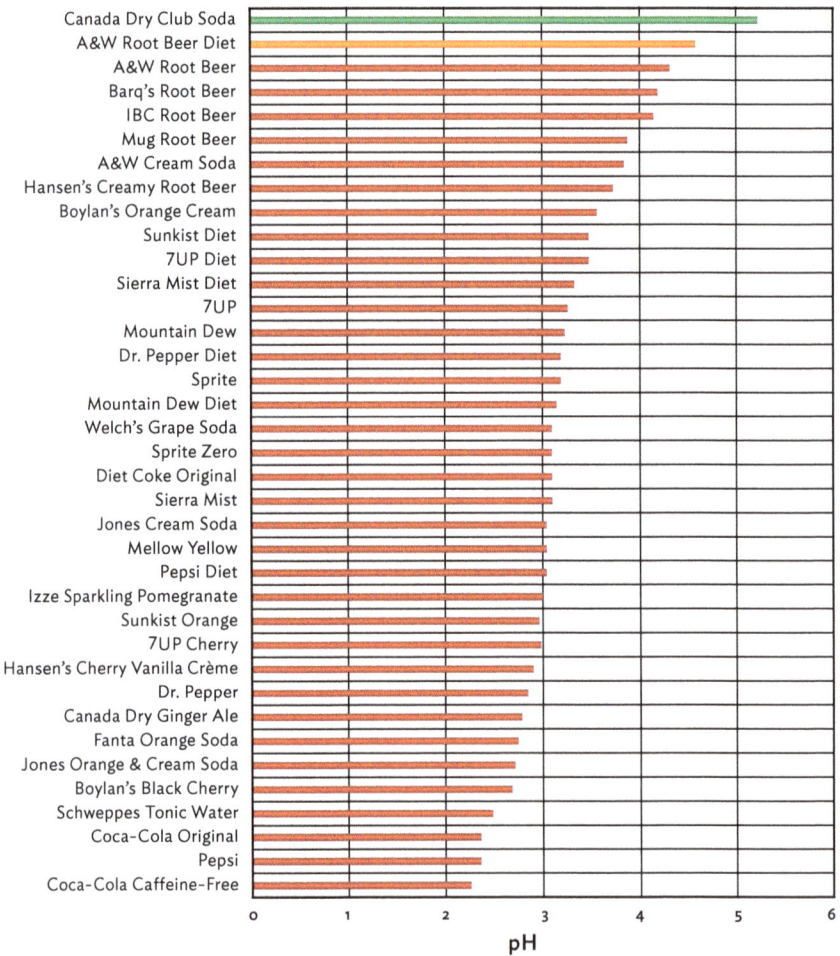

Figure 6.16. pH of various carbonated sodas (for more selections see [338]). Colors are shown to help approximate pH regions that may present relatively high (pH < 4), moderate (4 < pH < 5), or low (pH > 5) risks for dental erosion.

Figure 6.16 reveals that most carbonated beverages have pH less than 4, rendering them particular risky for dental erosion [164,339–341]. Canada Dry® Club Soda, which does not contain small organic/inorganic acids but does contain sodium and phosphate, is the only drink in this listing that manifests a pH above 5, while a few root beers exhibit pH above 4. Notably, tonic water and ginger ale are fairly acidic, having pH less than 3. And, in the sugar-free beverages, the diet variety seems to have relatively higher pH values (though this is modest): while still presenting erosive risks, the relative lack of adhesion to tooth structure by the sugar-free beverages suggests saliva may help reduce erosive potential [199,339]. Importantly, saliva may manage free-flowing formulations more effectively than more concentrated (i.e., more viscous or 'sticky') ones [339,342]. So in addition to low-pH concerns, what acids are present in these bubbly beverages?

Figures 6.17 thru **6.19** highlight the type of small organic/inorganic acid within various carbonated beverages sold by Coca-Cola®, PepsiCo®, and Dr Pepper Snapple Group®.

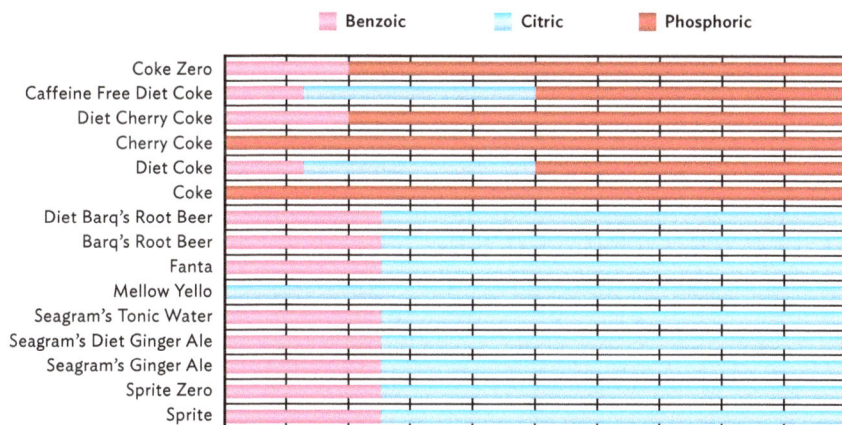

Figure 6.17. Small acids present in various Coca-Cola® brand carbonated sodas. Colors are used to help demonstrate acid strength (e.g., **Figure 5.1** and **Table 5.1** from the preceding chapter) among benzoic (including the benzoate salt form), citric and phosphoric acids.

With respect to Coca-Cola® and PepsiCo®, the carbonated beverages comprise benzoic (or, the benzoate salt form), citric, and/or phosphoric acid, with the use of the latter acid for the dark, nonroot beer colas (i.e., Coke® and Pepsi® brands); in contrast, the more translucent colas, along with the root beers, generally have citric acid, along with some benzoic acid.

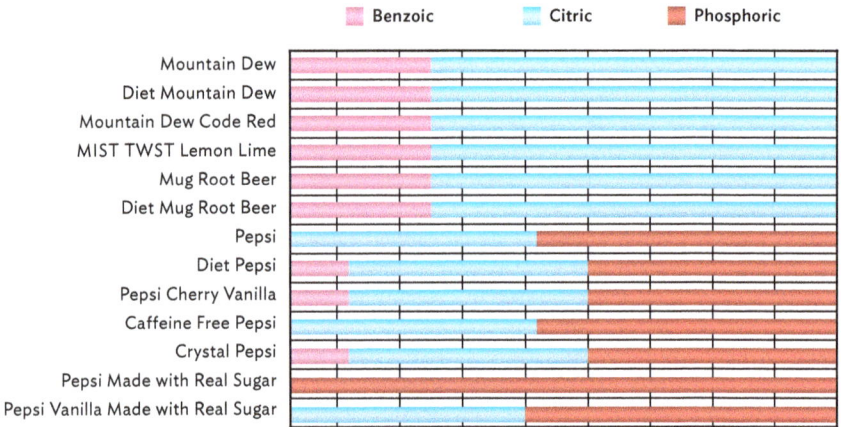

Figure 6.18. Small acids present in various PepsiCo® brand carbonated sodas. Colors are used to help demonstrate acid strength (e.g., **Figure 5.1** and **Table 5.1** from the preceding chapter) among benzoic (including the benzoate salt form), citric, and phosphoric acids.

The presence of malic acid for Diet Canada Dry® Ginger Ale and Diet A&W® Root Beer, along with benzoic acid (or its salt form) for regular A&W® Root Beer, are notable distinctions relative to the Coca-Cola® and PepsiCo® brands. In fact, relative to other root beers that contain citric acid, A&W® Root Beer and its diet analog do not contain citric acid and are less acidic (i.e., **Figure 6.16**).

So why are phosphoric, citric, malic, and benzoic (or, its salt) acids present in beverages anyway and does the taste profile really matter? While the answer to the latter question may be subjective, it helps to consider why these acids might be used. Recognizing that it is the second strongest acid among the four listed in **Figures 6.15** thru **6.17**,

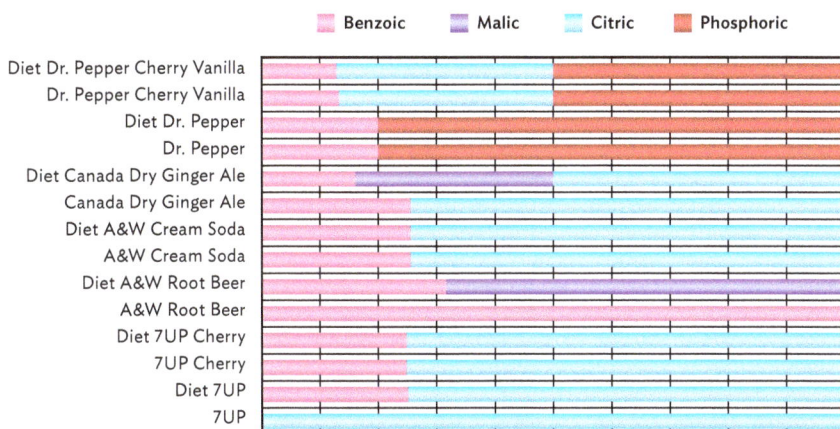

Figure 6.19. Small acids present in various Dr Pepper Snapple Group® brand carbonated sodas. Colors are used to help demonstrate acid strength (e.g., **Figure 5.1** and **Table 5.1** from the preceding chapter) among benzoic (including the benzoate salt form), malic, citric, and phosphoric acids.

citric acid is utilized in many (if not most) beverages for purposes that include an appealing taste profile (i.e., acidic burst), as well as preservative and antibrowning properties [309,310]; similarly, malic acid is used when flavor bursts are not desired, to increase palatability, and may help extend flavor intensity while masking potentially undesirable aftertastes; additionally, it also provides preservative properties [310,343]. Benzoic acid (or, the benzoate salt form) is typically included for antimicrobial purposes, although it is also found in minor amounts in various fruits [344]. Phosphoric acid is commonly found in colas (as observed here), cottage cheese, and beer, and is used primarily as an acidulant that confers sharp, tart flavors (e.g., for the cola 'bite'); it is also used for preservative (e.g., in cheese) and gelling (e.g., for jams and fillings) purposes [345].

pH and organic/inorganic acids of waters (e.g., sparkling, flavored, etc.)

The steady rise in bottled water consumption in the US finally coincided with the intake of carbonated beverages in 2016 [334], but this doesn't necessarily mean consumers are making healthier or tooth-friendly choices: the bottled water category includes several subcategories, with many waters presenting dental erosion risks at least as great as carbonated beverages. While plain bottled water certainly poses less risk for enamel demineralization, often these waters are formulated with citric and other acids to improve the taste profile. The following figures assess several categories of bottled (or canned) water, including still (i.e., noncarbonated), sparkling (i.e., carbonated), flavored, mineral, and coconut, as well as community tap water.

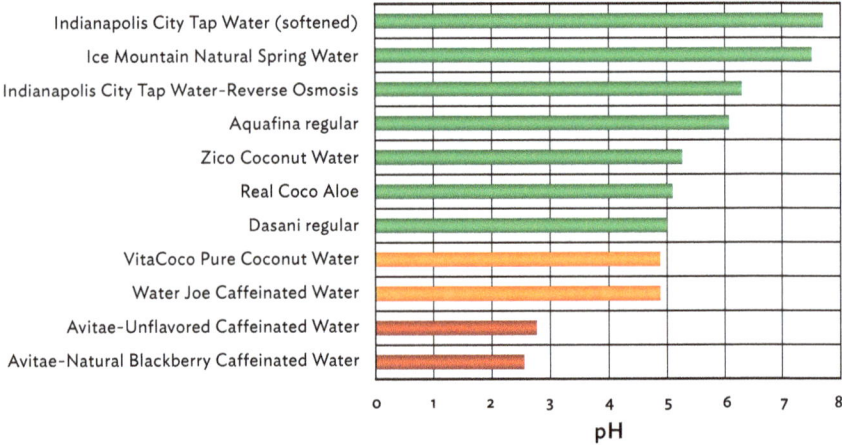

Figure 6.20. pH of various waters, including still (i.e., noncarbonated), caffeinated, and coconut waters, along with tap water from Indianapolis, Indiana (both the Dasani® and Aquafina® still bottled waters were measured elsewhere [338]). Colors are shown to help approximate pH regions that may present relatively high (pH < 4), moderate (4 < pH < 5), or low (pH > 5) risks for dental erosion.

The pH of still, caffeinated, coconut, and Indianapolis (Indiana, US) community tap water are presented in **Figure 6.20**. These data demonstrate the variation in water pH: even among still waters, Ice Mountain® presents the highest pH relative to Aquafina® or Dasani®. The Indianapolis community tap water pH is reduced by about one pH unit upon reverse osmosis. The coconut waters exhibit pH hovering around 5, while the pH of caffeinated water pH is less than 5, with the Avitae® brand demonstrating even lower pH (i.e., less than 3).

The range in pH is, however, narrower for flavored waters as shown in **Figure 6.21**, with all of them bearing relatively higher risks for dental erosion. Most of these waters have pH values that are comparable with the carbonated colas and beverages shown in **Figure 6.16**, and thus are a stark contrast to the noncarbonated, nonflavored bottled waters: for example, while unflavored Dasani® bottled water has pH near 5, the flavored Dasani® waters typically have pH near 3 (e.g., lemon or strawberry flavored). Thus, the appealing taste characteristics of these waters are complimented by lower pH, which, therefore, present increased dental erosion risks.

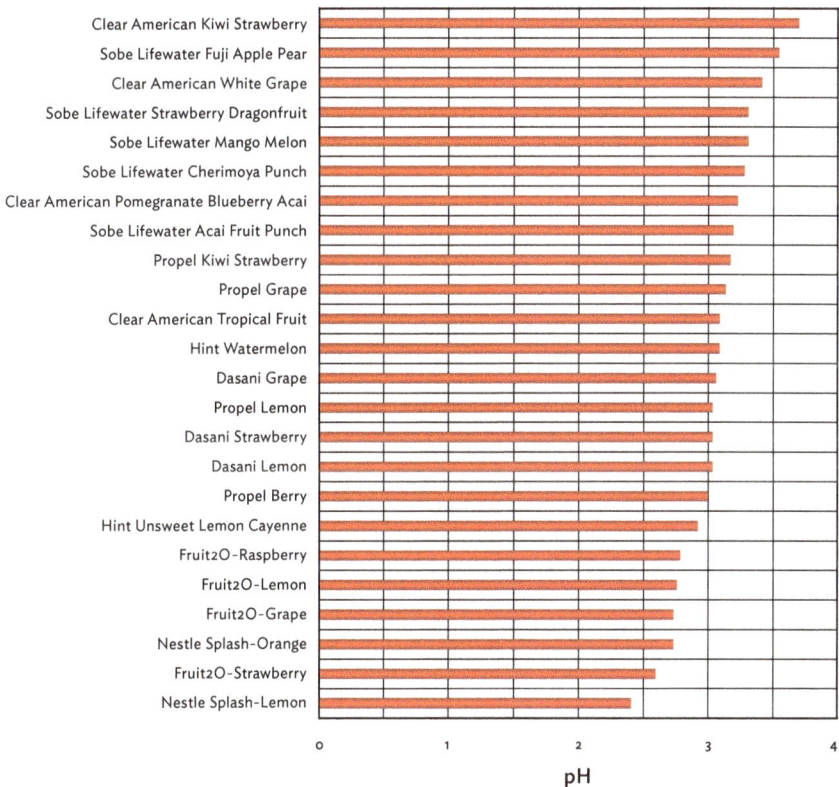

Figure 6.21. pH of various flavored waters (about half of these data are from [338]). All waters in this category present relatively high (pH < 4) risks for dental erosion. For even more flavored water data, see [338].

What about sparkling (or carbonated) waters? As shown in **Figure 6.22**, there is great variation in pH relative to noncarbonated flavored waters: the natural mineral waters, S. Pellegrino® and Perrier®, exhibit the highest pH, including those that are flavored. (Note: between these two carbonated mineral waters, Perrier® is infused with natural carbonation from one of the three deep aquifer veins [346], while external carbonation is introduced for the S. Pellegrino® sparkling waters [347]. Importantly, both of these bottled mineral waters comprise calcium.)

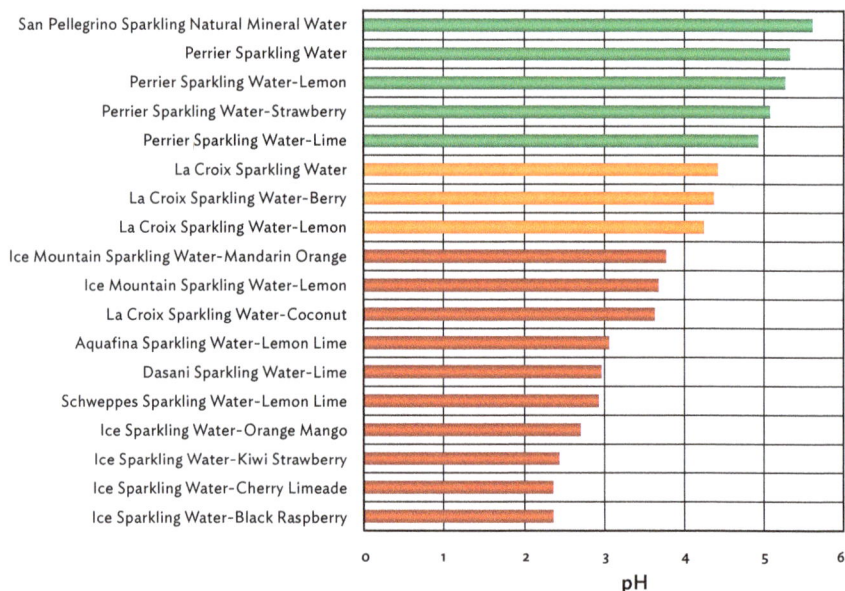

Figure 6.22. pH of sparkling (i.e., carbonated) waters (San Pellegrino® water was measured elsewhere [338]). Colors are shown to help approximate pH regions that may present relatively high (pH < 4), moderate (4 < pH < 5), or low (pH > 5) risks for dental erosion.

Most of the other sparkling waters, however, are fairly acidic, including those from La Croix®, Dasani®, Ice Mountain®, Aquafina® and Schweppes®. Contributing, at least in part, to the relatively acidic nature of these waters, is the presence of benzoic (or benzoate), citric,

and/or phosphoric acids as shown in **Figure 6.23**. Notably, the Dasani®
flavors constitute all three acids (benzoic, citric, and phosphoric),
while the others usually comprise citric acid. Similar to the carbonated
beverages discussed above, these acids impart specific flavor characteristics that contribute to taste appeal. Other flavor inclusions may
derive from distillation techniques that, while possibly described as an
'essence' (obtained from the rind or peel, for example), often remain
manufacturer secrets (e.g., La Croix®) [348].

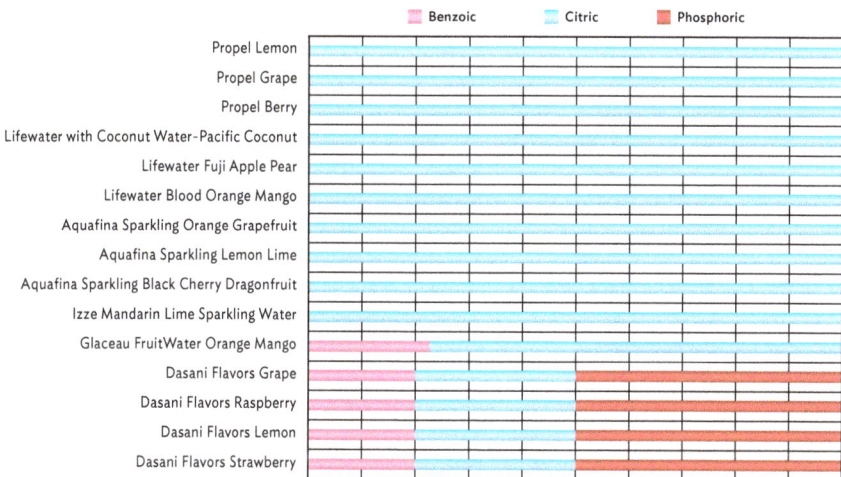

Figure 6.23. Small acid content of various bottled waters. Colors are used to help
demonstrate acid strength (e.g., **Figure 5.1** and **Table 5.1** from the preceding chapter)
among benzoic (including the benzoate salt form), citric, and phosphoric acids.

Although one may think these relatively clear liquids are harmless
(especially if they are zero-calorie and/or sugar-free), an acidic pH and
the presence of acids present erosive risks. Still, if imbibition is desired,
then this should be done without swilling or prolonging the contact
of these drinks with the teeth, since the retention of these small acids
can remain on the surfaces of teeth, even with limited exposure (e.g.,
[299]). In my opinion, based on the relatively benign pH, lack of small

organic/inorganic acids, the presence of calcium, and the availability of some flavor variations, sparkling mineral waters are healthy and fun options. And while 'plain' bottled water still presents a healthy choice, if one wants to incorporate some flavor into the water, perhaps adding a slice of fruit or its juices (keeping in mind to limit contact with the teeth) and adding a health-minded sweetener (e.g., xylitol or stevia) may help satisfy taste-sensory desires.

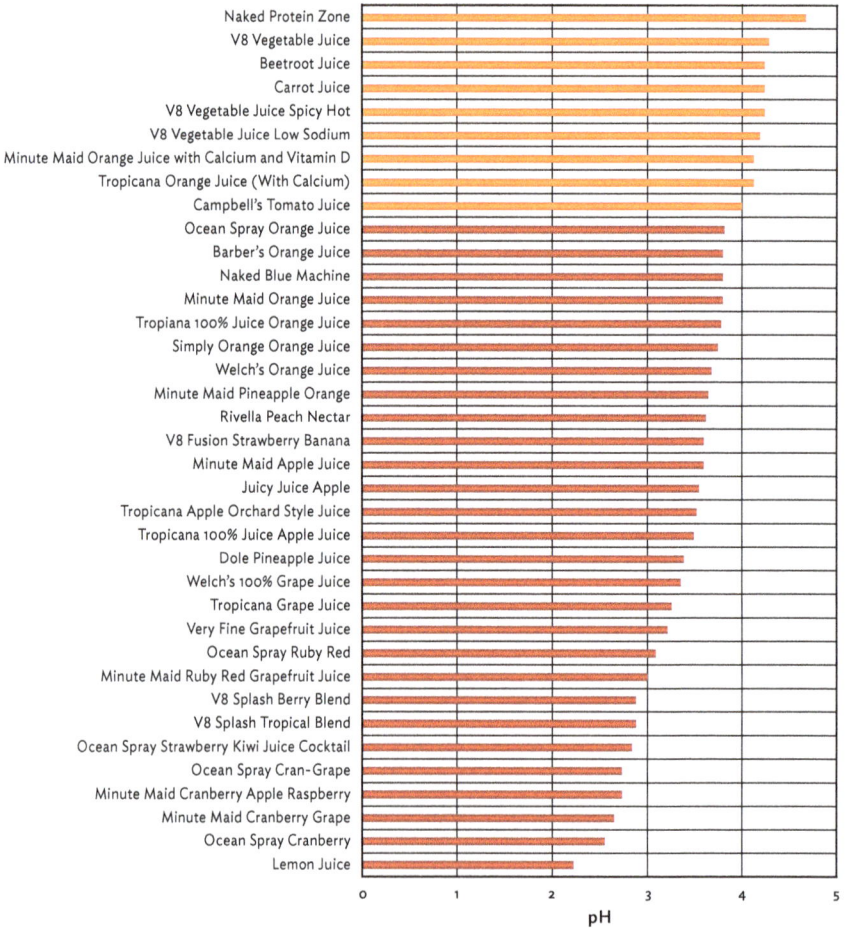

Figure 6.24. pH of juices. Most are selected from [338], except for carrot juice and peach nectar [342], and beetroot juice [164]. Colors are shown to help approximate pH regions that may present relatively high (pH < 4) or moderate (4 < pH < 5) risks for dental erosion. For even more juice data, see [164,338,342].

pH of juices and juice drinks

Juices and juice drinks, although a relatively modest expenditure (less than 2% for SNAP and non-SNAP US households in 2011 and ranking about 17th out of the 30 food subcategories [318]), are nevertheless recognizable and a popular form of refreshment (e.g., orange or apple juice) throughout the world. As one might expect based on the fruit and vegetable pH and acid content detailed previously, these types of beverages generally have a more acidic pH (usually less than 4), and, therefore, bear on dental erosion [339–341,349]. Similar to carbonated beverages, the presence of sugars and the 'stickiness' of the drink impart additional erosive risks [339,342]. **Figures 6.24** and **6.25** detail some popular versions and brands of juice and juice drinks available in the US.

A key difference between juices and juice drinks is that the latter is infused with real juice and/or added small organic acids (e.g., citric, malic, etc). Between either juices or juice drinks, the ones comprising fruits are most acidic, especially those comprising the more acidic citrus (e.g., lemon and grapefruit) and/or berry (e.g., cranberry) fruits. The dominant acids in juices are similar to that in fruits: for example, malic acid and citric acid are dominant in apple and orange juice, respectively, while grape juice comprises mostly tartaric and malic acids; also, pineapple juice has high citric acid content but also contains malic acid [350]. In general, vegetable juices present relatively less erosive risks (by virtue of higher pH), although they still comprise citric, malic, and/or other acids [351]. Interestingly, the protein beverage Naked® Protein Zone (**Figure 6.24**) is buffered by protein (whey and soy), which helps to offset the fruit juices. Still, this beverage type presents moderate erosion risks, especially as this may be relatively more viscous (which can present retentive risks [342]) compared to more free-flowing drink options.

pH and small organic/inorganic acids of sports drinks

Within the very popular sweetened beverage category (which accounts for about $3 billion in 2011 US family expenditures [318]) are sports drinks such as Gatorade®, Powerade®, and vitaminwater®. The pH and acid content of some of these popular sports drinks brands in the US, along with Red Bull® energy drink, are shown in **Figures 6.26** and **6.27**.

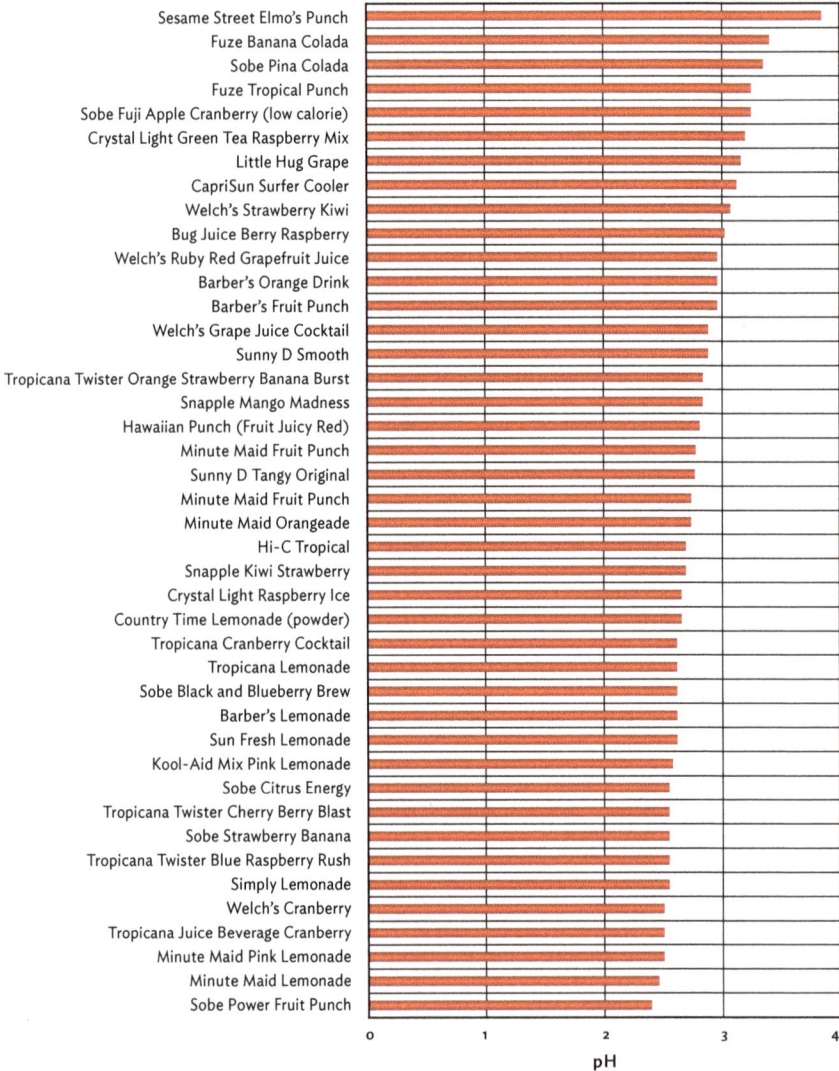

Figure 6.25. pH of juice drinks (selected from [338]). All drinks in this category present relatively high (pH < 4) risks for dental erosion. For even more juice data, see [338].

Similar to the fruit juices and fruit drinks, the pH of these are all less than 4, and when combined with their popularity, these may present significant dental erosion risks [340,352,353]. The formulations of sports drinks include ascorbic, citric, and/or phosphoric acids, as shown in **Figure 6.27**. In particular, even the sugar-free versions of vitaminwater® contain all these acids and have pH near 3, while the sugared versions lack phosphoric acid but generally have pH also near 3 (except for the fruit punch version). In contrast, the carbonated beverages typically resulted in diet versions having slightly higher pH (i.e., less acidic) relative to the sugar

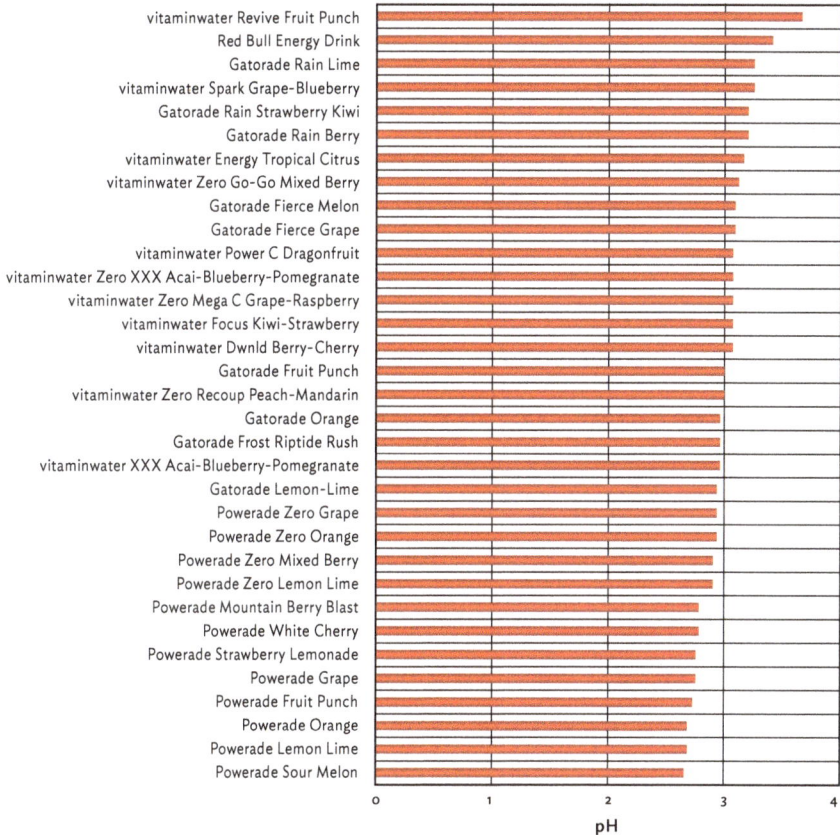

Figure 6.26. pH of sports drinks (selected from [338]) and Red Bull® energy drink [342]. All drinks in this category present relatively high (pH < 4) risks for dental erosion. For even more sports drink data, see [338].

version. Despite the absence of phosphoric acid, Powerade® typically had the lowest pH values. Gatorade® lacked ascorbic acid, although all versions seemed to maintain pH near 3, with some containing phosphoric acid.

Given that viscosity of these formulations may be comparable, some sports drinks, by virtue of pH and/or acid content, present elevated risks for dental erosion [282,304]. However, like the causal relationship between sugar and caries, not all who imbibe sports drinks are subject to dental erosion (e.g., [354], and references therein), so genetic susceptibility, habits, drinking behavior, nature of the sports drink, and so on all bear on an individual's ultimate risk level. And, certain sports may be more demanding on the dentition and thus factor into destructive processes: for example, in a study where cyclists and swimmers all exhibited dental wear, the cyclists exhibited much greater prevalence of advanced wear into dentin [355]. Recently, a dose-response relationship was observed for sports drinks and dental erosion among 16-17-year-old adolescents [282]: sports drinks present elevated dental erosion risk factors, especially when consumed three or more times per week.

Although perhaps useful for replenishment of lost fluids and electrolytes (e.g., when body mass is reduced by 2% or more), many who are exercising even on a regular basis would find water to be sufficient [164,353,356,357]; still, sports drinks can improve recovery relative to other fluid formats [356]. A primary reason to choose a sports drink (instead of, for instance, a carbonated drink) for rehydration after an exercise bout is related to its osmolality, which should constitute a low, but effective, level [358]. For instance, carbonated beverages and fruit juices (e.g., apple, orange, etc.) have relatively high (e.g., more than double) osmolality relative to milk, Gatorade®, Powerade®, or Lucozade® Sport [356]. This is important, since absorption of carbohydrates and electrolytes is encumbered when osmolality is high. Furthermore, fluid and carbohydrate absorption (through the colon) are significantly improved in the presence of sodium, which may make this the most important electrolyte for post-exercise recovery [356].

The use of sports drinks, however, is not limited to systemic ingestion: more recently, studies are highlighting the benefits of short bouts of mouth-swishing (e.g., five seconds over a one-hour endurance period) with a sports drink as a means of improving performance and/or recovery [359–363]. Some of these sports drinks may or may not include caffeine which, as shown in **Figures 6.20** and **6.26** (e.g., Avitae® and Red Bull®, respectfully), typically are found in acidic drinks. Though five seconds may not sound too alarming, as discussed previously, a single rinse with a citric acid solution led to sustained levels of citric acid along the upper anterior teeth [299]. Even further, dental erosion manifests over repeated exposures to acids, so even casual athletes routinely participating in this behavior may be elevating their erosive risks [138,165,169,170,199,277].

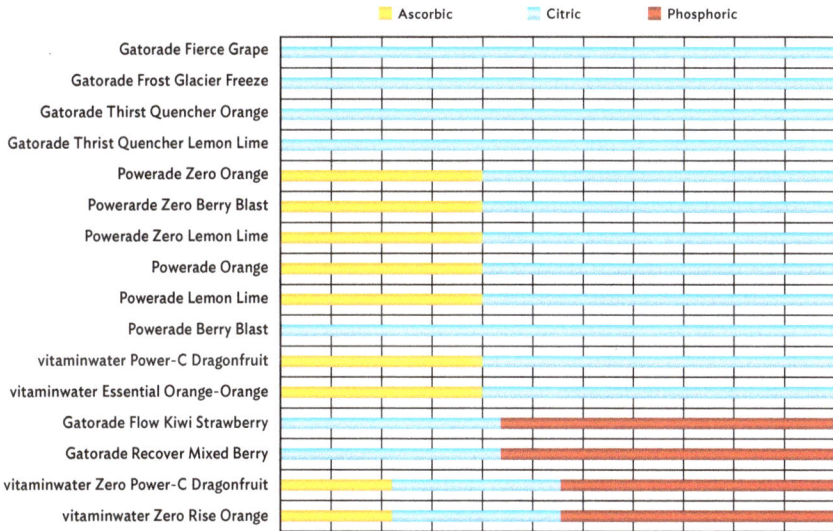

Figure 6.27. Small acid content of various sports drinks. Colors are used to help demonstrate acid strength (e.g., **Figure 5.1** and **Table 5.1** from the preceding chapter) among ascorbic, citric, and phosphoric acids.

As discussed previously, athletes may develop elevated risks for infection and/or dental decay due to mucosal reductions [96–99,169].

When the professional athlete is observed rinsing and spitting with a sports drink, this behavior can trickle down to viewers, including kids, children, and teenagers participating in athletics. In fact, when posted on popular websites and blogs (e.g., [169]), readers with avid interests in the sport may be prone to incorporate—and adapt—such behavior to fit their needs. Given the competitive landscape that exists in various sports at various different levels, it is clear that routine rinsing and spitting certainly may contribute to risks for dental erosion. To be sure, these risks are not solely related to the professional athlete: dental erosion has already been observed among physically active adults (male and female, between 18 and 32 years of age) who regularly attend fitness centers [169].

Recent research on exchanging or supplementing milk-based or milk-derived products for carbohydrate-electrolyte sports drinks during exercise or for post-exercise recovery appear to confer performance and/or recovery benefits. This extends to chocolate milk (with fat) [364] as well as skim milk [365], and may reduce exercise-induced muscle damage [366]. And, experimental sports drinks supplemented with milk-derived proteins also show promise due, in part, to the effect of proteins on water retention [367]. The prospect of using milk has tooth-friendly advantages and will be discussed later in this chapter. In the meantime, for those seeking to gain a performance edge, there exist alternate and/or complementary strategies that still support athletic prowess while mitigating risks for dental erosion.

pH and small organic acid content of some beer, wine, spirits, and vinegars

A distribution of pH values for vinegar and various alcoholic beverages, including beer, spirits, and wines is presented in **Figure 6.28** (from [164] and [342]). Among those listed, wine, vinegar (including salad dressing), lemon-flavored alcoholic drinks, vodka, and cocktail drink yield the lowest pH and, therefore, present the greatest demineralization risks. Noncitrus flavored beers seem to provide moderate risks, while the syrupy/sugary beverages (i.e., limoncello and Cointreau) are least risky from a pH perspective.

Recalling **Figure 6.7**, the pH values of sugar and syrups are about 5, and likely contribute to the relatively higher pH of limoncello and Cointreau liqueurs. With respect to limoncello, the lemon flavor is obtained through using lemon oils (which is obtained from peel scrapings known as 'zest') instead of lemon juice (which is rich in citric acid), a feature which also helps to keep a relatively high pH; this process is likely mirrored with the orange-flavored Cointreau liqueur.

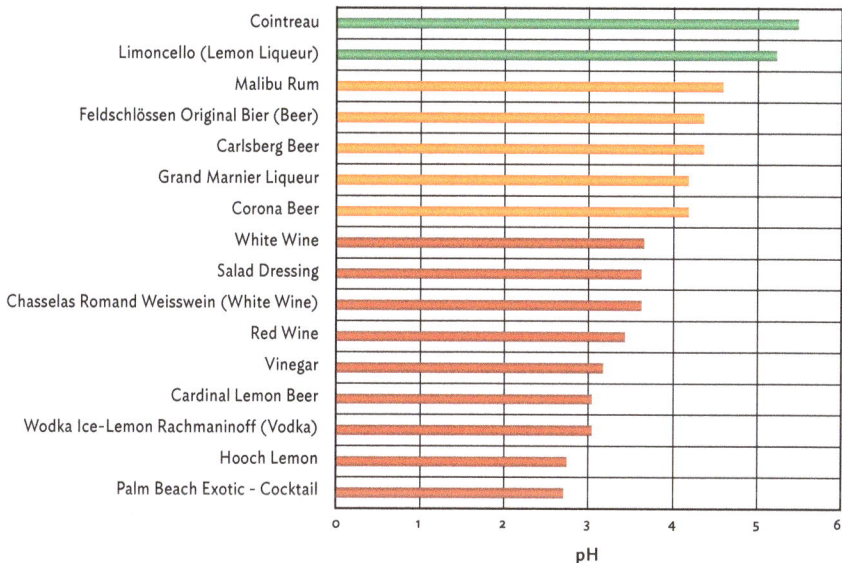

Figure 6.28. pH of some alcoholic beverages and vinegar (from [164] and [342]). Colors are shown to help approximate pH regions that may present relatively high (pH < 4), moderate (4 < pH < 5), or low (pH > 5) risks for dental erosion.

With respect to wines, the acid content between red and white wines varies considerably, as noted in **Figures 6.29** thru **6.31**, with acetic, succinic, lactic, malic, citric, and/or tartaric acids identified in various wines from different regions and/or brands [350,351,368–370]. In these three figures, all are arranged with respect to decreasing acetic acid content. As tartaric, malic, and citric acids are common in grape juice [350], sensibly these are also observed in wines; however, the relative abundance varies widely due to fermentative processes, which helps evolve acetic and succinic acids. In essence, these data support the vinicultural and enological character that helps shape the unique sensory profile of a given wine.

Though quite enjoyable, wine manifests a potent dentition-damaging combination of low pH and small organic acids. Despite the robust buffer capacity of saliva, it can readily be overcome by wine (and can impart even more damaging effects on those with encumbered salivary flow) [371]. So it is not surprising that professional and amateur wine tasters, as well as casual and habitual drinkers, are prone to dental erosion: for the former, this is usually related to frequent swilling/rinsing events for taste evaluations (e.g., [372]), while protracted drinking in private or social settings is usual for the latter (e.g., [373]).

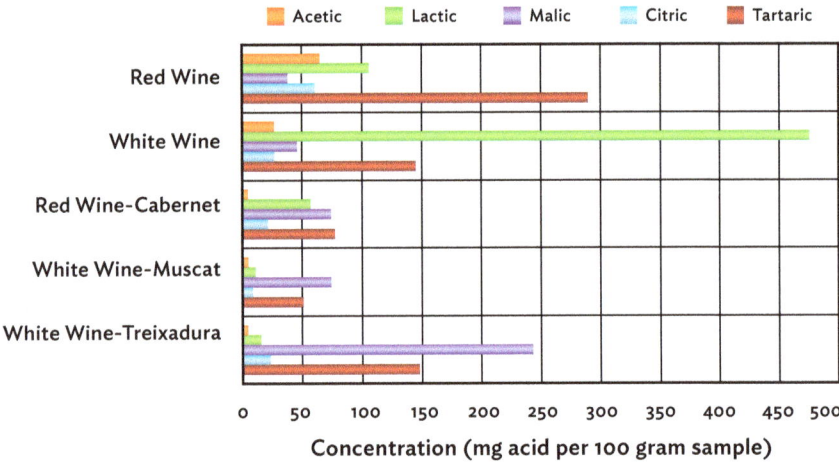

Figure 6.29. Small acid content (mg of acid or sugar per 100 gram sample) of wines, including Muscat and Cabernet wines [351], red and white wines sourced from a store in Spain [350], and a sample of white wine from Treixadura [368].

Fermentation of wine by acetic acid-generating bacteria (e.g., *Acetobacter aceti*, as described by Thomson in 1852 [374]) produces vinegar. While the pH of vinegar reported in **Figure 6.28** is around 3.2 (and the pH of salad dressing is only slightly higher), other studies on plum, grape, rice, and apple vinegars reveal pH as low as 2.4 (for plum vinegar)

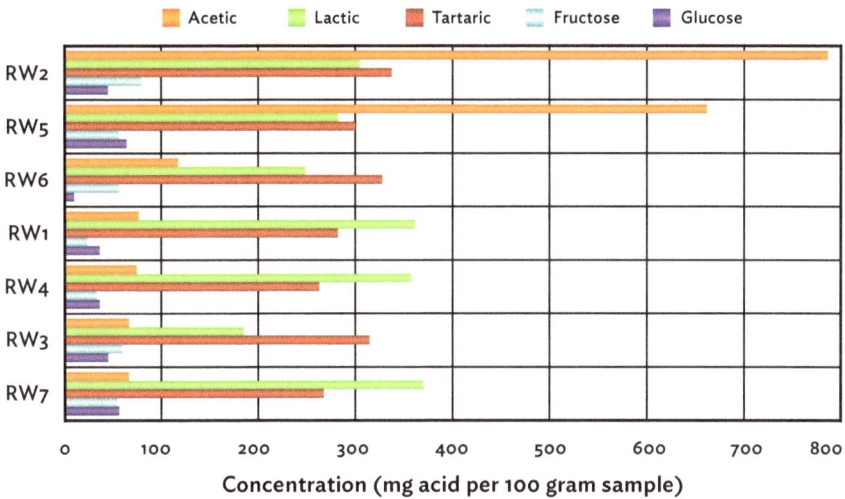

Figure 6.30. Small acid and sugar contents (mg of acid or sugar per 100 gram sample) of seven different Austrian red wines arranged in order of decreasing acetic acid content (from [369]).

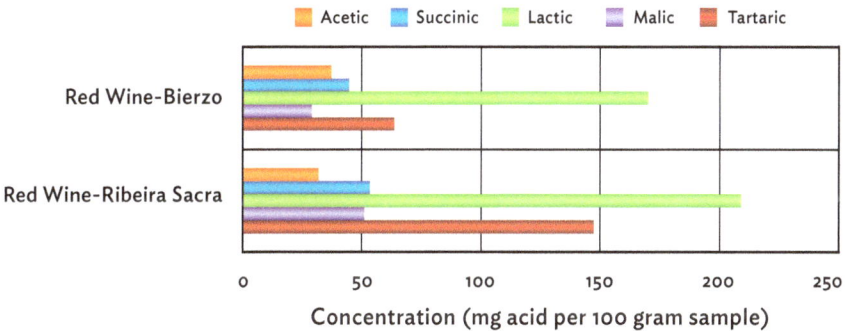

Figure 6.31. Small acid content (mg of acid per 100 gram sample) of two regional Spanish wines (from [370]).

[375]; as apple vinegar has the highest pH (pH ~ 3.2), the pH values (listed in increasing order) of white, rice, wine, raspberry wine, balsamic, grape, and apple cider vinegars lie in between these limits [375]. While acetic acid is common in all vinegars, white vinegar has the least amount (at about 5% [375]); in contrast, aged balsamic has about 75% acetic acid content (along with ~ 16% malic acid), while higher concentrations are found for nonaged balsamic vinegar (~91% acetic acid, plus ~5% malic

acid), apple vinegar (~ 92% acetic acid, plus ~ 6% malic acid), and wine vinegar (~ 96% acetic acid, and less than 1% malic acid) [309].

Regardless of acid content, however, pH remains a primary factor in tooth demineralization, so while white vinegar, which is commonly used in culinary recipes, may have only 5% acetic acid, its pH is among the lowest of all the vinegars and, therefore, presents relatively greater risks for dental erosion. And while prolonged contact between teeth and white vinegar may seem unlikely, consider this: when ingested at bedtime, white vinegar may provide health benefits to those with Type 2 diabetes [376]. Like wine, the low pH of vinegars can gradually erode tooth mineral over time so provisions must be in place in order to successfully thwart dental erosion.

Although spirits (including rums, whiskeys, brandies, vodkas, etc.) comprise many acids, relative to wine, the acid content is usually lower. But, similar to wine, the type and concentration of acid varies. For example, Brazilian sugarcane-derived spirits (e.g., caninha or cachaça), manifest high acetic acid content (e.g., having, on average, about 2x as much acetic acid relative to whiskeys, with content in some brands exceeding 100 mg per 100 gram sample) [377]), while cognac (a type of brandy made from white wine), has about 4x as much lactic acid compared to acetic (where acetic acid is present in less than 1 mg per 100 gram sample) [351]. And while spirit consumption usually contrasts with wine imbibition, the pH of these liquids still presents risks for dental erosion; in fact, these risks become elevated as the drink becomes more appealing when combined, for instance, with low-pH juices (including fruit and vegetable) and/or cocktail mixes (e.g., the Palm Beach Exotic Cocktail drink shown in **Figure 6.28**).

Similar to wine and spirits, as shown in **Figure 6.32**, a range in organic acids naturally exists among beer brands [378]. Usually lower in alcohol relative to spirits and wines, beers also appear to manifest lower contents of acids: for instance, among the beers in **Figure 6.32**, the beer with the most lactic acid (i.e., B3) comprises 10x less lactic acid relative to the Ribeira Sacra red wine shown in **Figure 6.31**. While the fermenting processes used in making bread, beer, spirits, and wine typically involve the same fermenting agent (i.e., the yeast species *Saccharomyces cerevisiae* [379,380]), the nature of the feedstock (e.g., grains and grapes), the presence of other microbes, and general fermenting conditions (e.g., mashing or musting, pitching rate, temperature, time, etc. [381]) clearly influence the acidic and alcoholic output. The pH of the lager beers in **Figure 6.32** ranges between 4.2 and 4.6, and is consistent with the nonlemon flavored beer pH reported in **Figure 6.28**. Thus, concomitant with relatively higher pH, beer manifests less acid content relative to spirits and wine (unless, of course, acids and/or juices are introduced for flavor purposes). Drinking behavior aside, these combined characteristics render beer capable of producing dental erosion, albeit to a relatively lower degree compared to wine and spirits; additionally, beer presents less erosive risks compared to carbonated colas, fruit juices/drinks, and sports drinks.

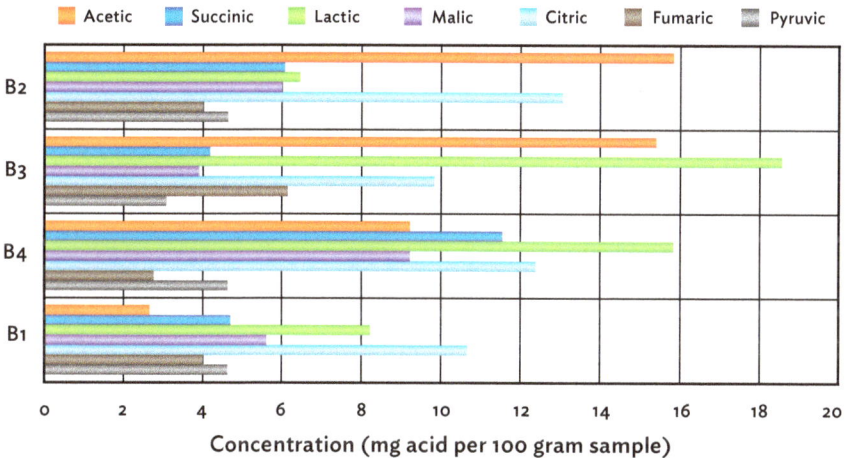

Figure 6.32. Small acid content (mg of acid per 100 gram sample) of four regional Italian lager beers arranged in order of decreasing acetic acid content (from [378]).

pH and small organic acids of some dairy and nondairy milks, health-based drinks, and creamers

The milk segment of food and drink expenditures ranks about ninth on grocery lists of SNAP and non-SNAP households (3.5 and 3.8%

135

of all grocery expenditures, respectively) [318]. While not as popular as meat, fruits, vegetables, and sugary beverages, this category (which generated $1.5 billion in 2011) is not only familiar but also is exploding in product diversity [382].

In general, citric acid predominates small organic acid content in mammalian milk, regardless of fat content (i.e., skim or whole) and state (i.e., liquid or powder), with powdered milk products generally having higher concentrations [383]. Compared to other dietary selections, citric acid content in liquid milks is generally higher than those in beers and many vegetables, but is similar to some red wines and fruits (e.g., ~ between 80 and 200 mg per 100 gram sample); however, the powdered versions can be several times greater compared to the liquid analog.

In contrast, sour milk, buttermilk, sour cream, yogurt, whey (including powdered), kefir, and cheeses generally have an abundance of lactic acid [383]. Whey and buttermilk (including powdered product) generally comprise both citric and lactic acids: however, while the citric and lactic acid contents are similar in whey (with slightly more citric than lactic but both having around 120 mg acid per 100 gram sample), buttermilk is rich in lactic acid and contains little citric acid; additionally, buttermilk also has about 8x more acetic acid compared to citric acid.

Excluding whey and cheese, these other dairy products generally comprise minimum levels of lactic acid starting around 600 mg per 100 gram sample. For cheese, the lactic acid concentration can vary widely: for example, the lactic acid contents in Muenster (i.e., with 50% fat content), Limburger (i.e., with 40% fat content), and cheddar cheese (i.e., with 50% fat content) are 70, 285, and 1,330 (in units of mg per 100 gram sample), respectively [383]. Despite the acid content, these foodstuffs provide at least two major benefits to the oral environment that help counter caries and/or erosive processes: calcium and a benign pH. Consistent with the pH values shown in **Figure 6.7**, an augmented list of bovine-based milks (including sour, whey, fermented, flavored, and lactose-free), human milk, and liquid eggs, is shown in **Figure 6.33**. With the exception of whey, buttermilk, fermented, and sour milk, the remaining liquids all have pH greater than 6. Of particular interest, fat content, flavor variations, and the absence of lactose (i.e., the Lactaid® milks) do not lend to lower pH values, regardless of the brand. Also, prepared liquid eggs have pH consistent with values albumen [386], and do not present tooth demineralization risks.

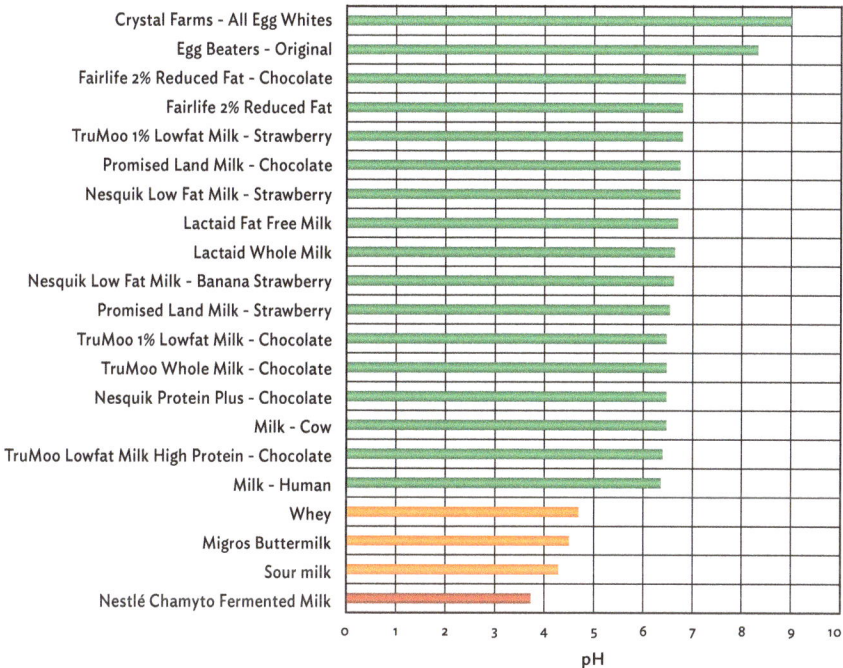

Figure 6.33. pH of liquid eggs or milks, with pH from sour milk and whey [164], buttermilk [342], fermented [384], and human and bovine milk [385]. Colors are shown to help approximate pH regions that may present relatively high (pH < 4), moderate (4 < pH < 5), or low (pH > 5) risks for dental erosion.

As noted above, the concentration of lactic acid is pronounced in fermented milk, sour milk, buttermilk, and whey, and may contribute to lower pH values; however, the calcium content helps buffer the relatively low pH so tooth demineralization risks are reduced compared to similar pH systems lacking calcium. In fact, sour milk, yogurt (which has pH between 4 and 5), and cheese (especially cheddar, which has a pH approaching 6) are good sialagogues, contain calcium, and can strengthen weakened enamel [164,387,388]; while these effects are attenuated in whey [164] and buttermilk [342], fermented milk, which is the only liquid in **Figure 6.33** having pH less than 4, presents elevated risks for tooth erosion [384].

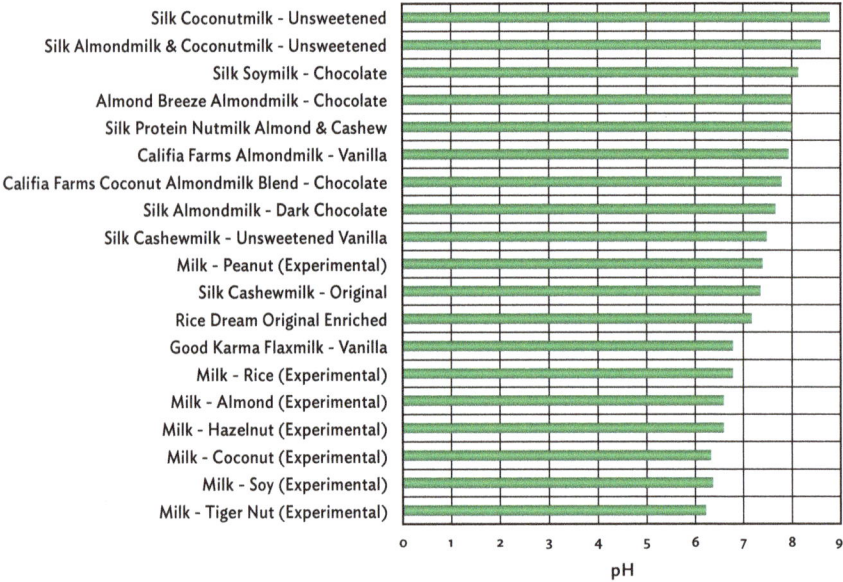

Figure 6.34. pH of commercially available plant-based milks, along with the following 'experimental' milks: peanut and rice [391]; almond [392]; hazelnut [393]; and coconut, soy, and tigernut [394]. All pH values are relatively high, indicating relatively low (pH > 5) risk for dental erosion.

And what about nondairy options? Plant-based milks have long been familiar (e.g., almond milk was especially common during the Medieval Period [389]), with soy among the first nondairy milk substitutes available in Western commercial markets [382]. As manufacturers evolve efficient processes to capture variations of plant-based sources, in turn, options for consumers (especially in the United States) continue to emerge. So in addition to 'as is' nuts and seeds or nut butters [390], plant-derived milk alternatives are now readily available, including rice, flax, coconut, almond, cashew, and more [382].

With respect to small organic acids, usually these milks comprise relatively low amounts, if at all, with some exceptions noted for the inclusion of ascorbic acid to help meet dietary recommendations. In general, these plant-based sources are low in small organic acids, but contain rather abundant amino acids and phytochemicals [313,316]. In fact, many of the plant-based milks available in the US contain more calcium than dairy milks due to the addition of calcium (e.g., calcium carbonate). However, there are exceptions: for formulas adhering to 'natural-only' ingredients, often calcium is lacking in these 'organic' plant-based milks.

pH values of various plant-based milks are shown in **Figure 6.34**. All milks are above pH 6, indicating they pose minimal risk for tooth demineralization. In general the 'experimental' milks are those devised in the laboratory and not commercially available: these milks tend to have lower pH values compared to commercially available milks (e.g., Silk®, Califia®, Rice Dream®, and Good Karma®). Most of the commercially available milks also have a fair amount of calcium with recommended intake at typically around 45% (which is higher than that found in dairy milk). Though these milks are available as 'unsweetened', the 'sweetened' varieties usually contain added sugars; however, the amount is usually modest and may actually be less than dairy milks. Even so, like dairy milks and yogurts, the potential caries-related risks due to sugar content are offset by pH and calcium content (assuming, of course, the usual and appropriate oral hygiene measures are in place). Thus, the combination of low organic acid content, high calcium content, and benign pH render these milks beneficial (i.e., presenting minimal, if any, risk) to the dentition.

To meet nutritional needs, protein milks are sometimes used to supplement the diet. pH values of several brands of protein milks are shown in **Figure 6.35**, with all of the milks demonstrating relatively low risk for dental erosion. Protein sources include dairy milks (MET-Rx® and Special K®), dairy milk proteins only (Muscle Milk® and Premier®), or soy (Advant Edge®) and pea (Evolve®) proteins. Protein milks vary in macro- and micronutrient profile according to brand and functional design, with some high in sugar while others may be sugar-free. These present relatively low demineralization risks, especially compared to protein drinks that have lower pH (e.g., Naked Protein Zone® in **Figure 6.24**) and contain fruit juices and/or high organic acid content. In addition to healthy pH, these protein milks also comprise calcium and phosphate, which can help offset erosive risks.

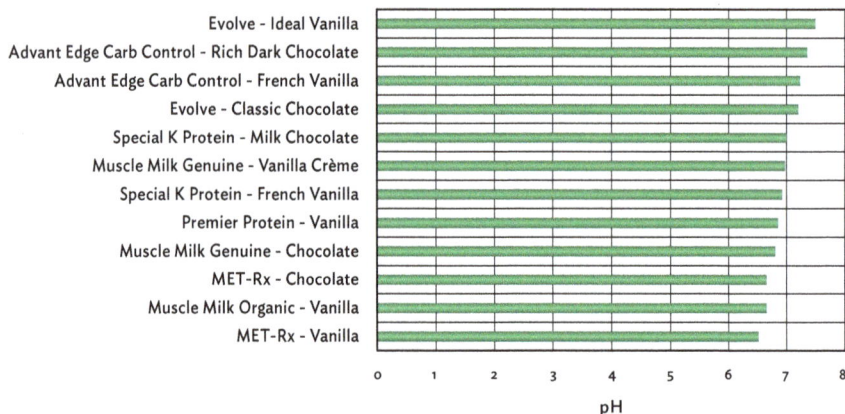

Figure 6.35. pH of several commercially available protein milks. All pH values are relatively high, indicating relatively low (pH > 5) risk for dental erosion.

The pH of several drinks designed for specific populations are shown in **Figure 6.36**. With exception of Pedialyte® Mixed Fruit, these drinks contain dairy milk proteins and are designed to meet nutritional needs of children and/or adults, including those with diabetes (i.e., Glucerna®), those experiencing challenges meeting daily nutritional needs (e.g., Ensure®), or those seeking a more amenable body weight (e.g., SlimFast®). Each of the listed drinks has a diverse nutritional profile, though ascorbic acid is present in most of them, along with citrate salt. Similar to the protein and nondairy milks, these specialty drinks (with the exception of Pedialyte®) also contain calcium and phosphate to help meet recommended daily intakes. Excluding Pedialyte®, these formulations have tooth-friendly pH and present little (if any) risks for dental demineralization.

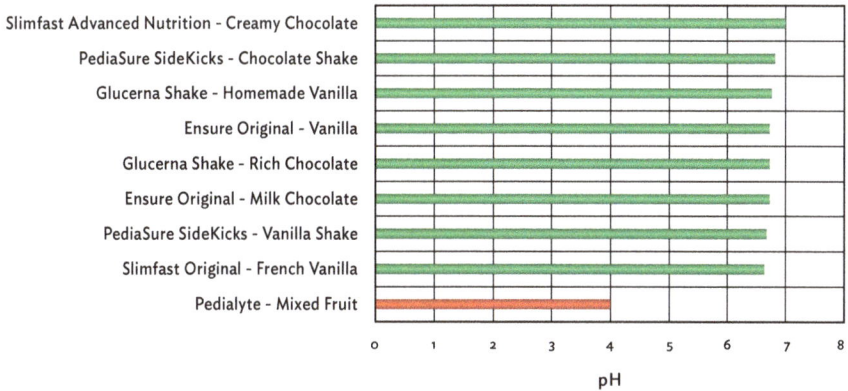

Figure 6.36. pH of several commercially available specialty drinks. Colors are shown to help approximate pH regions that may present relatively high (pH < 4) or low (pH > 5) risks for dental erosion.

While comprising micronutrients such as potassium, sodium, and zinc, Pedialyte® lacks calcium and presents relatively higher risks for dental erosion due to its pH and citric acid content. Pedialyte® is designed to rehydrate due to sickness, travel, or exercise, and, by virtue of its mineral composition, claims to be a 'more effective' option for replacing electrolytes [395]. The appealing flavor, which is flavored in part with citric acid, is meant to facilitate rehydration; however, this drink may also present elevated demineralization risks (especially for kids) if, in accordance with Pedialyte® recommendations, the drink is frequently sipped [395].

And, with respect to dairy and nondairy creamers, the pH values (**Figure 6.37**) are all above 6. Notably, the almond-based creamers typically have the higher pH, followed by coconut milk creamers. The Meijer®,

Nestlé®, and International Delight® creamers are made with oils (vegetable and/or soybean) and milk protein derivatives, while the Land O'Lakes® creamers are made with dairy milk. Additionally, the Land O'Lakes® dairy creamers also contain calcium, while none of the creamers contain small organic acids. Altogether, these creamers present low risks for dental erosion.

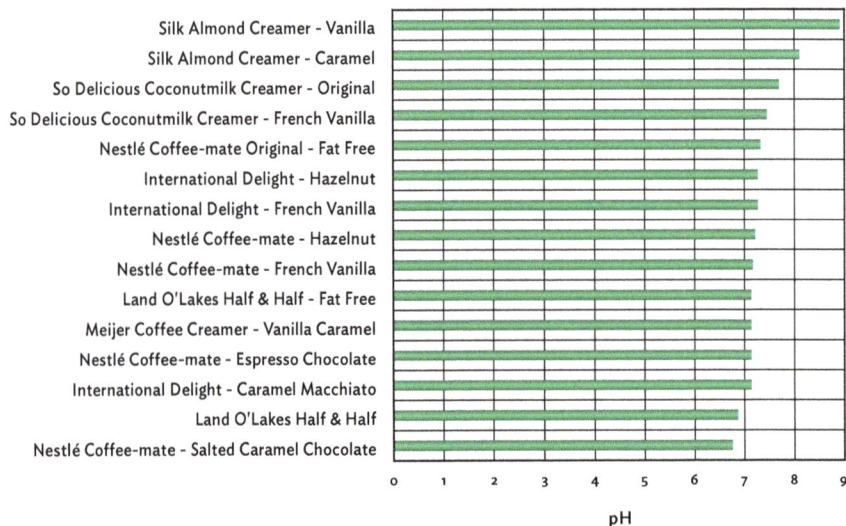

Figure 6.37. pH of several commercially available dairy and nondairy creamers. All pH values are relatively high, indicating relatively low (pH > 5) risk for dental erosion.

pH and small organic/inorganic acids of coffees and teas

The *Camelia* genus of tea plant is indigenous to China and India, both of which continue to be both the world's largest tea producers and consumers [396,397]. Seemingly popular since time immemorial, tea is presently the world's most consumed drink, followed closely by coffee [396,397]. Key advantages driving the popularity of tea include taste and culture variations (e.g., white, green, oolong, black, pu-erh), relatively low barriers to brewing (e.g., infusions of two or three leaves compared to percolation of about 10 grams of roasted, ground coffee beans), and the many health benefits (especially those effected by green tea, including oral health benefits) [396–403]. Separately, native to the Red Sea region

(Yemen and Ethiopia, in particular) and long-invigorating Ottoman armies, English and Dutch traders eventually sprung the coffee trade doors wide open, with many now enjoying some version of coffee on a daily basis [404,405]. Out of about 100 species of *Coffea*, the two most prevalent forms of coffee enjoyed by consumers worldwide are robusta and arabica [405,406]. Together, tea and coffee dominate as the world's most popular drinks so it is highly relevant to explore their pH and small acid content. And although not discussed here, the reader is strongly encouraged to check out the references used in this section to learn more about tea and coffee, including variations, compositions, and purported health benefits.

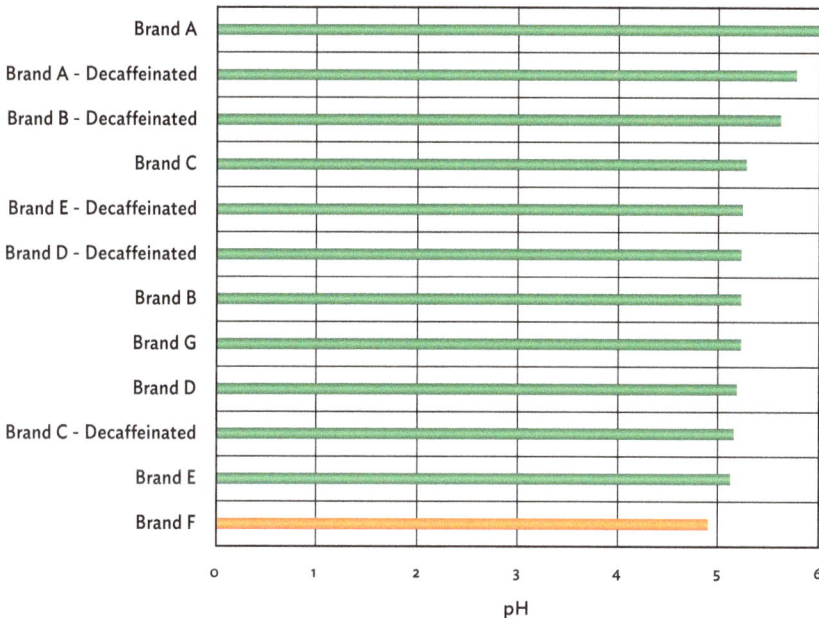

Figure 6.38. pH of brewed coffee (from experiments on caffeinated and caffeine-free commercial brands available in the US [407]). Colors are shown to help approximate pH regions that may present relatively moderate (4 < pH < 5) or low (pH > 5) risks for dental erosion. On average (and within standard variability), the pH of brewed coffees is higher than 5.

Coffee beans are fruits of *Coffea* plants, and manifest a bevy of constituents that give rise to the properties of the particular species of fruit or seed. Thus, the often bitter taste of coffee is due to a complex blend of components including caffeine (which itself is quite bitter), small organic acids (e.g., succinic, acetic, malic, citric, etc.), and phytochemicals (which includes chlorogenic acids, quinic acid, ferulic acid, and so on).

As shown in **Figures 6.38** and **6.39**, the pH of brewed coffee hovers around 5, and this is consistent with ready-to-serve coffees (i.e., those already brewed and bottled such as the bottled Starbucks® Medium Roast Coffee); in contrast, brewed and bottled coffees incorporating milk blends (or milk proteins) result in a higher pH, usually over 6. Thus, if creams or milks are added to a given coffee (freshly brewed or previously bottled), one can expect the pH to elevate.

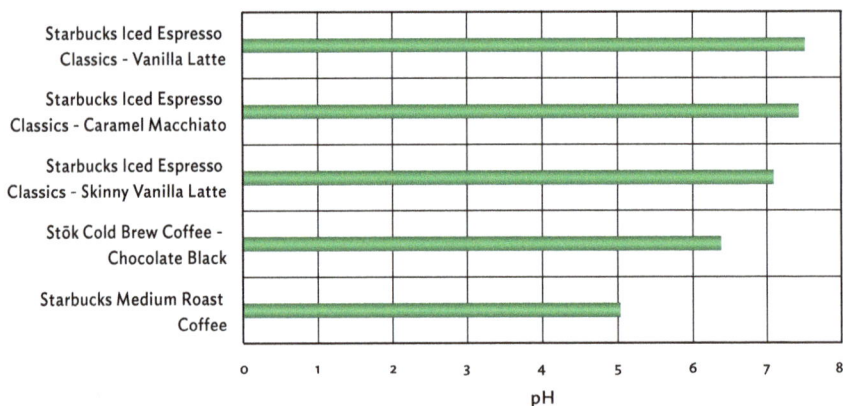

Figure 6.39. pH of ready-to-serve coffees available in the US (Starbucks® Medium Roast from [338]). All pH values are relatively high, indicating relatively low (pH > 5) risk for dental erosion.

While coffee pH does not vary widely (unless spiked with agents, e.g., milk or cream), the acid content is dependent on the nature of the bean (e.g., arabica vs. robusta), roasting (e.g., light, medium, or dark) and preparation (e.g., percolation vs. espresso) conditions. For example, one study demonstrated that both arabica and robusta green coffee beans lose their ascorbic acid but gain acetic acid during a roasting

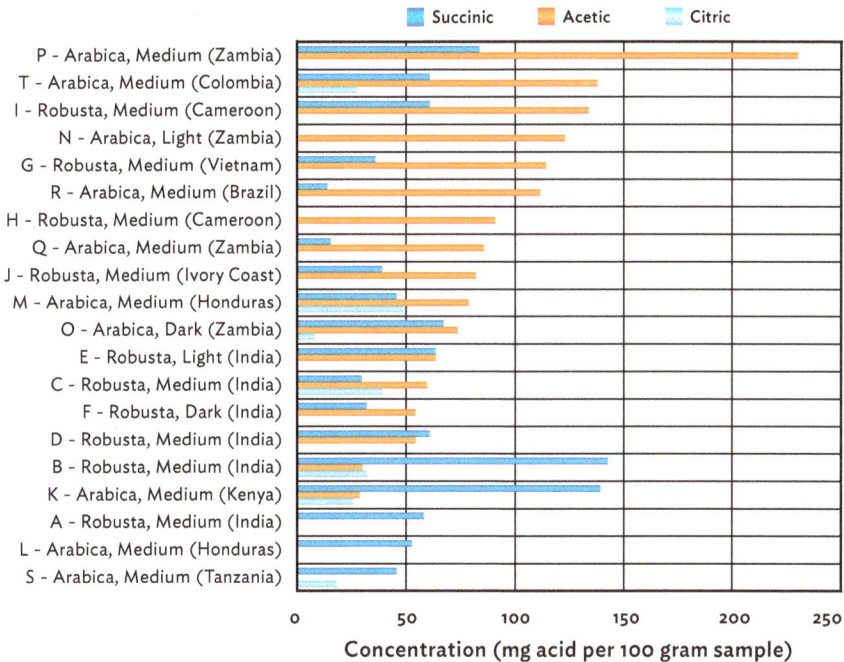

Figure 6.40. Small organic acid content (mg of acid per 100 gram sample) of 20 arabica or robusta coffees (light-, medium-, or dark-roasted) from different countries (from [406]). These are the three major small organic acids detected, and data are presented in order of decreasing acetic acid content.

procedure [408]. Separately, expressions of small organic acids were not predictable among 20 different arabica and robusta beans sourced from different origins of the world (**Figure 6.40** based on data from [406]): for example, **Figure 6.40** reveals that while some medium roast arabica beans yield high acetic acid content (e.g., P—Zambia), other arabica beans had none (e.g., S—Tanzania); and, this unpredictability extends to light, medium, and dark roasting conditions regardless of the origin and coffee bean type. In these examples, the citric acid content, which can be among the most damaging to tooth structure, is not present in high quantities. And while sweeteners may help improve the palatability of coffees, these do not seem to elevate dental demineralization risks—in fact, adding sugars may elevate pH and help stimulate saliva, both of which may help create commensal biofilms (e.g., non-acidogenic plaque) while clearing carbohydrates from the oral environment; and, when combined with milks that contain calcium (and/or phosphate), the already low risk of demineralization potential is further depressed due to saturation and/or buffering effects.

In contrast to coffee pH, the many variations of tea lead to a greater pH range for both brewed and ready-to-serve teas (**Figures 6.41** and **6.42**, respectively). In **Figure 6.41**, the three highest-pH teas from the US do not contain added acids, while the remainder of the teas (including both US and Brazil) are all flavored with added acids (e.g., malic, citric, phosphoric, or even fruit juices) [338,409]. For example, the Coca-Cola® Matte Leão Black Tea Peach Flavor available in Brazil includes citric and phosphoric acids, while the Feel Good Green Tea (Brazil) includes ascorbic and citric acid along with lemon juice. Snapple® Raspberry Tea and Arizona® Green Tea with Ginseng are each flavored with citric acid, while several of the US brands also comprise more than one acid: regular and diet versions of Lipton® Green Tea with Citrus contain ascorbic, citric, and phosphoric acids, while NESTEA® Red Tea Pomegranate Passionfruit contains citric and phosphoric acids.

The presence of phosphoric acid in bottled tea might be surprising, as this acid has the dubious distinction of being present in carbonated beverages (and is sometimes referred to generally as 'food acid'). In fact, the presence of this aggressive acid can diminish the perception and value of an otherwise seemingly healthful beverage option, especially since bottled tea made with this acid has been shown to soften enamel [410]. From an oral health respective, as teas (including ready-to-serve) are generally not guzzled but are frequently sipped, it is important to understand differences among brands and formulations in order to minimize potential damage to the dentition. So with respect to ready-to-serve teas, unless the teas do not contain any added acids, they are on par with many of the carbonated and juice-type beverages and therefore present elevated risks for demineralization.

Among brewed teas in **Figure 6.42**, fruit teas (e.g., orange, apple, lemon, rosehip, and blackberry) pose the greatest potential for dental erosion, including demineralization of both enamel [416] and dentin [417]. While brewing conditions may vary, **Figure 6.42** suggests white, green, black, oolong, and herbal teas present moderate-to-low risks for tooth demineralization; however, given the deleterious effects of fruit teas or even ready-to-serve flavored teas (e.g., even black tea infused with acidulants such as citric and/or phosphoric acid) as discussed above, infusions produced from tea (e.g., herbal, green, white, etc.) comprising citrus flavors may yield lower pH, and, therefore, present elevated risks for demineralization.

With respect to tea popularity, black tea is a favorite in the Western world (although green tea is quickly catching on), while the East imbibes white, green (which has long been a staple in China, Japan, Korea, and Vietnam), oolong, and pu-erh (which involves storage of green tea leaves for periods of 10 years or more and is especially popular in China) teas [396–398]. Similar to the roasting of coffee beans, the processing of tea from green to black [408] leads to steep reductions in ascorbic acid content (i.e., even to the point where content is below apparatus detection limits) [398]. Given that both brewed tea and coffee produce an abundance of phytochemicals [400,408], the relatively higher pH values for teas (excluding fruit teas) may be related to relatively low levels of small organic acids: as shown in **Figure 6.43** [418], all infusions, including lemon-flavored teas, yield acid content much less than those from roasted coffee beans (**Figure 6.40**).

The processing of leaves (e.g., from green to black), also leads to large reductions in sugar content (including sucrose, fructose, and glucose): for example, fructose content is reduced by almost 50% in black tea compared to green tea [398]. Additionally, the processing (i.e., oxidation) of leaves en route to black tea is accompanied by the creation of large polyphenolic molecules (e.g., condensation of catechins, which are in high abundance in green tea), resulting in darker-colored infusions [398]. As such, minimally processed (e.g., white or green tea) or semiprocessed (e.g., yellow or oolong tea) teas tend to have higher total phenol content relative to processed teas (e.g., black or pu-erh) or herbal teas [397,398,401].

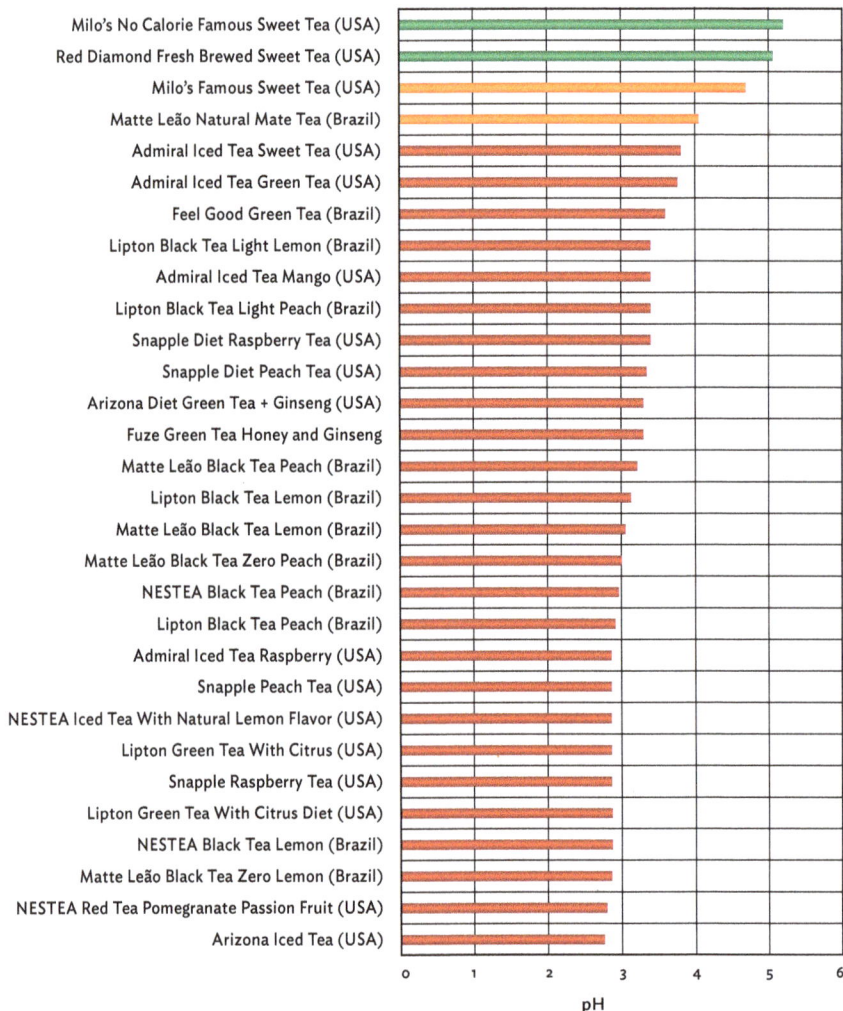

Figure 6.41. pH of ready-to-serve teas (US beverage data are based on [338], while Brazilian teas are based on [409]). Colors are shown to help approximate pH regions that may present relatively high (pH < 4), moderate (4 < pH < 5), or low (pH > 5) risks for dental erosion.

In contrast to the drop in total phenol content with tea processing, the inverse is true for fluorine content as shown for black (**Figure 6.44**), green (**Figure 6.45**), and nonblack and nongreen tea infusions (**Figure 6.46**) [419]; additionally, ready-to-serve teas also contain fluoride (**Figure 6.47**) [419]. Taken into the plant from the soil, fluorine ultimately deposits into tea leaves: as such, fluoride content is sensitive to the degree of tea leaf processing [419,420]. In general, it seems black teas (**Figure 6.44**) have the widest fluoride range (from 0.3 to 4.5 ppm), with most having content higher than 1 ppm, and is likely due to differences in geographical or horticultural differences, as well as processing conditions; in

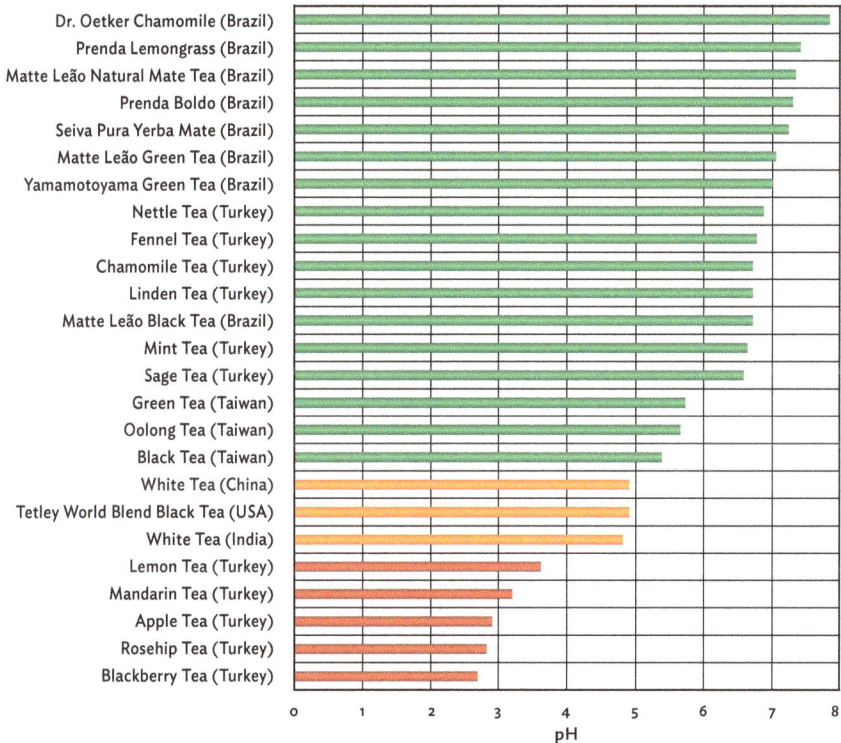

Figure 6.42. pH of brewed white, green, black, oolong, fruit, and herbal teas (from [398,409,411–415]) sourced from various locations, including Brazil, China, India, Taiwan, and Turkey. Colors are shown to help approximate pH regions that may present relatively high (pH < 4), moderate (4 < pH < 5), or low (pH > 5) risks for dental erosion.

149

contrast, the range for green tea (**Figure 6.45**), which enjoys minimal processing, is narrower (with most ranging between 0.6 to 1.6 ppm). Oolong and pu-erh teas (**Figure 6.46**) both entail some processing, and are similar to green tea in fluoride content (ranging between 0.4 and 1.7 ppm), while white (which is the least processed) and herbal (which manifest different phytochemical profiles and general plant characteristics) teas generally have fluoride content less than 1 ppm (**Figure 6.46**). These results mirror those separately obtained for black, green, and herbal teas [420]. With respect to prepared teas (**Figure 6.47**), fluoride content may vary in accordance with tea type (as shown here), and is likely to be further influenced by ingredient selection and manufacturing processes.

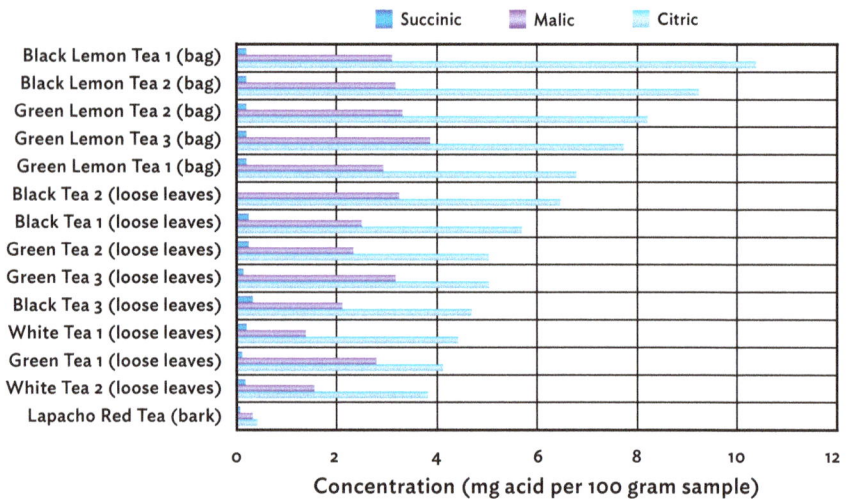

Figure 6.43. Small organic acid content (mg of acid per 100 gram sample) of several infusions from white, green, black, lemon-flavored teas, along with herbal Lapacho Red bark tea (from [418]). These are the three major small organic acids detected, and data are presented in order of decreasing citric acid content.

Interestingly, those teas manifesting fluoride content near 1 ppm mirrors that found in communities with water fluoridation [421], and would support approaches that encourage low levels of topical fluorides in the oral environment [34]. Because it is impractical for families to assess fluoride content of a given tea, it would seem that for children with developing dentition (i.e., those less than 12 years of age) black tea should be avoided in order to minimize fluorosis concerns [419,420]. However, for those with permanent dentition, partaking in a postmeal tea or afternoon tea break may not only help offset potential effects from the accompanying cookie (especially for tea tempered with a touch of milk), but may also help promote oral health [400,402,403].

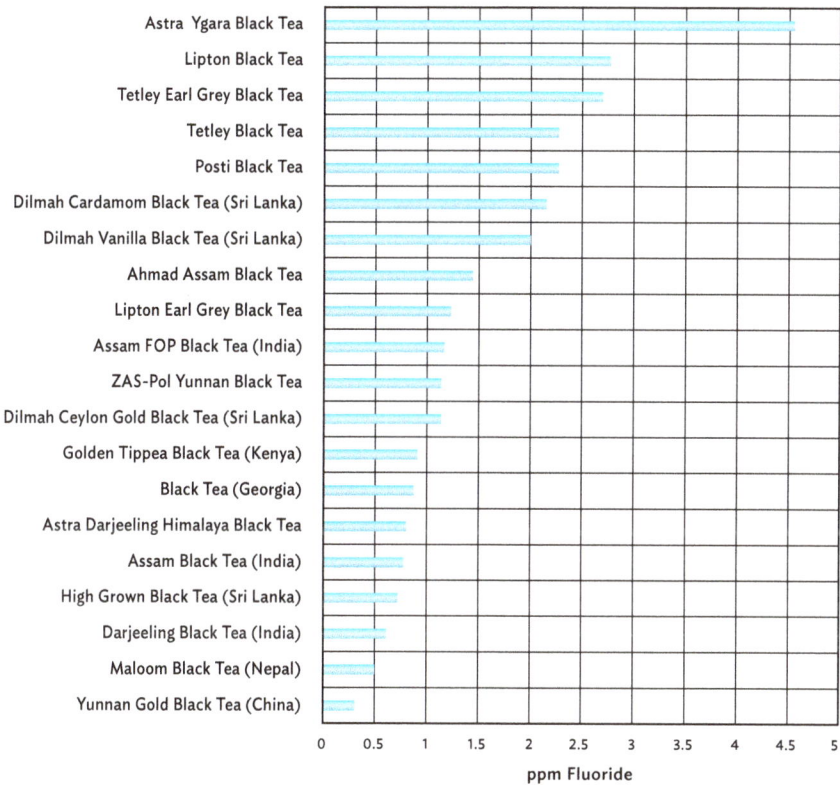

Figure 6.44. Fluoride content (ppm) of black tea infusions (from [419]). Data are presented in order of decreasing fluoride content.

pH and small organic acids of some candies

In 2011, the candy segments ranked 15th among food categories in both SNAP and non-SNAP households [318]. While this may not sound like much, consider this: combined expenditures for candy (~ $840 million) were higher than beans, nuts, and seeds combined ($772 million). Contrary to modern viewpoints [422,423], tooth decay was rampant in two distinct pre-Industrial Revolution populations: on one hand, it was the upper crust, who had the privilege of enjoying multiple dining courses, of which usually involved sugary substances; and, for the second, the 'southern islanders' who consumed 'acid liquors and fruits' in abundance (i.e., it has long been known that acids from vegetables and fruits promote dental erosion) [319]. Helping to dispel the myth that foods with poor nutritional quality are mainly overrepresented by those with lower socioeconomic status (SES) [422,423], in addition to spending more money on low-nutritional foods, non-SNAP households also dished out a higher fraction of total grocery expenditures for these

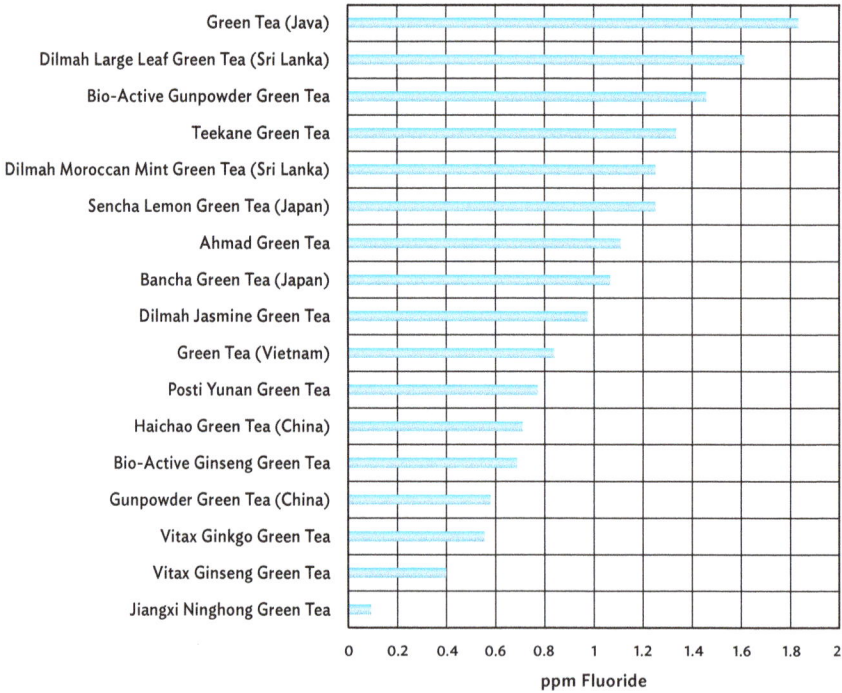

Figure 6.45. Fluoride content (ppm) of green tea infusions (from [419]). Data are presented in order of decreasing fluoride content.

sugary goodies: non-SNAP and SNAP households spent 1.47% and 1.44% of their respective "Solid Fats & Added Sugar" allocations on nonchocolate candy (note: when factoring in chocolate candy, including seasonal chocolate varieties, non-SNAP households spent even more) [318]. Just as fast food is enjoyed by virtually every SES in America (with middle SES enjoying just a touch more than everyone else)

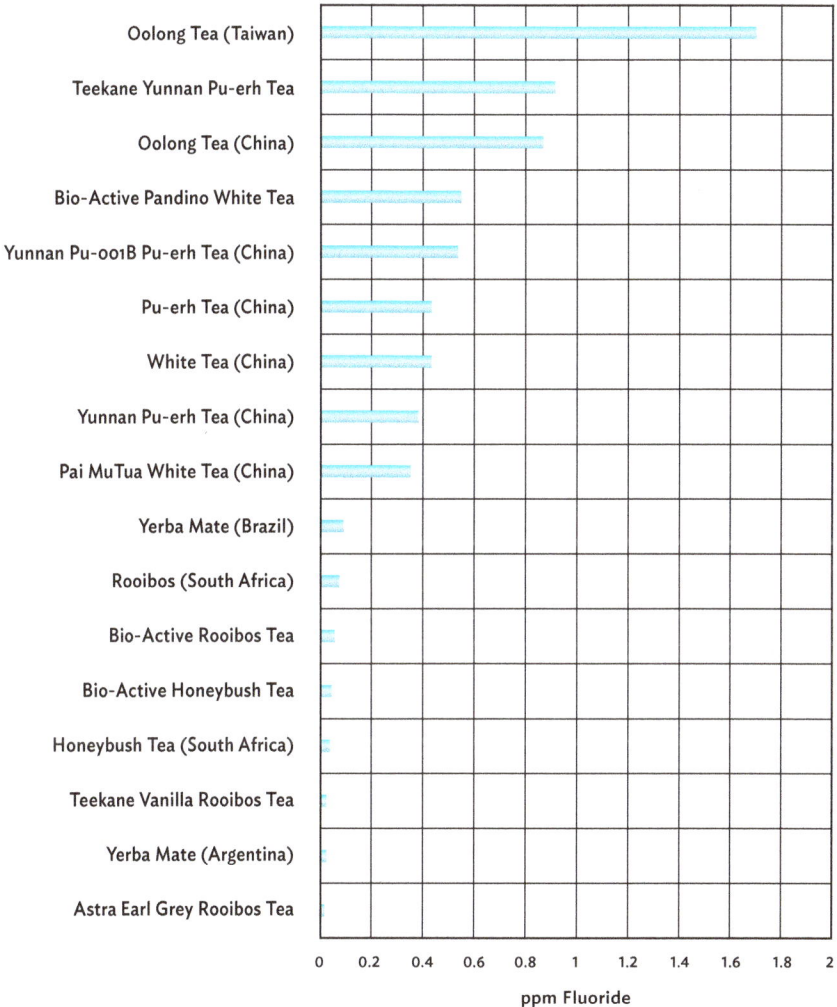

Figure 6.46. Fluoride content (ppm) of nonblack and nongreen tea infusions (from [419]). Data are presented in order of decreasing fluoride content.

[424,425], the desire for a low-nutritional 'fix' is often too tempting to resist, affecting all levels of society [318,424,425]. To that end, as stated by a former president of the New England Manufacturing Confectioners' Association almost 100 years ago: 'everyone eats candy' [426].

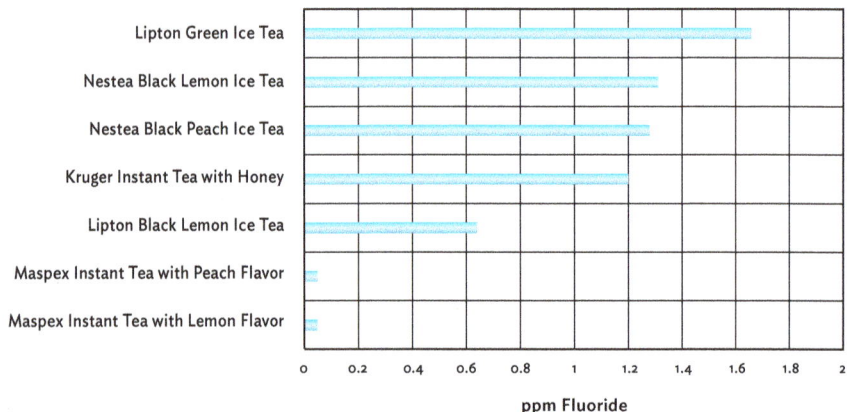

Figure 6.47. Fluoride content (ppm) of ready-to-serve (i.e., brewed and bottled) tea (from [419]). Data are presented in order of decreasing fluoride content.

Regardless of demographic and economic status, nonchocolate candies present elevated risk factors for dental erosion. As recently analyzed in 16-18-year-old adolescents, more than three sour sweets in a given week led to greater erosive wear [282]. **Figure 6.48** presents a compilation of pH values for various nonchocolate candies, most of which are sour [427–432]. The predominant acids present in these formulations are malic and citric, with the latter most common by far. This includes the sugar-free Flopi Florestal® candies (all flavors, including the higher-pH Ginger and Lemon Balm varieties), which include citric and ascorbic acids [428]; thus, while sugar-free options may sound promising from a caries perspective, the presence of small organic acids (e.g., citric acid), which is likely coupled with an acidic pH, renders such formulations high-risk for dental erosion. From an erosive perspective, the sour varieties are most damaging relative to the nonsour counterpart (for example, the Life Savers®, Twizzlers®, and Jolly Rancher® candies [431]), with long-lasting and/or hard candies (e.g., jawbreakers) sustaining acidic oral environments [433]. Among the candies shown, erosive risk exceptions include the Tic Tac® Mint, Cinnamon, and Extra-Strong flavors, which in addition to exhibiting the highest pH values, do not contain the small aliphatic acids [427]; and although they contain sugar, these likely present limited caries risk as long as proper oral hygiene is in place.

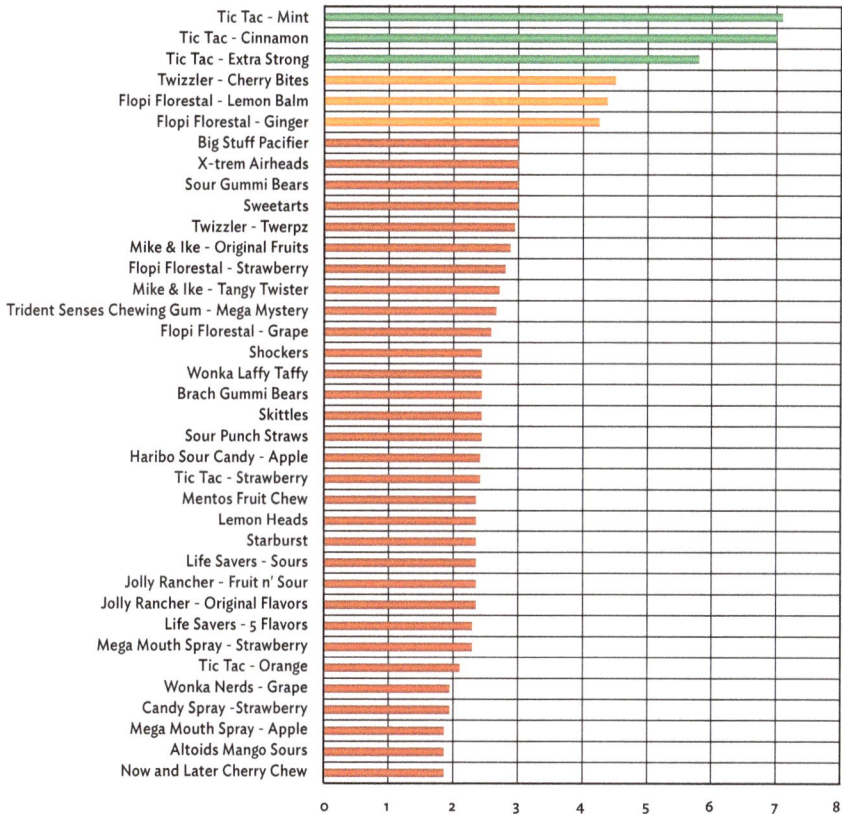

Tic Tac - Mint
Tic Tac - Cinnamon
Tic Tac - Extra Strong
Twizzler - Cherry Bites
Flopi Florestal - Lemon Balm
Flopi Florestal - Ginger
Big Stuff Pacifier
X-trem Airheads
Sour Gummi Bears
Sweetarts
Twizzler - Twerpz
Mike & Ike - Original Fruits
Flopi Florestal - Strawberry
Mike & Ike - Tangy Twister
Trident Senses Chewing Gum - Mega Mystery
Flopi Florestal - Grape
Shockers
Wonka Laffy Taffy
Brach Gummi Bears
Skittles
Sour Punch Straws
Haribo Sour Candy - Apple
Tic Tac - Strawberry
Mentos Fruit Chew
Lemon Heads
Starburst
Life Savers - Sours
Jolly Rancher - Fruit n' Sour
Jolly Rancher - Original Flavors
Life Savers - 5 Flavors
Mega Mouth Spray - Strawberry
Tic Tac - Orange
Wonka Nerds - Grape
Candy Spray -Strawberry
Mega Mouth Spray - Apple
Altoids Mango Sours
Now and Later Cherry Chew

0 1 2 3 4 5 6 7 8

Figure 6.48. pH of candy items from various locations including Brazil (Tic Tac® [427] and Flopi Florestal® [428]), Netherlands (Mega Mouth® and Candy Spray [429]), Switzerland (Haribo® and Trident® [430]), and US (Jolly Rancher®, Twizzler®, Mike & Ike®, and Life Savers® [431], along with the rest [432]). Colors are shown to help approximate pH regions that may present relatively high (pH < 4), moderate (4 < pH < 5), or low (pH > 5) risks for dental erosion.

Actionable solutions to help reduce damaging potential of acidic foodstuffs and drinks

The damaging potential of a number of foodstuffs and drinks based on pH and small acid content has been presented. So what can one do to counter the deleterious effects of acidic foodstuffs (including candies) and liquids? Healthier options exist (and continue to evolve), especially as consumers become more knowledgeable and demand healthier selections. Some effective options include:

✓ calcium-containing foodstuffs and liquids;

✓ sugar-free sweeteners; and,

✓ fluoride.

Other options may also exist, but here, I will focus on these three, with some commentary on each, although an expanded discussion of fluoride is reserved for Chapter 8.

Calcium

First, one should consider acidic drinks or confections (i.e., candies, mints, and gums) that contain calcium, provided such choices exist. Although most candies do not contain calcium, those that do can limit the damaging effects brought about by pH, small organic acids, and/or the combination of these by virtue of helping to change the degree of super-saturation in the oral environment [250,340,434,435]. When candies are supplemented with calcium, the erosive potential is dramatically lowered, and, depending on the calcium content, may neutralize erosive risks altogether [435]. Another example is orange juice: that which contains calcium presents lower erosive risks compared to that without [340,434]. Thus, for those appealing beverages or candies presenting elevated risks for erosion, whenever possible, choose options comprising calcium. Additionally, phosphate may also provide buffering effects that can help reduce acidic potential [349]. But since tooth mineral is especially susceptible to the effects of H^+ and small organic acids, when acidic solutions comprise calcium, demineralization effects are greatly reduced [204], with some often accompanied by a relative increase in pH (i.e., less acidic) [340,434].

Sugar-free sweeteners

Second, consider sugar-free options in the form of sugar alcohols, or more generally, polyols. Two of the most popular sugar-free options are sorbitol (six-carbon polyol) and xylitol (five-carbon polyol), with the former having about 60% sweetness compared to sugar (i.e., sucrose) [436]; in contrast, xylitol, though more expensive, is just as sweet as sugar, is naturally produced by the human body, is a major component in yellow plums, and is also found in strawberries, bilberries, cauliflower, raspberries, lettuce, spinach, onions, and endives [437–439]. Increasing in popularity, erythritol (four-carbon polyol) has about 70% sweetness of sugar, has greater chemical stability than sucrose, xylitol, and sorbitol, and improves the mouthfeel and nonflavor attributes of foodstuffs and liquids [438–441]. All three of these have demonstrated noncariogenic activity, and, therefore, can reduce the incidence of dental decay [438,441,442]. In addition to these sugar alcohols, other sugar alcohols include mannitol, maltitol, and more, and are commonly found in a variety of foods and drinks; additionally, they are often used in baking as sugar-substitutes [438]. Sucralose (synthetic) and stevia (natural) are also forms of sugar alcohols, and are characterized by being low-calorie, super-sweet sugar substitutes; in contrast, aspartame (synthetic) and saccharin (synthetic) are not sugar alcohols but are also nonfermentable zero-calorie sweeteners with sweetness greater than sugar [438].

Although sorbitol has long been used as a standard sugar-free option [443], xylitol has an advantage in that it is not readily consumed by pathogenic aerobic microbes (e.g., *S. mutans*) [444], and, therefore, has been positioned as a better noncariogenic sweetener option [437,442,445].

Xylitol can help stimulate the growth of anaerobic gram-positive microbes (e.g., bacilli, cocci, and *Veillonella*) [446], which are especially prominent in the gingival sulcus but to lesser extents along the gingival margin, tooth surfaces, cheek, tongue, and saliva [447]: such microbial sensitivity may be one reason why xylitol confers some efficacy against root caries (e.g., 40% reduction over a three-year period!), but remains ineffective for coronal caries [448]. But demonstrating sugar alcohols are not a panacea for caries, for adults (i.e., ages 21 thru 80) with caries experience and already using fluoridated toothpaste, supplementation with xylitol does not appear to provide enhanced protection [449]. In general, however, both sorbitol and xylitol are most effective when frequently (e.g., more than six grams daily and ideally consumed between meals [445]) used in sugar-free confections that stimulate the saliva [437,438], especially chewing gum [90,450,451]. Particularly effective as a postmeal refreshment or between-meal confection, comestibles incorporating xylitol or sorbitol can help promote saliva's natural remineralization benefits [90,445,450,451]. And, these effects may be magnified even further as emerging evidence suggests erythritol may have even greater anticaries potential (and at least the same cariostatic activity) than either xylitol or sorbitol [442,452,453].

Whether the action of these sugar alcohols alters plaque constituency, inhibits microbial acid production, or simply facilitates saliva production, these sugar-free components can play an important and critical role in the management of oral health.

As shown above, even if sweetened with sorbitol, the sugar-free Florestal® candies still present elevated demineralization risk factors by virtue of its low pH; as such, it is important to understand that simply having a sugar-free comestible does not reduce demineralization risks. Ideally, a convenient and fun troche, mint, gum, etc. ought to be sugar-free and either have calcium or be free of strong acids (e.g., citric or phosphoric)—of course, a pleasing color and great flavor are necessary, too!

Importantly, like any new food or diet modification, gastrointestinal (GI) changes and possible (but temporary) discomfort may arise as the gut flora adapt to the change in food source [446,454,455]. This is normal [455]. Because everyone manifests unique gut biomes and/or absorption characteristics, tolerance to certain sugar alcohols or alternatives will be individually based. It is important to be patient with one's body as the gut adapts to the change in feedstock—this should occur within a four-week period (more or less, of course, depending on an individual's microbial adaptability [446]), and quite possibly much sooner than that. In any case, the short-term, mild discomfort to effect long-term, meaningful benefits is likely worth it.

Fluoride

Finally, perhaps one of the easiest methods to counter potentially damaging foodstuffs and drinks is to ensure fluoride is available in the oral environment [34,456]. Fluoride has been shown to be an effective strategy in managing dental erosion [457–459], and when incorporated at low levels (e.g., ~ 2 ppm fluoride) in a juice, can stave off dental erosion and/or caries [460]. In fact, green or black tea (both ready-to-serve and/or freshly brewed) may be an excellent adjunct to a given diet, given that they have low levels of fluoride commensurate with that in community fluoridated water. Further details about the fluoride mechanisms of action and applications are the subjects of Chapter 8.

In closing out this chapter, for those seeking additional tips on countering potentially damaging foodstuffs and drinks, consider the following 11 suggestions:

✓ Review your oral health and options with a dental professional, including possibly seeking more than one opinion since, like many questions or situations, there can exist more than one recommendation: a trained dental professional can help assess your status and risk level for dental erosion, decay, or other potential problems.

✓ Ensure topical fluorides are part of your daily oral hygiene, keeping in mind neutral formulations (i.e., not acidic rinses or toothpastes) may be more amenable to the delicate oral environment—when used appropriately, fluoride is safe and effective. More on fluoride is presented in Chapter 8.

✓ Recognize that certain foods and liquids may present risks for dental erosion—the pH and small acid type data presented here help to highlight the relevance of these factors.

✓ Avoid certain foods completely—though perhaps not preferable, this is a sure way to eliminate risky food. If one chooses to pursue this path, then to help make this suggestion more palatable I recommend initially swearing off only a few foods (keep it simple!) as part of an 'off-limits' list (instead of swearing off entire categories of foods). Doing so may help reduce potential anxiety, confusion, or even binge behavior that often results during the course of strict dieting. Gradually, as understanding and comfort in these lifestyle changes become routine, the 'off-limits' list can be expanded as needed/desired.

✓ Limit or reduce the frequency and/or duration of consuming acidic comestibles, liquids, or other foodstuffs. Recognize that sticky foods rich in sugar and/or sour-flavored present additional risks due to protracted contact with the teeth.

✓ If enjoying acidic foods or liquids, incorporating higher-pH foodstuffs and liquids may help counter demineralization risks. Some sialagogues such as cheese or milks may provide additional benefits without risk for tooth wear; others, however, such as peanuts or salty crackers, may present risks for tooth wear if consumed in conjunction with acidic food/drink/candy.

✓ When using a straw with the beverages (and this is true especially for children), avoid biting and/or 'aiming' the straw at the tooth as these typically lead to more erosive damage.

✓ Do not brush teeth immediately after imbibing an acidic drink—wait at least 30 minutes. If a fresh mouth is desired, then rinse with fluoridated water or saliva substitute (having pH greater than 6) to help improve remineralization activity.

✓ Be aware that saliva may not be able to successfully protect the teeth if acidic liquids or comestibles are consumed before bedtime, late in the night, or in other situations where salivary flow may be minimal such as immediately after aggressive exercise, or as a side-effect from certain medications or therapies.

✓ Whenever possible, opt for foodstuffs and liquids that include calcium—just as proteins are key to those with diabetes, calcium is key to those with elevated demineralization risk factors; and,

✓ Incorporate sugar-free options that have a healthy pH as part of a postmeal or between-meal supplement. Comestibles touting sour flavors are probably too acidic. Additionally, options that comprise calcium can provide further benefits. Bonus points for selections made with xylitol and/or erythritol. Choose wisely!

The above strategies are designed to help reduce demineralization risks while still enjoying food and drink!

And while fluoride is called forth as an important component to prevention-minded approaches, what other strategies have been proposed to help clean the teeth and/or otherwise thwart decay? This is what the next chapter is all about.

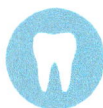

CHAPTER SEVEN

A Glimpse into the Past: Pre-Fluoride Preventives

RECORDS AT LEAST AS OLD AS THE EGYPTIANS of antiquity demonstrate that clean, let alone white, teeth have long been desired and prized: as such, myriad approaches and recommendations have been devised and tried [298]. One of the oldest and simplest cleaning methods involves the expulsion of food particles from the teeth by use of slivers of wood or shrub (i.e., a toothpick), including cypress or those with styptic properties such as pine, aloe, juniper, and rosemary; of course, those examples were especially preferred but any twig or implement can suffice, with metallic toothpicks (e.g., from silver or gold) favored by the affluent. And as relayed by ancient Roman and Arabian health specialists, spiced mouth rinses were often used after toothpick cleanings, with sage, cinnamon, rosemary leaves, juniper seeds, moschata (i.e., pumpkin or squash), cubeb (i.e., Java pepper), and cedar-flavored mastic (i.e., translucent resin found on Mediterranean trees, whose shapes were originally described by Hippocrates as 'tears').

The following chapter presents a glimpse into some historical examples of preventive care for the teeth prior to the advent of fluoride. And although this treatment is not meant to be exhaustive, stimulated readers can learn more through the referenced material used in constructing this chapter (e.g., these references are particularly insightful [298,461]). I have highlighted many documented examples for perspective and interest, from antiquity up through the mid-1950s. Of particular relevance, some of the approaches now used in the 21st century, including the concept of elevating oral pH, have been explored previously, and supports the view that history is oft likely to repeat itself. Even so, appreciation of past approaches and experiences can allow for new insight that may spark or streamline research and development efforts.

So let's begin with the Pharaohs.

Dental preventives in antiquity

Hieratic characters found on papyrus detail favorite tooth-strengthening medicaments of the ancient Egyptians, including the use of bluish-green copper patina (i.e., verdigris) combined with green lead chlorophosphate (pyromorphite) and scented with various gums and spices; in other formulations, absinthe or saffron might be used [298]. In ancient Rome, Emperor Nero's Greek physician Andromachus of Crete improvised a form of theriac (which was long known in ancient Greece and usually included opium as the primary therapeutic along with many other components, especially snake flesh) as the de facto treatment against poisons and ailments, including dental maladies; Galen also utilized a form of theriac in treating Emperor Marcus Aurelius [298].

Dental preventives in the 14th through 18th centuries

In the 14th century, Guy de Chauliac's *Chirurgia magna* was widely circulated throughout Europe (all hand-written copies, however, as the printing press was yet to be invented): as perhaps the Middle Ages' most prominent surgeon, he recommended preventive treatments consistent with Arabian doctors, which included those comprising burnt salt and honey, with perhaps some vinegar or pulverized cuttlefish bone admixed therein [298]. Throughout most of the ancient, early, and Medieval epochs, dentifrices and powders usually were comprised of finely powdered substances including chalk (calcium carbonate) and gypsum (calcium sulfate), shells (snails, clams, oysters, and cockles), or animal bones and horns, including both the horn substance itself, which was usually burnt, along with distillations of horn oils, such as hartshorn, which also produced ammonium carbonate salts [298]. The use of aqua fortis (i.e., nitric acid) and oil of vitriol (i.e., sulfuric acid) were regularly used to exenterate decay from carious teeth for several centuries, and were also promoted as effective tooth-whitening agents by the 15th (e.g., by the Italian physician and professor Montano), 16th (e.g., by the Dutch doctor Foreest), and 17th centuries (e.g., by the respected French surgeon and professor Rivière). In the 16th century, Ambroise Paré, a seasoned and respected master barber-surgeon who ultimately cared for four French kings and who embodied palliative treatment, proffered the virtues of oxycrate (i.e., water plus vinegar solution), along with professionally applied instruments to aid in cleaning and tartar control [298]. In addition to recommending pulverized burnt bread as a capable dentifrice (which essentially is a form of charcoal, and would be revisited in the 20th century), he advised the careful use of aqua fortis to achieve better cleaning results when tartar and blackening failed to be removed with instruments [462]. While toothbrushes (made of animal hairs) or linen might be used to apply the dental powder or dentifrice, Pierre Fauchard, an 18th-century French dentist and regarded as a father of modern dentistry memorialized through his seminal book *Le Chirurgien Dentiste* [298,463], advocated the use of sponges, or the roots of the marshmallow or alfalfa plants as alternatives, coupled with plain water, or whenever possible, aqua vitae (i.e., alcohol); indeed, he also encouraged the use of powders, dentifrices, and mouthwashes to maintain proper dental health.

Pasteur & Lister

While diachylum (a plaster-like composition comprising plant juices, lead, and oils extracted from animals) has been used since antiquity to help protect and improve the healing of wounds, the separate but pioneering works in the mid-19th century of Louis Pasteur and Josef Lister forever changed medicine and dentistry.

Known for fermentation theory [48], Pasteur was responsible for demonstrating that microbes (a term coined by the French military surgeon Sédillot) existed on the surfaces of all substances (including animate and inanimate) and manifested aerobic and fermenting faculties, processes which could be performed simultaneously and were controlled by the presence of oxygen or sugar feedstocks: when oxygen levels are high, the microbes (e.g., yeast, which was routinely studied by Pasteur) exhibit great activity, including population growth and mobility; but when oxygen is reduced (a situation described as 'anaerobic', as coined by Pasteur), they assume a dormant state. And when yeast was presented with sugar, by virtue of fermenting action, carbonic acid gas and alcohol were produced. While these characteristics forever affected beer- and wine-making, they also provided a basis for understanding the origin of suppurations of injured flesh as well as the communicable nature of microbes (of which were particular interest to the French physician Savaine) [464]. Ultimately, these results helped shaped Dr. Willoughby Miller's steadfast view [11] that dental caries develops "*in the mouth by fermentation of carbohydrates*"; Dr. Miller continues, stating that "*micro-organisms do not exert a direct influence on normal enamel; their action upon the enamel in the first state of decay is, therefore, indirect—that is, they act by means of the acids which they produce.*"

Crediting Pasteur's enlightenment on the activity of microbes, the English surgeon Josef Lister opined that a treatment that could destroy or somehow inactivate these microbes (even if they were dormant), would then stave off infection and decomposition of injured tissue. Lister's panacea was carbolic acid and when applied to the injury (either misted by pump or washed with linens) would reduce inflammation, therefore improving the likelihood of healing and recovery [465]. As such, Lister is credited with devising a modern form of antiseptic that facilitated surgeries, including abscesses and compound fractures, which, by virtue of sepsis, would have otherwise necessitated amputations [466]. And, as early as 1862, carbolic acid was recognized as a possible therapeutic for use in dentistry due to its nonodorous and high water solubility characteristics [467]. And, tipping a marketable hat to Josef Lister, 'Listerine' was launched as an antiseptic (both body and mouth) by the Lambert Pharmacal Company in the late 19th century and into the 20th century (e.g., see **Figure 7.1** for example ads [468]). But how effective was carbolic acid, or even Listerine, in controlling the microbes attributed to dental decay? In his book published in 1890 [11], Dr. Miller ranked Listerine (then a combination of various components including oil of eucalyptus, borobenzoic acid, wintergreen oil, and more) as a mild but effective antiseptic, working in less than 30 seconds, a timeframe that was comparable to salicylic and benzoic acids; for reference purposes, carbolic acid 'devitalized' microbes within 15 minutes and was on par with 10% hydrogen peroxide solution.

Powered by the advent of and rapidly evolving technologies surrounding steam-driven ships, coal-fired engines and machines, and kerosene illumination, the advances put forth by Pasteur and Lister (and others) were soon percolating throughout the world. So during this revolutionary time period, what were some of the existing dental preventives available to and used by consumers in the mid-to-late 19th century?

As reported by one troubled dentist in 1860 [469], the use of charcoal to clean the teeth was so destructive to the gums that they loosened teeth to such an extent they fell out (the dentist lamented he had replaced entire sets of teeth in several people); additionally, such repeated use also blackened the gum tissue in some of his patients. His reasoning for why people would use charcoal is akin to those today: *"What the public seem to demand in this age of steam, is something that will* <u>whiten</u> *the teeth at once, no matter how long they may have been neglected.*" Instead, he prescribed the following solution that did not involve a toothbrush but retained the use of boles: use a wedge-shaped slice of red cedar, orange, or hickory wood, along with some fine chalk, and gently polish the teeth, careful to not irritate the gumline—and, to do so not more often than two or three times per month [469].

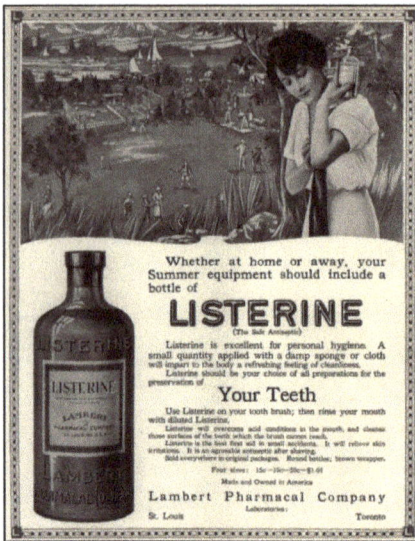

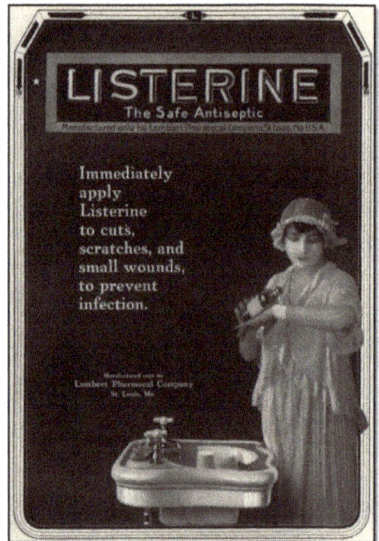

Figure 7.1. Listerine advertisements from 1915 (left) and 1917 (right) promoting cleanliness of the mouth, as well as superficial body wounds and cuts (from [468]).

Several years later, a separate recipe called forth the virtues of toothbrushing with his unique dentifrice formula: Castile soap, Peruvian bark, crushed cuttlefish bone, chalk, orris, cinnamon, wintergreen oil, and sugar (for palatability, of course) [470]. Although this is just one of myriad 'expert' recipes (not to mention homemade recipes), this formulation comprises essential components found in virtually all other dentifrices: chalk, soap, and flavoring (e.g., orris and wintergreen oil). As noted in the 1873 annual American Dental Association (ADA) meeting, Japanese were noted to have very clean teeth (as did the Chinese), and utilized the bark of the willow tree as toothpicks; additionally, Japanese dentists (who were very well-regarded) did not perform restorations [471]. Also at the ADA meeting, condemnation regarding the patent nostrum 'Sozodont' (which was a red liquid dentifrice introduced several years prior and comprised nearly 40% alcohol [461]) was made in response to purported deleterious and/or nonbeneficial effects in the mouth [471]; these views clashed with its marketing claims, including those initially published in the American Quarterly Church Review that stated 15 New York City clergymen as well as *"hundreds of others . . . are convinced of its excellent and invaluable qualities"* [472]. An example of an advertisement for 'Sozodont' is shown in **Figure 7.2** [473].

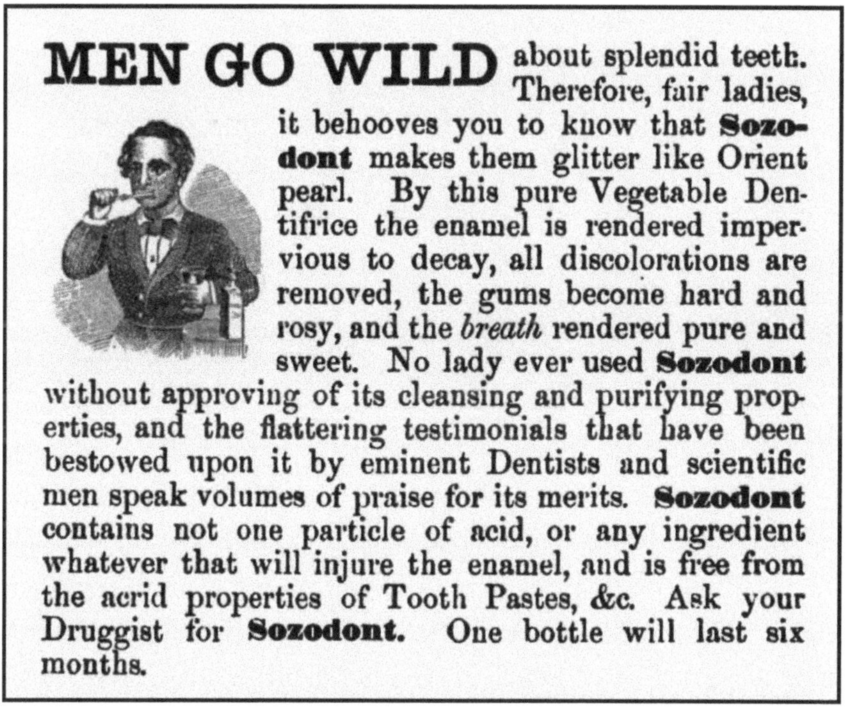

Figure 7.2. An 1878 Sozodont advertisement appealing to 'fair ladies'(from [473]).

In addition to commercial liquid dentifrices (e.g., Sozodont), commercially available tooth powders, like the best-selling Dr. Lyon's brand of Tooth Tablets (which were compressed tooth powders) and Tooth Powder, were also embraced by the public. As the advertisement for the 'perfect' Tooth Powder in **Figure 7.3** relays, just wet your toothbrush, add some powder, and apply to your teeth for a cleaner mouth with 'purified' breath.

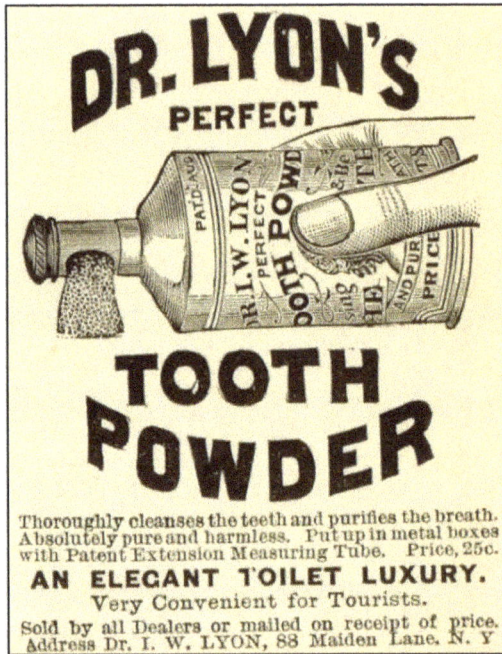

Figure 7.3. An 1891 advertisement for Dr. Lyon's 'perfect' Tooth Powder (from [474]).

Besides liquid dentifrices and tooth powders, dental creams were also available, although the single container of cream (often a ceramic or metallic jar) into which various family members would stab their toothbrushes rendered this relatively unhygienic [461]. But as paints and some foods were packaged in convenient, travel-friendly tubes, why not toothpaste? The first dental cream (or dentifrice) marketed in a tube was Doctor Sheffield's Crème Dentifrice, with advertisements appearing in many trade journals and mainstream magazines, such as that appearing in 'The Theater' as shown in **Figure 7.4** [475]. Although

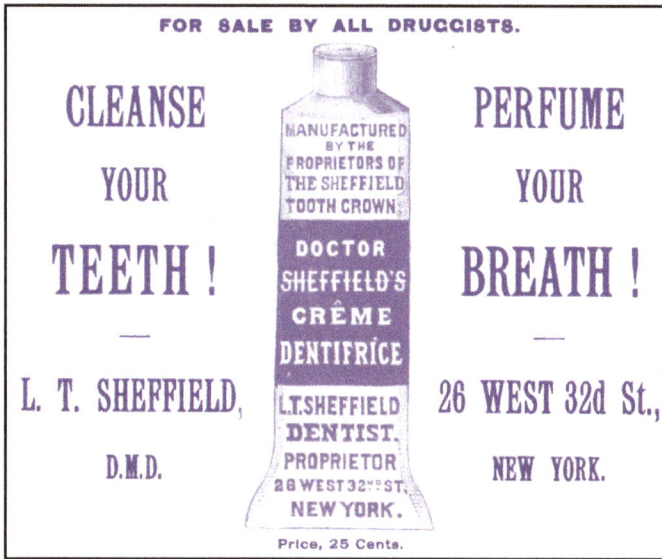

Figure 7.4. An 1886 advertisement for Doctor Sheffield's tube dentifrice (from [475]).

the formula was not publicly disclosed, a similar dentifrice of consistency was achieved using Castile soap, chalk, and glycerine [476].

Finally, another notable late-19th century product was very common in the dental office, and also met a welcoming public: salts of cocaine. The primary use? As shown in the 1885 advertisement (**Figure 7.5**) [477], one purpose was to 'cure' toothaches, presumably by numbing the afflicted region. With chemical extractions and purifications practically perfected by the late 19th century (e.g., **Figure 7.6** from [478]), cocaine was commonly injected by dentists to numb the region requiring surgical intervention: cocaine anesthetics were either prepared by the dentist from various salt forms (e.g., dissolving cocaine phosphate and cocaine hydrochlorate salts in various solvents [478]), or purchased from commercial sources including such brands as Dorsenia (~ 20% cocaine content), Weinmann's (~ 5.5% cocaine content), Eureka (~ 3.3% cocaine content), or Dental Surprise (~ 1.5% cocaine content) [479], with the latter perhaps aptly named since the relatively low cocaine content might fail to provide sufficient numbing prior to aggressive intervention. In any event, the widespread use of cocaine during this period of history certainly leaves an impression.

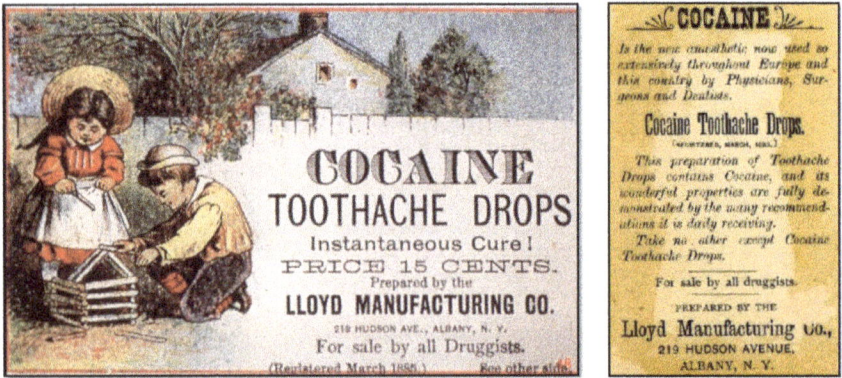

Figure 7.5. 1885 advertisements for toothache drops containing "cocaine and its wonderful properties" (from [477]).

Figure 7.6. An 1895 advertisement for various manufactured alkaloids, including quinine and cocaine (from [478]).

Dental preventives in the early 20th Century: Tube toothpaste & toothbrushes

Several years later in the early 20th century and just prior to World War I, Colgate and Kolynos introduced dental creams in a tube (for example, see **Figure 7.7** [480]). Following the lead of Sheffield, these products rocketed to the top of the dentifrice market based on the familiarity of Colgate, a leader in sanitary products (they were previously known for soap and detergents) [481], while Kolynos enjoyed support from the dental community [482,483]. While Colgate's ribbon-shaped delivery and subsequent lay-flat performance on the toothbrush was an improvement over existing tube dentifrices, the recipe for Kolynos' success was based on its founder-dentist, a well-known dental researcher (Dr. N.S. Jenkins) who was known throughout the dental community as the inventor of the porcelain inlay [483]. Dr. Jenkins was inspired by Dr. Willoughby Miller's research that acidogenic bacteria produce tooth decay, so he devised an antiseptic toothpaste (of which comprised many known antiseptic ingredients including benzoic acid, alcohol, eucalyptus, and peppermint oils) called 'Kolynos' (which is also the eponymous name of the company and is an amalgamation of Greek words meaning 'disease preventer') [484]. When launched, the popularity of Kolynos was enormous: *three million* samples were requested (i.e., door-to-door marketing was not performed) and profitability was achieved within 16 months [483]. After World War I, Kolynos introduced an improved method of maintaining cap compliance by having a portion of it affixed permanently to the tube, apparently solving the struggle of maintaining cap-tube integrity [485].

In addition to Colgate and Kolynos, two other major tube toothpaste entrants also emerged prior to 1920 that are worthy of comment: Pebeco and Pepsodent. Pebeco is notable because it did more than identify that a clean mouth was necessary: as shown in **Figure 7.8** [486], it called forth the problem 'acid-mouth', and, using paper pH test strips that it supplied (which was creative in its own right), purported to neutral-ize the said 'acid-mouth' condition through the stimulation of saliva (which, in essence, practically all flavored toothpastes inherently do).

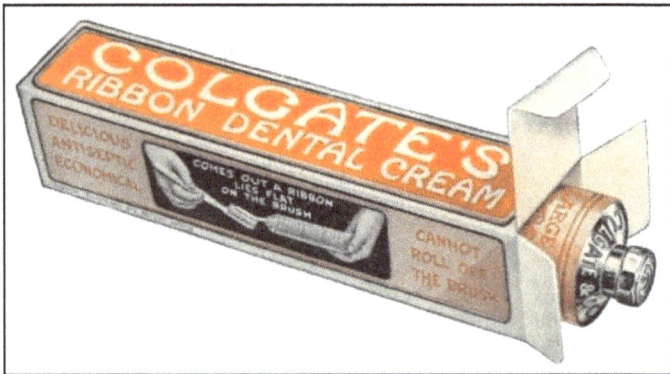

Figure 7.7. Colgate's ribbon dental cream advertised in 1912 (from [480]).

The product of brilliant marketing strategies from two prominent admen, Pepsodent eventually rocketed to the number two toothpaste behind Colgate. Led by the team of Albert Lasker (considered a found-ing father of modern advertising) and Claude Hopkins (regarded as one of the original and most creative admen of his era and whose book *Scientific Advertising* is still in use today), the men expertly deployed 'reason-why' copy to win eager consumers. If these two names do not sound familiar, perhaps you may have heard of at least one of these other products that either one or both of the men worked on: Palmolive soap, Sunkist oranges, Lucky Strike cigarettes, Goodyear tires, or SunMaid raisins. As explained in the advertisement shown in **Figure 7.9** [487], the admen touted the removal of the mucin-based biofilm that resides naturally on the teeth by virtue of the pepsin component in the toothpaste. Helping to triple its sales, Pepsodent sponsored the 'Amos 'N' Andy' radio show beginning in the late 1920s, and then used Bob Hope, then a relatively new comedian, to help further the brand by the late 1930s [461].

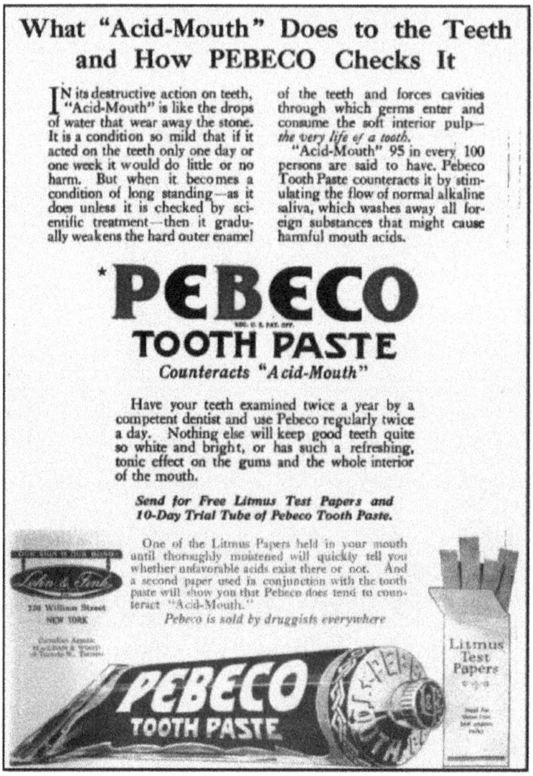

Figure 7.8. Pebeco's advertisement in the May 1920 issue of Good Housekeeping (from [486]).

The market size of the US dentifrice market was more than $60 million annually in the 1930s, and to carve a corner in this competitive segment, marketing efforts usually highlighted 'acceptance' by the dental profession (e.g., **Figure 7.9** [487]). But were these formulations truly therapeutic and did dentists really support them? Here is one comment regarding dentifrice efficacy by the American Dental Association (from [461]): *"Dentifrice has in itself no magical or chemical power to clean, and the best mouthwashes are warm water or a solution of common table salt."* Additional examples are even more pointed: the titles and conclusions of two dental research papers published just prior to the 1920s and then another published in 1927 said it all:

✓ Regarding the falsity of published claims, Taylor et al. provides examples involving the marketing of Kolynos, Pebeco, and Pepsodent (among others) and title their paper 'Highfalutin Dupery' en route to addressing the various questionable and/or unscrupulous claims [488];

✓ About the special ability of Pepsodent to digest mucin-based films that reside on the teeth? Experiments indicate these marketing claims are "*wholly unwarranted*" [489]; and,

✓ Regarding reduction in oral microbes, Veader & Frier concluded that "*None of the forty-one toothpastes examined can be dependent upon to accomplish this disinfection.*"[490].

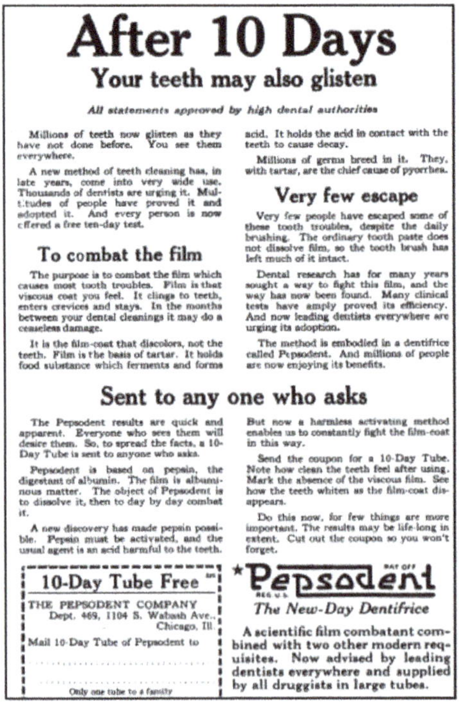

Figure 7.9. Pepsodent's advertisement in the June 1920 issue of Good Housekeeping (from [487]).

Despite professional protestations to marketing claims, the daily practice of toothbrushing with dentifrices or powders was destined to become stricture. But while the above toothpastes may have been questionable, the device used to apply the toothpaste to the teeth (i.e., the toothbrush) underwent a major innovation. In the early 20th century, hog hair was the principal brush material used in toothbrushes, with much of it sourced from China, as well as India and Russia [461]. Concomitant with the 1937 onset of the Second Sino-Japan War, which affected the extent of Chinese hog hair exports, DuPont announced a breakthrough synthetic material with properties similar to nylon and that was ideal for toothbrush bristles, especially as it practically doubled the lifespan of the bristles relative to hog hair. The shortage of hog hair combined with the rather robust DuPont material began a trend toward synthetic bristles that essentially quenched the animal hair market. The first company to introduce the new DuPont material (called 'Exton') was Weco (which already enjoyed a commercial relationship as DuPont manufactured the Weco brand of hog hair toothbrushes) in 1937 and this appeared in their 'Dr. West' brand; after a few years when the DuPont exclusivity expired, other oral care companies launched toothbrushes with synthetic bristles (with many utilizing nylon) [461].

Moving further into the 20th century, three major 'actives' in dentifrices competed for consumers' desires for cleaner, healthier mouths: antienzymes, ammonia, and chlorophyll. Along the way, a notable improvement in general dentifrice formulations was also achieved: the agricultural giant, Monsanto, patented a dentifrice base in 1944 that incorporated sodium lauryl sulfate, which helped improve dentifrice flowability (e.g., claim 1) [491].

Dental preventives in the early 20th Century: Antienzymes strategies

Digestion begins in the mouth [92], with enzymes such as amylase responsible for hydrolyzing cooked starches into simpler carbohydrates (i.e., amylolytic activity), which in turn serve as feedstock for acidogenic bacteria [45]. Saliva's digestive action was formally observed by Erhard Leuchs in 1831, and shortly thereafter amylase (or, ptyalin, as initially named by Berzelius in 1840) was identified as a major enzyme responsible for saliva's action [492]. Whether the enzymes are secreted by salivary glands or by the myriad microbes residing in the mouth, the production of acids has implications for dental decay [493–495]. Among the acids produced, which includes both weak (e.g., acetic and propionic) and strong (e.g., pyruvic and lactic) acids [84,208,218,496], it has been shown caries-free people have lower levels of strong acids relative to those susceptible to caries [84,496]. As such, strategies that target inhibition of enzymatic activity, which would, therefore, inhibit acid production, would seem scientifically sound: in fact, such 'anti-enzyme' strategies were among those employed in earnest by researchers (especially Fosdick) beginning in the 1940s [497–500].

But despite finding some potent 'actives' that could inhibit amylolytic activity (most notably, quinones having vitamin K-like structure), something was missing: the inability to penetrate into and/or remain in plaque [501]. In fact, this inability frustrates virtually all antimicrobials (including chlorhexidine [53]), with the exception of fluoride (which is discussed in great detail in the next chapter), as noted by Fosdick in 1948 [502]. While Fosdick promoted the use of a vitamin K-like agent in chewing gums as a means of neutralizing food acids produced during a meal (much to the consternation of dental researchers as the Fosdick 'vitamin K' didn't exhibit properties characteristic of vitamin K familiar to scientists, such as prothrombin activity [502]), efficacy was ultimately limited by regions of undisturbed plaque (i.e., plaque traps) as discussed in Chapter 1.

Thus, while neutralizing acids (e.g., via antienzyme strategies) may be important, there were two main drawbacks: firstly, ensuring effective administration of the antienzyme agent at or near the same time of carbohydrate consumption remained challenging; and secondly, penetration and/or disruption of plaque, including frustrating bacterial/

plaque attachment to the dentition, appeared to be the rate limiting step. With Fosdick still at the forefront in this area of research [503], strategy pivoted, thus renewing antienzyme excitement in the 1950s, which, in turn, resulted in several commercial formulations based on the following two prominent antienzyme agents:

✓ Sodium N-lauroyl sarcosinate: synthesized and patented by Colgate in 1954 [504]; and,

✓ Dehydroacetic acid (DHA): synthesized and patented by Warner-Lambert in 1956 [505].

While both conferred some anticaries benefits, in rat studies conducted by the National Institute of Dental Research, sarcosinate was more effective against smooth-surface caries while DHA had a better occlusal-caries benefit; however, DHA also produced the most systemic damage [506]. Importantly, while sodium lauryl sulfate may sound similar to sodium N-lauroyl sarcosinate, these two molecules are distinct, with the former demonstrating greater foaming action but negligible reduction in caries incidence or activity [506]. And, despite its limited efficacy, that didn't stop several companies from utilizing it as an 'active': the 'active' ingredients corresponding to 'WD-9' (Bristol-Myers' Ipana), 'Irium' (Lever Brothers' Pepsodent), and 'GL-70' (Procter & Gamble's Gleem) were all essentially sodium lauryl sulfate; separately, the 'active' for 'Gardol' (Colgate) was sodium N-lauroyl sarcosinate, while 'Antizyme' (Warner-Lambert's Listerine) contained DHA [507]. Examples of print advertisements extolling the benefits of toothpaste with these 'actives', include those for Ipana (**Figure 7.10**), Gleem (**Figure 7.11**), Listerine (**Figure 7.12**), and Colgate (**Figure 7.13**). And, as the popularity in television grew, dentifrice advertisements evolved in response, such as an advertising jingle for Colgate with Gardol (which can be viewed via the weblink in [512]).

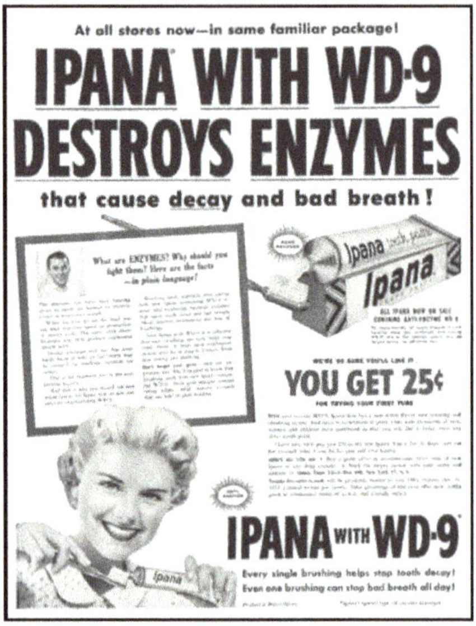

Figure 7.10. Advertisement for Ipana with WD-9 antienzyme dentifrice appearing in 1953 issue of LIFE (from [508]).

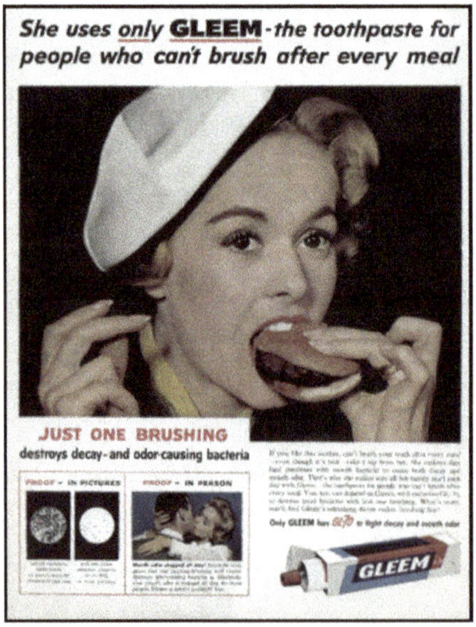

Figure 7.11. Advertisement for GLEEM with GL-70 antienzyme dentifrice appearing in 1958 issue of TIME (from [509]).

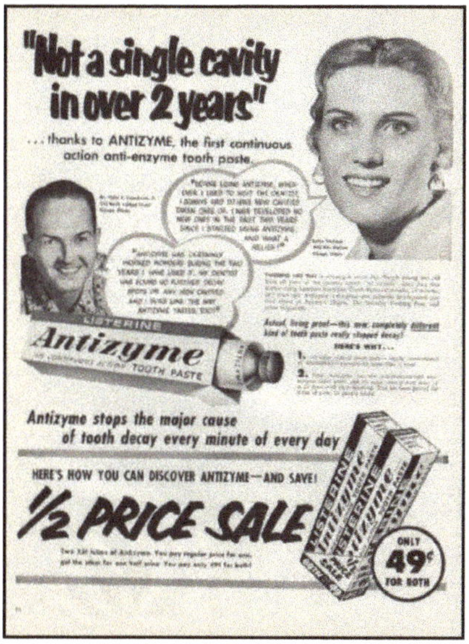

Figure 7.12. Advertisement for Listerine antizyme dentifrice appearing in a 1955 issue of LIFE (from [510]).

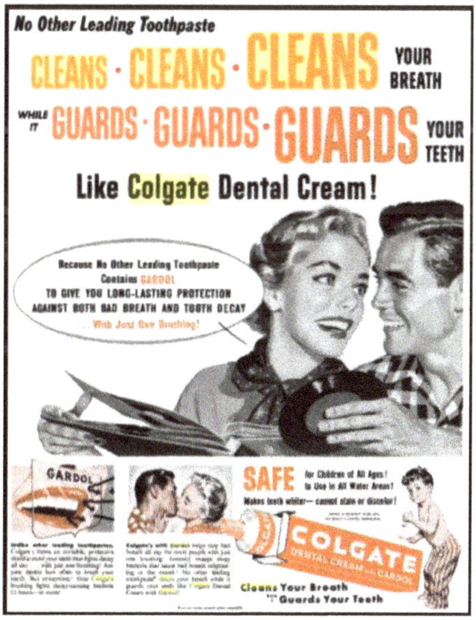

Figure 7.13. Advertisement for Colgate with Gardol dentifrice appearing in a 1957 issue of LIFE (from [511]).

But these formulations, at least based on advertised claims made to the public, still failed to win dentist support. With deepening dentifrice disdain, the American Dental Association maintained that manufacturers' marketing claims were still unwarranted and charged government agencies with passivity [513]. For example, in a bid to compel federal agencies to manage toothpaste claims, expert dentist testimony stated that regarding Colgate's Gardol there was "*not substantial reduction in decay . . . and it certainly is not stopping decay*" [507]. So despite the bevy of manufacturer and university research efforts, advertising claims for dentifrices comprising antienzyme agents were targeted for deception and recklessness [513]. But such criticism extended beyond antienzyme agents, to include other 'actives' as well.

Next, another approach for providing anticaries benefits that mirrors some present-day research efforts is presented: ammonia production.

Dental preventives in the early 20th Century: Ammonia production

In order to better understand why ammonia-producing techniques might be considered a viable approach in the management of dental caries, it's important to explore the scientific backstory. And presently, research in salivary ammonia production is enjoying renewed attention, including the availability of dentifrices (and other topical formats), just like those from the 1940s and 1950s that sought to counter caries activity.

The many-microbe causative view of dental caries emphasizes the damage that dissimilar bacteria can effect when working together, and underlines the weakness of targeting individual microbial pathogens [45,51,66,67]. In fact, due to the rather complex interplay among the various species, this may be one of the reasons why Dr. Willoughby Miller never pointed to a single dominant microorganism as the caries culprit [11].

But a disease condition derived from pathogenic activity but lacking a prime pathogen conflicts with conventional reasoning and medical expectations: after all, the basis for vaccine efficacy is predicated on identifying the pathogen (e.g., smallpox or polio). Because many diseases can be linked to a single source and very often 'mitigated' (or perhaps even eliminated), it is logical to identify a primary pathogen for a given disease in order to thwart its possible effects.

Prior to the now-popular many-microbe ecological view [45,51,66,67], the primary pathogen for dental caries was linked to *Streptococcus mutans* [44], due in large part to its pulpal prominence in a carious tooth [514]. But prior to *S. mutans*, attention was focused on *Bacillus acidophilus* (now referred to as *Lactobacillus acidophilus*), since this species was commonly found in relative abundance in those with caries experience (especially in active caries lesions) compared to those without [515,516]. Efforts to determine which species (i.e., *S. mutans* or *L. acidophilus*) might present the greatest caries threat led to a compromise of sorts: *L. acidophilus* is especially prominent in the superficial layers of enamel, while *S. mutans* is typically prominent deeper in enamel and certainly into dentin [517].

Realizing that *L. acidophilus* is a common microbe in the mouths of caries-susceptible people, producing lactic acid from fermentable carbohydrates that, in turn, leads to decalcification, attention turned promptly to developing an immunization therapy, an effort which would last more than 30 years. Though several experiments involving animals and humans were conducted, the results were mixed at best: similar to vaccination trials involving *S. mutans* [518], ultimately no immutable relationship developed between *L. acidophilus* counts and dental caries [519–521]. In short, the failure to achieve clear immunization benefits underlines the multimicrobial nature of the caries process and supports the view made by Dr. Robert G. Kesel in 1943 (and arguably still holds true today) that *"the more we know, it seems, the less we understand about the whole process."* [522].

While efforts to develop passive immunization were underway, other researchers sought to counter acidogenic activity head-on. In the early 1940s, Stephan published on the pH fall that ensues from exposure to a glucose rinse [306,523]; logically, it follows that expediting the return to a more neutral pH environment would limit decalcification and, therefore, thwart the caries process [524]. Years previously, Chicago dentists Grove and Grove surmised that partaking in an alkaline diet can help stimulate ammonia production [77]. However, those results couldn't be replicated, and, in fact, revealed that ammonia production was practically unchanged and perhaps even depressed regardless of whether proteins, fruits, vegetables, or even bicarbonate were consumed [76]. And while restricting carbohydrate foodstuffs is fraught with inherent difficulties [522], elevating mouth pH (i.e., saliva and plaque fluid) without special dietary considerations may be more practical and effective [522,524,525]. But how might this be accomplished? One possibility involved supplemental ammonia production.

The purpose of ammonia production is believed to help neutralize acidogenic activity [526]. In the oral environment, evolution of ammonia can naturally occur via at least two mechanisms: the hydrolysis of urea (i.e., ureolytic processes that also evolve carbon dioxide) or the deamination of amino acids (e.g., arginine) [527,528], with the former generally producing relatively less ammonia [529]. In 1943, Stephan understood the potential of the conversion to ammonia by salivary urease activity [525] through the action of commensal bacteria (e.g., *S. salivarius*, which is perhaps the most ureolytic organism in the mouth) [527,528,530]. Additionally, several amino acids (e.g., arginine, alanine, and aspartic acid) present in saliva also contribute to ammonia production [527,528,531]: microbial examples of amino acid digestion through enzymatic activity include oral *Streptococcus* species (e.g., *S. sanguinis* [70]) [532,533], as well as some *Actinomyces* and *Lactobacilli* species [45].

For existing insults and infections (i.e., incipient lesions and frank caries), the plaque material is decidedly acidic with the pH hovering near 4 [523], despite the presence of amino acids that might otherwise serve to elevate pH via natural salivary ammonia production [531]. It has been observed that those manifesting virtually little to no caries experience tend to harbor microbiota amenable to ammonia production [37,38,40,41,529,530]. In turn, those naturally caries-resistant have oral ecologies that do not sustain acidic plaque pH, and are, therefore, able to overcome acid challenges produced from carbohydrate fermentation. So while the energy requirement to overcome an established infection by virtue of salivary ammonia is too demanding, what about neutralizing plaque pH to prevent caries incidence or progression through topical supplementation (i.e., as a preventative intervention) [522,524,525,531,534,535]?

With respect to amino acid deamination pathways, recent approaches to improve ammonia output have been based on arginine supplementation via topical formats (e.g., arginine-containing toothpaste) [536,537]. But is arginine supplementation improving anticaries benefits of those most susceptible to caries? Consistent benefits are primarily attained when arginine is combined with fluoride [538,539], the latter of which is the ultimate anticaries agent and is discussed in detail in the next chapter. In fact, some argue there lacks compelling evidence for arginine supplementation, especially for those with higher risks for dental caries (i.e., those who need it most) [540]. Contributing to this perspective, observations reveal that lactic acid production is dramatically and undesirably elevated shortly after cessation of arginine use [72]. Ultimately, even with an abundance of arginine present, the 'right' composition *and* activity of microbes (i.e., commensal, nonacidogenic, or nonaciduric) are needed to produce sufficient amounts of ammonia to overcome an acidic environment. With respect to active caries, the levels and/or activity of ammonia-producing microbes are swamped by the action of acidogenic species in the plaque biofilm, despite seemingly higher levels of amino acid feedstock (e.g., [531]). Importantly, the most abundant amino acids in saliva include proline, glycine, serine, and glutamic acid [541], with the first two commonly serving as osmoprotectants for microbial species (including pathogenic species such as *S. mutans* [74]); additionally, as these four are not generally involved in deamination, these factors contribute to the inherent difficulties in influencing microbial ecology. And demonstrating that ammonia production may not be the best factor in caries control (and, therefore, not 'the' anticaries solution), the levels of ammonia produced between caries-susceptible and caries-free people are not always disparate, as observed in the similar arginolytic activity of eight-year-old children with and without caries experience [529].

But prior to the use of arginine, the original pH-elevating mechanism driving ammoniated dentifrice innovation in the 1940s and 1950s was principally based on a one-two punch combining ammonium phosphate salt and urea, with the content and hydrolysis of the latter regarded as the key factor [522,525]. Biologically, saliva contains relatively low levels of urea [525,529], so introducing additional urea to help stimulate ammonia production and stave off acidogenic activity seemed like a logical approach [525]. Indeed, experiments revealed that high concentrations (e.g., 50%) were found to elevate plaque pH [525], shrink the pH drop due to a glucose challenge [525], and facilitate penetration deeper into plaque material [495]. Separately, the use of ammonium phosphate was based on several factors including its ability to inhibit *L. acidophilus* counts and to provide buffering effects via phosphate; importantly, it is also odor-free [531].

While urea and ammonium phosphate were initially proposed as separate antiacid agents, the combination of the two seemed to work best [534]. In fact, two independent groups patented dentifrice combinations comprising both agents, both of which resulted in commercial dentifrices: Dr. Robert Kesel led a team at the University of Illinois [80], while Dr. Chester Henschel, a New York dentist and director of a nonprofit foundation, led another [78]. But because the patents were essentially covering the same technology, litigation ensued, resulting in forfeiture and transfer of the rights of the Henschel patent covering an ammoniated dentifrice (initially licensed to by F.W. Woolworth Co. and later acquired by Block Drug Co.) to the University of Illinois Foundation (UIF), which already had license agreements with Colgate, Pepsodent, Kolynos, Walgreens, and others [542]. An example of a print advertisement for an ammoniated dentifrice is shown in **Figure 7.14**.

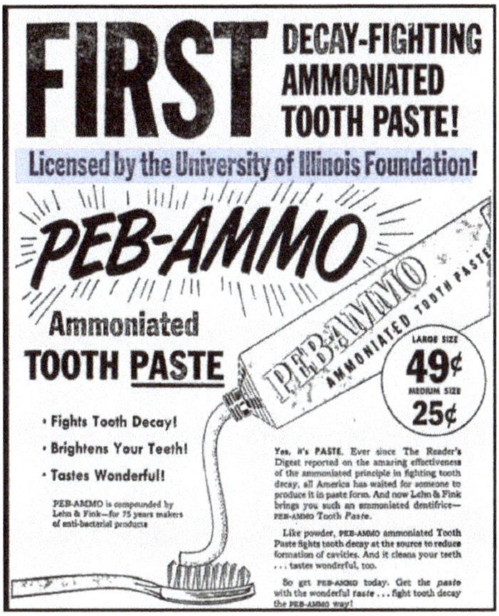

Figure 7.14. Advertisement for Lehn & Fink's PEB-AMMO ammoniated dentifrice appearing in 1949 (from [543]).

Contributing to its antibacterial properties (e.g., [525] and references therein), urea is particularly effective in denaturing proteins and lowering solution viscosity (as initially observed by Spiro in 1900) [544,545]; in fact, these properties help explain how urea is able to penetrate through aggregated plaque [495]. But despite high urea loading and concomitant lower *L. acidophilus* counts, these effects did not translate into convincing clinical caries reductions [81,82,534]. While casual correlations were made between reductions in *L. acidophilus* and the 'likelihood' of caries [524,525,527,531,534], there was a dearth of well-designed, placebo-controlled trials [535,546]. When independent laboratory studies (i.e., those without perceived or actual commercial conflicts of interest) were conducted to assess the impact of ammonia on *L. acidophilus*, the results not only could not confirm the putative benefits of ammonia but also pointed to several other factors that can bear on the relationship, including the lack of uniform experimental techniques, composition of growth medium, hydrogen ion concentration, size of the bacterial sample, and relative quantities of ions present [547,548]. In fact, these researchers confirmed that any ureolytic action observed was not through bactericidal mechanisms but due primarily to denaturing effects on proteins, which was an established observation [495]. And because potassium is important in microbial activity (especially among lactic acid-producing bacteria [549,550]) and is found in abundance in the oral environment (e.g., at least 10x the level of urea [102]), for ammonia to exert a comparable benefit against lactic-acid producing bacteria its levels would have to greatly exceed those of potassium under neutral pH conditions [548,549]. Altogether, the lack of a strong and consistent caries-reducing effect (even at high urea content) appears to derive from a combination that includes the relatively potassium-rich oral environment and the relatively acidic and ammonia-deficient plaque environment. These intrinsic reasons may account for present-day observations that there remains no link between plaque urease activity (i.e., microbial composition) and caries status [551].

As such, variations in experimental techniques, understanding, and expectations frustrated efforts in developing consistent and impactful ammonia-based therapies. Bypassed, forgotten, or simply unaware, prudent present-day researchers pursuing etiological or developmental efforts focusing on evolution of ammonia in the oral environment should bear in mind these important historical studies.

Dental preventives in the early 20th Century: Chlorophyll

Lastly, while medicine men have long-used (for centuries, if not millennia) plant material for medicinal purposes, the development of chlorophyll, which was first identified in the early 19th century, as a potential anticariogenic agent exploded in the 1940s. So what made this possible?

Worthy of the 1915 Nobel Prize in chemistry and creating a watershed moment in botany [552], Dr. Richard Willstätter pioneered the extraction of high-purity, high-yield chlorophyll from leafy plant matter

[553]; even further, Dr. Willstätter demonstrated that when combined with an alkali salt (e.g., KNO_3), the large, green, scepter-shaped pigment (chemical formula $C_{55}H_{72}O_5N_4Mg$, with the magnesium ion situated in the center of the chlorin ring) became water-soluble [553]. Research soon thereafter confirmed the commonality between chlorophyll and hemoglobin, where both molecules manifest base porphyrin structure and contribute respiratory functions to the living system in which they are found [554]. Moreover, animal studies demonstrated that chlorophyll supports red blood cell generation, thus linking the importance of leafy plant matter to sustenance: in studies with anemic rabbits, those fed a combined diet of iron pills plus leafy plants achieved normal hemoglobin content more quickly than those fed either iron pills or leafy vegetables alone [554].

Although other researchers had been exploring the use of chlorophyll prior to 1940, Dr. Benjamin Gruskin appears to have jumpstarted a domino effect with his initial 1938 patent covering chlorophyll-containing ointments, solutions, salves, and unguents [555]. In addition to fighting colds, his 1940 seminal studies demonstrated benefits in treating acute and chronic suppurative conditions involving many bacterial infections as they relate to proctology, gynecology, surgery, dermatology, and the upper respiratory tract (emphasizing those in the ear, nose, and throat) [556,557]. So popular was the chlorophyll craze that even the Ford Motor Company patented chlorophyll-containing medicaments [558].

The benefits of chlorophyll include rapid healing and sustained proliferation of healthy tissue cells, along with the inhibition of bacterial action [556,559]. Though not considered a bactericidal, numerous studies demonstrated a clinically observed bacteriostatic effect [559,560]. And while a detailed mechanism remains a mystery [561], the oxygenation produced by chlorophyll appears to confer action on proteins and cells of anaerobic bacteria [556,560] (e.g., possibilities include generation of singlet oxygen (a high-energy form of oxygen), superoxide radicals (O^{2-}), and/or hydrogen peroxide [562,563]), and even on insect

larvae when stimulated with light [563]. Since myriad anaerobic microbial pathogens reside on mucosal membranes throughout our bodies,
the appeal for a nontoxic, efficacious, and easily available therapeutic
is clear. In short time, applications of chlorophyll broadened to include
anemia, ulcers, tumors, cysts, burns, carcinoma, and dental maladies
[559]. Interestingly, observations also suggested antibiotic action can
be improved when combined with low levels of chlorophyll [564].

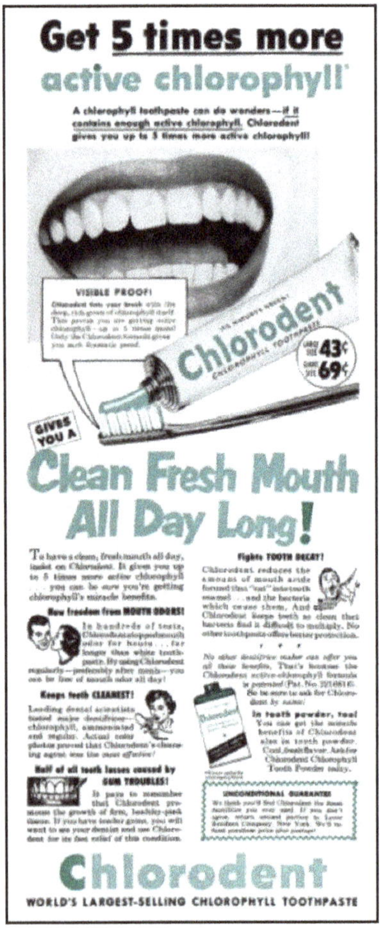

Figure 7.15. Advertisement for Chlorodent
dentifrice with chlorophyll appearing in
the early 1950s (from [570]).

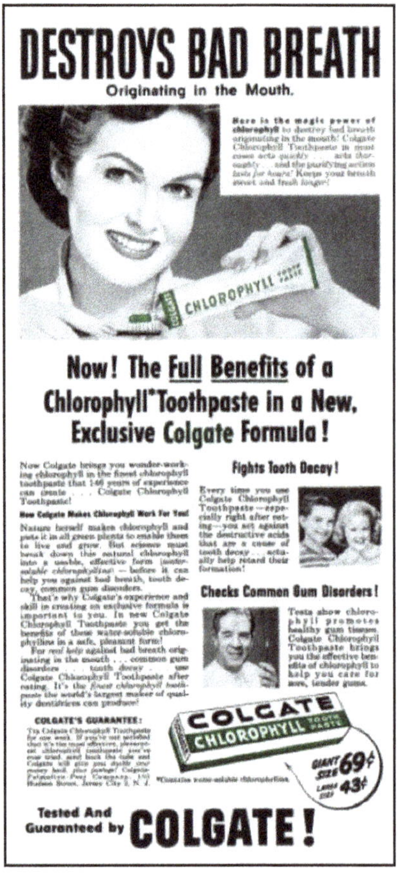

Figure 7.16. Advertisement for Colgate
dentifrice with chlorophyll appearing in the
early 1950s (from [572]).

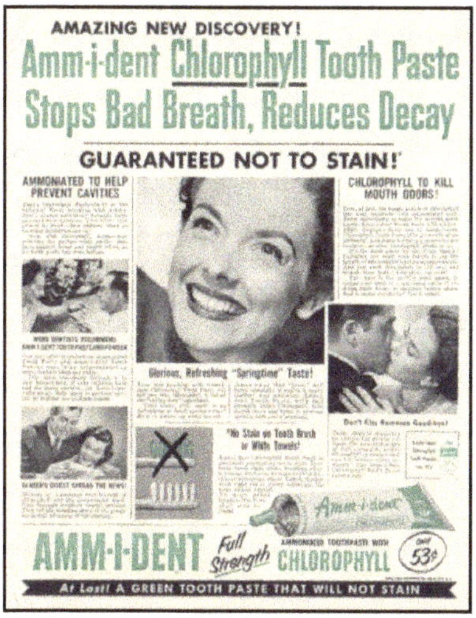

Figure 7.17. Advertisement for Amm-i-dent dentifrice with chlorophyll appearing in the early 1950s (from [573]).

Anticipating consumer demand for chlorophyll, the Rystan Company was formed in 1941 by two admen (O'Neill Ryan Jr. and Henry Stanton Jr. [461]), who subsequently secured rights to Gruskin's patents [555,565]. En route to patenting their own formulations, Rystan introduced the first commercial topical medicaments, referring to their chlorophyll salts as 'Chloresium' [566]. And with respect to dental issues, chlorophyll found a niche in battling soft tissue maladies, including bad breath and gingivitis [559]. With respect to cariogenic bacteria, significant reductions in *L. Acidophilus* (and other oral microbes) observed from independent research groups confirmed the bacteriostatic properties of chlorophyll [564,567–569]. Rystan subsequently licensed chlorophyll technology to other companies for dentifrice use, including Lever Bros. (makers of Pepsodent) [566], who marketed the 'Chlordent' or 'Mentasol' (in England) dentifrices (e.g., **Figure 7.15** [570]), and within two months of launch would soon trail only Colgate in commercial success [571]. In turn, Colgate denied Rystan's monopoly (legally or not [566]) and introduced their own version of chlorophyll dentifrice (e.g., **Figure 7.16** [572]). Other manufacturers soon introduced chlorophyll dentifrices of their own [461], including a version of Block Drug's Amm-i-dent toothpaste appearing in a 1952 advertisement in **Figure 7.17** [573].

Dental preventives in the early 20th Century: Segue to fluoride

For all the virtues of chlorophyll, it could not inhibit glycolysis (and, in contrast, could even increase acid production) [569], and some bacterial strains could develop some resistance to chlorophyll's effect [564]. Despite these limitations, without controlled clinical studies, and without acceptance from the American Dental Association (an organization which became increasingly vocal against dentifrice marketing practices), chlorophyll continued to dominate dentifrice innovation . . . that is, until a dentifrice was developed that could clearly demonstrate clinical caries reductions. While fluoride was a familiar decay prevention tool used by dentists [574], in a revolutionary turn of events that even the American Dental Association did not initially accept [575], topical fluoride would soon become available in a convenient dentifrice format, accompanied with the soon-to-be-famous tagline '*Look, Mom—No Cavities!*' [576]. Overlapping with calls to overhaul dentifrice marketing claims [577], the advent of a clinically effective fluoride dentifrice eventually brought 'order' to the seemingly 'wild-west' nature of dentifrice research and marketing practices. And because fluoride continues to endure as the predominant anticaries agent, the next chapter devotes full attention to how fluoride came about and why it works so well.

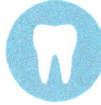

CHAPTER EIGHT

Fluoride: Thwarting Demineralization and Accelerating Remineralization

AND THEN THERE WAS FLUORIDE. Fluoride is the clinically proven gold standard in preventive dentistry and is regularly found in community water supplies as well as many preventive modalities including toothpastes, mouthrinses, and varnishes [578,579]. Its simplicity, economics, and efficacy against dental caries provided not only a significant advance in public health benefits but also helped vanquish many inconsistent or ineffective, albeit sometimes popular, products pushed by bold marketing that used limited (if any!) scientific research. But while fluoride is well-known, well-utilized by many dental practitioners, and is likely a part of daily oral care regimen, what is the backstory on

> *Fluoride is the clinically proven gold standard in preventive dentistry and is regularly found in community water supplies as well as many preventive modalities including toothpastes, mouthrinses, and varnishes.*

fluoride, why does it work so well in thwarting dental decay, and how is fluoride delivered today? In order to answer these questions, let's harken back to research from more than a century ago.

Geological fluorine sources and enamel mottling

From a geological perspective, elemental fluorine is commonly found in the earth's crust and oceans (~ 585 ppm and 1 ppm, respectively [210]), is a major component in fluorite (also known as fluorspar or calcium fluoride), and is commonly found in combinations with silicate or alumina, apatite, and even lead [580–583]. Minerals with fluorine usually appear white in color, although fluorine imbues crystals with greens, blues, and purple (e.g., fluorite cubes or wavellite spherulites) [580,581]. Typically, minerals comprising fluorine are often found among those with lead: in particular, galena (lead sulfide) deposits are usually in abundance with fluorite, with the latter considered gangue material [580,582]. Galena usually occurs with ores of silver, though the concentration of silver varies dramatically but is typically orders of magnitude smaller than lead content; an exception within the galena group is argentite, which is comprised mostly of silver [580,582]. Galena is usually found in granite, sandstone, and limestone rocks [580], all of which are in great abundance especially in the western United States' Rocky Mountain region [583].

As pegmatites (i.e., coarse, crystalline granite) are found in virtually every county in Colorado from Larimer County in the north to Custer County in the south [583], runoff from the Rocky Mountains contributes elements from these minerals, including lead and fluorine, into the natural spring waters. Spurred by local dentists reporting on discolorations in the enamel of the townspeople born and reared within this region, in 1916 Drs. McKay and Black reported on the mixed appearances of white, yellow, brown, and black enamel after personally visiting and investigating the situation. Through live and histological probing, the scientists understood the Rocky Mountain mottled teeth to be brittle, pitted, and grooved, but surprisingly resilient to dental caries [584]; however, the source of the mottling confounded the men and no explanation was proposed. Interestingly, such phenomena had been reported in the local populace by Italian dentists in and around the Naples region in 1901 [585]: there, the source turning the enamel black and spotted was assumed to be related to the volcanic gases diffusing into the local spring waters. Ongoing investigations published in 1930 demonstrated that certain communities throughout the United States were especially susceptible to enamel mottling, especially those founded to support mining operations [586]. Due to technological limitations during this time, robust and reliable water quality assessments were not yet possible; even so, manganese was detected and subsequently indicted as the cause for the brownish staining of enamel [586]. But the source of the other discolorations (e.g., the opaque or black spots) along with the physical deformities still remained a mystery [587]. So what might explain these observations?

Present-day scientific assessments confirm fluorine is found in the human body [24,588–594] in fractions higher than zinc and about half that of iron [593]. These results support 19th century knowledge, where calcium fluoride (i.e., fluorite or fluorspar) or fluorine of apatite (i.e., fluorapatite) had been known to be present in human teeth and bones [588-591]. In fact, fluorine had been detected as early as 1803 in animal bones [595], a finding soon thereafter confirmed by Berzelius, the noted Swedish chemist and, among other accomplishments, the 'discoverer' of silicon and selenium elements [24]. With the realization that fluorine is found in teeth and bone [588], and that fluorine levels in prehistoric bones are much higher than in modern day man and animals [589–591,595], it follows that absorption naturally ensues from spring and river waters residing near fluoride-rich mineral deposits, as well as from the sea [589–591,595]. Hence, the distribution of fluorine (where it is commonly in the ionic form of F⁻, or fluoride) in groundwater naturally varies according to geological characteristics

[596]. In addition to its ubiquity in vegetables, plants, and animals, fluorine was customarily introduced into foodstuffs for preservation and/or dietary purposes [595,597]. Even further, the incorporation of fluorine into bones or teeth seemed to suggest it was essential for good health [588,595].

But consistent with most substances found on Earth (including fluorine, oxygen, water, etc.), it is the level of the said substance (and not the substance itself) that dictates whether the effect will be positive or negative [598]; as such, when rats were fed a diet rich in fluorine (ingested 225 ppm NaF), deleterious effects on tooth and bone structure resulted: for instance, in addition to being brittle and susceptible to tooth wear, the incisors lacked the characteristic orange tint but were instead dull and opaque and lacked the natural polished appearance [597]. But while some enamel mottling was found in the rats consuming an enriched fluorine diet, this was also the case for those rats fed a normal diet; thus, while opacity, brittleness, and the presence of pits or grooves in teeth—characteristics which had been observed by Drs. McKay and Black [584]—may be linked to systemic ingestion of fluorine, darker enamel discolorations (i.e., from yellow to black) and mottling may not derive solely from fluorine (or fluoride).

As mentioned previously, fluorine is commonly found among lead deposits; so in addition to nearby mineral springs, rivers, and streams naturally comprising these components, enrichment of water sources may also occur due to routine mining operations (for lead, silver, fluorite, sandstone, limestone, etc.). Thus, it follows that if fluorine (or, fluoride) is present in water, there's a high probability that lead is present as well, along with other components such as sulfates, aluminum, etc. Expensive but durable, lead cisterns and pipes (including lead-only or lead-lined) were commonly used to store and deliver well, spring, and processed waters to a community [599,600]. Therefore, contributions from the leaden infrastructure could also contribute to systemic accumulation that, over time, may impart toxic effects. That teeth become blackened, yellowed, or browned, and were easily subject to fracture and wear is a well-documented effect of lead poisoning [601], and is consistent with the "ebony black" assessments of Drs. McKay and Black [584]. Therefore, it is imperative to understand enamel mottling, discolorations, and physical deformations develop not just from fluorine but from multiple sources including, and arguably the most damaging, lead. Chemically, the isomorphic substitution of lead for calcium readily facilitates its incorporation into dental and skeletal apatites [26,602–603]. In fact, the ability of topically applied solutions comprising lead or lead fluoride to reduce enamel solubility was suggested as a clinical tool for controlling dental decay [602].

Detecting fluoride content and water fluoridation

But while the presence of fluorine in teeth and bone could be identified using a variety of chemical techniques, quantifying fluoride levels in water, especially low levels, proved particularly challenging [589–591,595,597,605,606]. Obviously, the ability to provide reproducible measurements on fluoride content in water would allow for a fundamental understanding of the physiological risks and putative benefits of fluorine. Ultimately, the first accurate method of detecting fluoride in water (including below 1 ppm) was published by Churchill in 1932. One of the key findings was that fluoride was only detected in drinking water in states west of the Appalachian Mountains. Also, it was observed the fluoride content in drinking water could be remarkably different: for instance, 2 ppm fluoride was found in drinking water in Colorado Springs, Colorado, (which also has galena and fluoride deposits) while water in Bauxite, Arkansas, which supported industrial-level aluminum mining, had almost 13 ppm fluoride [607]. Importantly, the latter site was also one that had exhibited severe mottling and discolorations [607]. The advent of the colorimetric method published in 1933 introduced relatively facile and accurate analytical testing [606], enabling scientists to begin to explore the interrelationship among enamel mottling, presence of dental caries, and fluoride content in water [607–611]. Over an evaluation period between 8 and 10 years, it was observed that minimizing the fluoride content in 'new' sources of drinking water to no more than 1 ppm dramatically reduced the level and extent of white, opaque spotting now known as dental fluorosis [607,609–613]. The decline in fluorosis also reduced darker discolorations, suggesting possibly reduced uptake of other causative agents such as lead, aluminum, manganese, etc.

The ability to measure fluorine content overlapped with research on fluoride's anticaries benefits. Continuing the work with water fluoridation in the early 1940s [611], Dr. Dean led trials in 21 cities that probed the fluoride-caries relationship [609]. Around the same time, microbiological assessments demonstrated fluorine levels as low as 1 ppm influence bacterial activity [50], suggesting further benefits of fluoride. With the success of the initial 21-city evaluation in children, several independent fluoride-caries investigations were conducted with respect to each city's community water supply [609,611], and this also extended internationally [614]. The successful outcomes of these collective studies support water fluoridation (both from natural and artificial sources [615]) as an anticaries measure with minimal fluorosis risks at levels around 1 ppm [421,612,614,616,617].

Fluoride as an anticaries agent

Contemporaneous with the rollout of water fluoridation in specific communities (e.g., [611]), investigations on topically applied fluoride was beginning to take hold [618]. One of the landmark studies demonstrating the benefits of systemic fluoridation was the work by Armstrong and Brekhus, where teeth comprising higher fluoride levels exhibited less indications of caries [619]. But a watershed study detailing the promising benefits of topically applied fluoride was based on a year-long study in Indianapolis, Indiana: published in 1942, topical 0.1% sodium fluoride solution (i.e., 500 ppm fluoride) professionally administered every three months to children (ages between 4.5 and 6) led to almost twice as many caries-free tooth surfaces compared to the control group (i.e., fluoride-free) [620]. Echoing the promise of topically applied fluorides, a separate report also in 1942 highlighted a similar caries reduction in permanent teeth of children (ages between 10 and 13) receiving topically applied 0.1% sodium fluoride over the course of one year [621]. Importantly, from a toxicological perspective, topically applied sodium fluoride solutions did not demonstrate systemic absorption [622]. Such promising therapeutic and safety results encouraged and buttressed further research in this area, including the fluoride source, fluoride concentration, and frequency of application [623-627]. However, anticaries benefits were not yet realized from toothpaste or mouthwash [628,629], so unsupervised at-home use of fluoride would have to wait.

With the growing body of clinical benefits, research into fluoridated systems continued to expand, driven to understand how and why fluoride was helping to reduce tooth decay. Initially, it was postulated that fluoride must work in one of two ways: either incorporate directly into enamel structure, or mitigate the insults leading directly to decay [629]. For example, by chemical substitution (i.e., fluoride exchange with hydroxyl groups in enamel apatite) fluoride physically strengthens the enamel and reduces its susceptibility to acids [630]. And, supporting the laboratory study claiming inhibition of acid production [50], significant reductions in clinical bacterial counts were observed when using a twice daily sodium fluoride dentifrice (500 ppm and 1000 ppm fluoride, with the latter concentration conferring greater benefits) [631].

But in the 1940s, prevailing thought reasoned only children would benefit the most from water fluoridation due to incorporation of systemic fluoride prior to tooth eruption (primary or secondary) [626,629]. While topically applied fluoride demonstrated higher levels of fluorine incorporation into enamel and reductions in enamel solubility, the benefits were principally observed in relatively young (or, "chemically unreacted" [626]) teeth. Contributing to this rationale were the fail-ures of at-home fluoridated dentifrices (in liquid and paste formats) to provide significant anticaries benefits in young adults at low and mod-erate fluoride levels (i.e., up to 500 ppm fluoride) [628,632]. But rather than a failure in either the fluoridated format or compliance using the dentifrice, reductions in bioavailable fluoride due to undesirable reac-tions between fluoride and other agents in a dentifrice (e.g., calcium) were not yet appreciated. That is, until a 1954 landmark study forever changed fluoridated dentifrices.

In what famously became the original Crest® formulation with 'Fluoristan' [576], a stannous fluoride dentifrice (1,000 ppm fluoride) successfully demonstrated a significant caries reduction relative to a control dentifrice over a six-month period in children (ages between 6 and 15) in Bloomington, Indiana. Importantly, the at-home toothpaste was used in an unsupervised manner, and demonstrated a particularly strong benefit for the older kids [633]. The 'magic' ingredient improv-ing on dentifrice abrasive standards was the discovery of a new class of heat-treated calcium phosphate phases that, although still suscep-tible to binding with fluoride, achieved clinically effective levels of bioavailable fluoride for anticaries benefits [634]. Importantly, this study provided clinical validation to the growing volume of studies demonstrating topically applied fluorides can strengthen and/or reduce solubility of teeth.

Following on this success, the study was repeated on adults (ages between 17 and 36) enrolled at Indiana University (Bloomington, Indiana) [635]. For the first time, clinically significant caries reductions were obtained from a home-use fluoridated dentifrice in an adult popula-tion over the course of six months and a year; in particular, the benefits were boosted when the participants maintained routine brushing habits. This study was the first to demonstrate that fluoride dentifrice confers clinical benefits to mature teeth, and in doing so firmly debunked the view that only immature teeth were sensitive to fluoride [626].

Mineralization from topical fluorides

Most of the initial dentifrices were acidic formulations (~ pH 4), as these seemed to exhibit the greatest reductions in enamel solubility [626]. Fluoride mouthwash (e.g., stannous fluoride or acidulated phosphate fluoride) also conferred deposition of fluoride [636], with low pH formulations (e.g., pH 4 or lower) favoring greater delivery compared to neutral solutions [626.637]. Although certainly able to reduce solubility of enamel and provide protection, not all of the deposited fluoride integrates within enamel structure but remains adsorbed onto the tooth surface or within the plaque fluid.

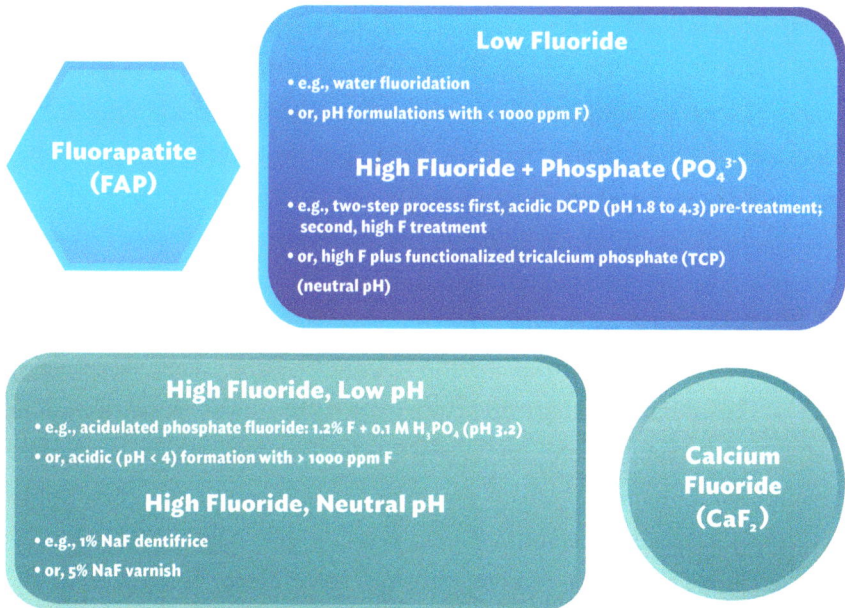

Fluorapatite (FAP)

Low Fluoride
- e.g., water fluoridation
- or, pH formulations with < 1000 ppm F)

High Fluoride + Phosphate (PO_4^{3-})
- e.g., two-step process: first, acidic DCPD (pH 1.8 to 4.3) pre-treatment; second, high F treatment
- or, high F plus functionalized tricalcium phosphate (TCP)

  (neutral pH)

High Fluoride, Low pH
- e.g., acidulated phosphate fluoride: 1.2% F + 0.1 M H_3PO_4 (pH 3.2)
- or, acidic (pH < 4) formation with > 1000 ppm F

High Fluoride, Neutral pH
- e.g., 1% NaF dentifrice
- or, 5% NaF varnish

Calcium Fluoride (CaF_2)

Figure 8.1. Conditions and some examples of topical treatments used effect formation of either fluorapatite ($Ca_5(PO_4)_3F$) or calcium fluoride-like mineral (with CaF_2 formula chosen for simplicity rather than preciseness), two fluoride-based minerals associated with enamel and anticaries benefits. With respect to the calcium fluoride mineral in the image: this does not only represent calcium fluoride, but rather a calcium fluoride-like mineral or agglomeration that may lack the typical cubic structure of CaF_2 and may exhibit spherical morphology. The point is that the calcium fluoride-like mineral is expected to function like a reservoir of calcium and fluoride when acted upon through hydration and/or acidic events [652–654].

Chemically, the introduction of fluorine into enamel produces fluoridated phases that exhibit reduced solubility compared to native tooth apatite, the mineral nature of which is largely comprised of either fluorapatite or calcium fluoride-like mineral as outlined in **Figure 8.1**.

NOTE:

With respect to calcium fluoride, though not exactly CaF_2, this is shown for simplicity and the true formula can be expected to depart from this 'perfect' stoichiometry; additionally, the appearance can also be expected to be less cubic and more spherical due to formation of calcium fluoride-like agglomerates.

In general, pH, concentration, and source of fluoride exert significant influence on the major mineral phase produced [636–643]. For example, water fluoridation (~ 1 ppm fluoride) and neutral sodium fluoride formulations having less than 500 ppm (and perhaps up to 1,000 ppm fluoride) generally favor fluorapatite formation [86,638-640,644,645]. In contrast, calcium fluoride is largely produced through topical application of acidulated phosphate fluoride [636], low-pH, high-fluoride gels or dentifrices [626,642], and other fluoride preparations generally having more than 0.5% fluoride [639–641,643]. An interesting exception is that of stannous fluoride, which by virtue of the stannous cation, does not seem to promote calcium fluoride or fluorapatite formation; rather, an amorphous apatite-fluoride phase appears to form [646], helping to increase resistance to enamel dissolution [647].

Based on the deep research pool of topical fluorides, neutral NaF formulations are among the best fluoride sources for the formation of fluorapatite [642,648]. Furthermore, frequent application of modest fluoride levels (< 1,000 ppm fluoride) and/or preparations that promote sustained-release characteristics (e.g., through reservoirs in plaque or saliva, as well as adhesion onto and penetration into the tooth surfaces) of fluoride seem to also favor fluorapatite formation [34,114,578,639, 640,643,649,650].

One criticism of acidulated fluoride systems (e.g., acidulated phosphate fluoride and/or low-pH dentifrices or gels) is that much of the calcium fluoride formed does not integrate with the tooth structure but adsorbs to the tooth surface or within the plaque. Due to the slow and/or limited conversion to fluorapatite from calcium fluoride (including calcium fluoride-like mineral phases) as well as nonmineralized adsorbed fluoride (e.g., association with plaque or saliva constituents), the risks for clearance from the oral environment are, therefore, increased by factors such as salivary action [636,640,642,651]. Some modern anticaries strategies favor calcium fluoride (or calcium fluoride-like) formation (instead of focusing only on direct fluorapatite formation), and is achieved by adjusting certain parameters, including the fluoride concentration, lowering the pH of the fluoride modality, and/or extending fluoride-tooth exposure [652–654]. These demands, some of which align with the low-level fluoride availability that encourages fluorapatite formation [34,578,643,649,650], have launched new avenues of research, including the following:

- ✓ Inclusion of phosphate salts to topical NaF solutions at neutral pH [655].

- ✓ Application of cavity liners and other coating agents following fluoride treatment, which directly led to the fluoride varnish modality [636,651,656–658].

- ✓ A two-step regimen comprising first an acid pretreatment with dicalcium phosphate dihydrate (i.e., brushite, $CaHPO_4 \bullet H_2O$), followed by high fluoride treatment [645,659,660].

- ✓ Another two-step regimen but this one involves a calcium pretreatment, followed by fluoride treatment [661,662].

✓ Split-compartment or water-free fluoride systems (often at acidic pH) for rapid precipitation of amorphous mineral from high concentrations of calcium and phosphate [663–668];

✓ Single-step, single-compartment system combining pH-neutral NaF and a customized β-tricalcium phosphate system engineered for sustained, low-level calcium release [114,139,160,181,183,650,669–675].

Topical fluorides: Water fluoridation and salts

The desire to deliver and extend exposure of teeth to fluoride has given rise to a number of different topical formats. In the US, a number of different product formats and fluoride concentrations have been approved to thwart the incidence of dental caries [149,676]. But given the variations in fluoride modalities, how does one format or fluoride concentration compare with another? Even in the 21st century and depicted in **Figure 8.2**, water fluoridation continues to provide a tremendous public health benefit, protecting against caries, on average, at least 27% and 34% of adults and children, respectively [677,678]. Sodium fluoride or fluorosilicate salts are usually incorporated in water fluoridation measures [612]. While water fluoridation appears more effective than fluoridated salt [679], fluoridated salt confers better benefits relative to no fluoride exposure [680]. But, drawbacks against fluoridated salt programs include conflicting messages regarding low-salt diets for health-based reasons along with individual's taste and dietary preferences, both of which can reduce compliance.

Topical fluorides: Rinses

Fluoride mouthwashes (or mouthrinses) were developed in the 1960s and 1970s as a public health measure to provide anticaries benefits and were thought to be especially appealing for those lacking access to other fluoride formats [648]. Originally developed for use in school-based programs (which, therefore, provide a high level of compliance), unsupervised use (i.e., at home) is now common, with daily (0.05% NaF) or weekly (0.2% NaF) fluoride mouthwashes approved for use by the Food and Drug Administration, along with acidulated phosphate fluorides [636,648,681]. The approximate efficacy of fluoride mouthwash is reported to be approximately 26% [682], although these are not meant for children less than six years of age due to swallowing risks [648]. Although enhanced effects may be marginal when combined with other fluoridated formats (e.g., use in combination with a dentifrice) [683], for those fitted with orthodontic brackets (which presents colonizing opportunities for bacteria and therefore increased risks for tooth decay), a daily-use mouthwash (i.e., 0.05% NaF) is recommended to help reduce white-spot formation [684].

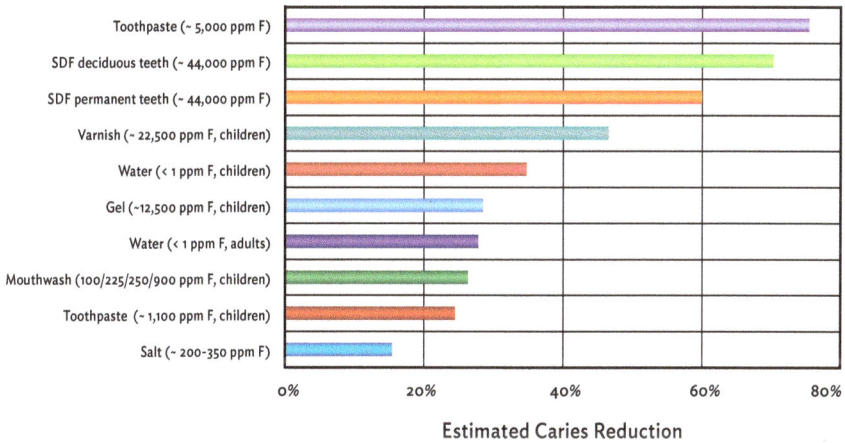

Figure 8.2. Estimated caries reduction relative to fluoride modality, including salt [679,680], mouthwash [682], water fluoridation [677,678], silver diamine fluoride (SDF) [728], toothpaste [736–738], fluoride gel [685], and fluoride varnish [685].

Topical fluorides: Gels

Fluoride gels typically have more than 10x the fluoride in standard over-the-counter (OTC) dentifrices. While some have neutral pH, most generally comprise acidulated phosphate fluoride (APF) and therefore have pH less than 5. Despite having 100x greater fluoride content, fluoride gels yield similar efficacy relative to fluoridated mouthwash [685], and this may reflect differences in frequency of use (i.e., gels are generally

DEMIN/REMIN IN PREVENTIVE DENTISTRY

an in-office treatment during regular dental visits, while mouthwashes are an at-home convenience). However, for daily-use fluoride gels, the efficacy can be much higher [686]. APF gel formats differ in viscosity but produce similar enamel fluoride uptake relative to APF solutions [686].

With respect to fluoride gels, there appear to be elevated risks with respect to children [687,688]. In addition to inadvertent overfilling by the clinician (e.g., usually trays hold 5 ml but due to tray-type and clinical error, the amount may easily swell to 12 ml), there are also serious risks for swallowing during the in-office treatment period (usually 20 minutes), with the range of ingesting ranging from 15% to 100% [688]. Given the high fluoride levels of gels do not necessarily translate into greater caries protection when other fluoride formats are available (e.g., water fluoridation, fluoride mouthwash, OTC fluoride dentifrices, or fluoride varnish) [685], the elevated ingestion risks should give clinicians pause—at least with respect to children whose permanent dentition has not erupted. [687,688]. The plasma fluoride levels in children after topical a 1.23% APF gel application were reported to be about 10x higher compared to ingestion after fluoride varnish application [687]. More recently, a clinical study involving 42 children six years of age revealed that a single treatment of a 2% fluoride gel produced an average increase in the amount of fluoride detected in urine of about 114% (i.e., from 0.0801 mg to 0.1721 mg fluorine); in contrast, a single application of a sustained-release 5% NaF varnish (Clinpro™ White Varnish with TCP) produced a significantly lower average increase of about 20% (i.e., from 0.0697 mg to 0.0835 mg) [689].

As the nature of APF systems is to deliver large amounts of fluoride, that which does not integrate directly with the tooth is expected to be adsorbed to various surfaces in the mouth, including on the tooth, the soft tissue (e.g., cheeks and gingiva), or even in plaque [636,642,648,651–654]. As such, salivary clearance of labile, non-integrated or even adsorbed fluoride may elevate safety risks [687]. To mitigate fluoride ingestion concerns, one can promptly rinse after the fluoride treatment (which is one reason young children are taught to rinse their mouths after toothbrushing with a fluoride toothpaste). But when rinsed with water immediately following gel treatment (for the purposes of removing residue and/or limiting systemic ingestion), additional fluoride is lost from the tooth, suggesting caries protection may be reduced at the expense of limiting safety risks [690]. Such risk-benefit analyses are contributing to the shift from fluoride gels to other dental formats: most notably, fluoride varnishes.

Topical fluorides: Varnishes

On average, fluoride varnishes afford about 46% caries reduction [685], which, in considering the improved safety profile of this format over gels [687] and its importance in pediatric programs [691,692], renders this a topical preparation worthy of further discussion. The problem of maintaining sustained exposure of fluoride to the teeth led to the development of fluoride varnishes in the 1960s and 1970s [648,657]. Recognized *a posteriori*, physical barriers were applied to the teeth after fluoridated treatment as a means of forcing fluoride retention to the enamel surface [636,651]. In effect, this approach created temporary thermodynamic isolation of the teeth from the oral environment [658], and proved successful in preventing bulk loss of fluoride after immediate treatment. Among the experimental barriers used were beeswax, nail polish, and cavity liner [636,651]. Backed with data demonstrating fluoride needed additional incentive to remain on the tooth, commercial innovations came shortly thereafter. Schmidt published on a water-insoluble resin system comprising 5% sodium fluoride, known as Duraphat® in 1964, with clinical efficacy realized soon afterward [657] (and later acquired by Colgate). And, the benefits of a novel polyurethane system comprising 1% difluorosilane, then known as Vivadent Fluor Protector (now known as Ivoclar Vivadent, with different versions available, including ammonium fluoride) were demonstrated in 1975 [656].

Currently, most marketed fluoride varnishes contain 5% NaF (~ 22,500 ppm fluoride), a level recognized by, for instance, the American Dental Association (ADA) [693]. The ADA recommends 5% NaF varnish applications given at least twice per year for children younger than six years of age, and also for children and teenagers up through 18 years of age. Additionally, 5% NaF varnish treatments are also recommended for prevention against root caries in adults when administered at least twice per year. In fact, many agencies and professional organizations recognize the anticaries benefits of fluoride varnishes, including the World Health Organization, American Academy of Pediatric Dentistry, the US Centers for Disease Control and Prevention, the American Dental Association, as well as other professional organizations in many countries (especially in Europe, where they were first introduced and used as a caries intervention) [656,657,693–696]. Recently, the US Preventive Services Task Force recommended "that primary care clinicians apply fluoride varnish to the primary teeth of infants and children starting at the age of primary tooth eruption" [696]. This statement not only demonstrates the importance of fluoride varnish for caries control but also highlights the role that clinicians on the medical side of healthcare (e.g., physicians, nurses, nurse practitioners, and physicians assistants) can play in helping to promote and provide preventive care [7]. To better serve children, there is evidence that dental clinicians would favor cooperation with medical personnel for preventive services, although there is some reluctance as well [697]. And from an aid-based perspective, fluoride varnishes implemented by nine months of age in the state of Indiana would facilitate Medicaid cost-savings relative to restorative costs within three years of implementation [698].

At this point I want to address some troubling marketing and design aspects of many fluoride varnishes, which I believe compromise the purpose of fluoride varnishes, potentially confuse clinicians, and elevate risks for pediatric patients. This is especially important since fluoride varnishes are applied after dental cleanings, meaning plaque reservoirs are not abundantly available to help retain and deliver fluoride, thus elevating risks for accidental ingestion.

Given the wide endorsements of fluoride varnish as an effective anti-caries measure, it is not surprising there are many commercial fluoride varnishes available today. Most of these varnish manufacturers appeal to dental/medical professionals on the basis of 'rapid (or fast) release', 'greater fluoride-ion release', or 'higher enamel (fluoride) uptake'. But important questions remain as to the safety and efficacy of these varnish systems. To that end, those manufacturers (which are many and include well-recognized names) relying on such claims unfortunately dismiss the purpose of a fluoride varnish, which is to prolong fluoride contact with the dentition; instead, such manufacturers are effectively creating what I consider to be a varnish-gel hybrid system that can be described as "rapidly releasing lots of fluoride, resulting in high fluoride precipitation and/or uptake". It is important to be reminded of the safety concerns of fluoride gels, as fluoride varnishes are thought to be a safer and more effective in-office fluoride alternative.

But if the varnish system is too fluid or too rapid in its delivery of fluoride, then it likely imparts elevated health risks (especially to children) given that the fluoride concentration in varnish is almost double that of fluoride gels. To that end, varnishes that promote 'rapid release' or 'thin films' may, in turn, sacrifice varnish durability, thickness, safety, and efficacy. Additionally, massive enamel fluoride uptake (or rather, surface adsorption, which is not generally addressed by the manufacturers) can create undesirable gradients that drive fluoride *from* the tooth. After all, teeth have limited fluoride absorption (which will be discussed later in this chapter): in practice, the outer layers of enamel accumulate fluoride [699,700], with much of it unable to be integrated effectively into the tooth due to the rapid and transient formation of calcium fluoride (and calcium fluoride-like mineral). In turn, this situation mirrors some limitations of APF mouthrinses and gels [636,642,648,651,687], and begs the question: where does all the excess fluoride go? Studies show that fluoride is retained largely in the outer enamel layers, and cannot readily diffuse more deeply into enamel [699,700]. So, one can surmise that much of the excess fluoride becomes cleared or swallowed, especially when applied to freshly cleaned teeth. Importantly, fluoride uptake is not necessarily a predictor of clinical caries benefits [642,647,701], so manufacturers constructing marketing claims should proceed with caution, while clinicians should be mindful to know the difference.

Similarly, varnishes that encourage adhesion of large amounts of precipitated, insoluble mineral to the enamel surface present similar issues. In these instances, insoluble minerals, which are transient just like deposited calcium fluoride (and associated calcium fluoride-like minerals), are subject to clearance and may not survive for diffusion into the enamel subsurface or incorporation into saliva and/or plaque. In the event, however, these do survive, other complications could develop such as poorly integrated enamel mineralization, soft tissue irritations, calculus accumulation, etc.

Thus, it is my opinion that dental and medical practitioners select a fluoride varnish format that displays the following properties [58]:

✓ Maintain a physical barrier for an extended period of time (e.g., at least 4, 8, even 12 hours); and,

✓ Provide controlled release of low-level fluoride to the dentition (e.g., steady exposure of low-levels of fluoride provide clinical benefits while manifesting reduced risk for fluoride ingestion; thus, rapid- and/or high fluoride-release properties do not mirror the purpose of a varnish and may pose unnecessary health risks); and,

✓ Encourage remineralization at and within the enamel surface and subsurface; incorporation of mineralizing agents into varnishes is OK provided they encourage precipitation of enamel-like or calcium fluoride-like mineral. Those that can integrate with enamel (i.e., formation of fluorapatite) are best.

With respect to the above, if fluoride-only varnish systems are desired, I suggest Duraphat® and Fluor Protector, mainly because these were among the first to be developed, and, therefore, remain true to the original purpose of a varnish, and have enjoyed clinical success over the last 30+ years. But for improved benefits, I recommend Vanish™ 5% NaF White Varnish with Tri-Calcium Phosphate [702] (or, outside the US, Clinpro™ White Varnish with TCP [703]), a clinically proven and popular varnish that is similar to Duraphat® but with notable improvements including color (i.e., it dries white/clear instead of yellow), sustained release of low-level fluoride commensurate with water fluoridation (~ 1 ppm fluoride) [704–706] and preventive protocols [34,692], and it comprises a customized calcium phosphate system designed specifically for the Clinpro™ (or Vanish™) varnish vehicle [672,707]. In addition to providing clinical protection against noncavitated carious lesions [708–711], this sustained-release system extends fluoride-tooth exposure [704,705], migrates into difficult to reach spaces in the dentition [704,705,712], effects surface and subsurface remineralization [713–723], produces acid-resistant remineralization [713–723], and is more effective in delivering fluoride to plaque fluid compared to other varnishes (including fluoride-only varnish, and another sodium fluoride varnish comprising amorphous calcium phosphate) [724]. Importantly, Clinpro™ (or Vanish™) also provides clinical relief from dental hypersensitivity [725]. Finally, from a safety perspective, Clinpro™ also confers significantly less risk for systemic ingestion of fluoride relative to other high-fluoride formats, such as shown clinically in a pediatric population relative to a 2% sodium fluoride gel [689]. As a further testament to safety, out of more than *ten thousand* (10,000+) varnish treatments delivered to more than 2,400 children (ages between 0 and 5 years old) up to a three year period (with each child receiving, on average, 4 varnish treatments), there were zero fluoride varnish-related adverse events [691]. Ergo, the 3M varnish systems (Clinpro™ and/or Vanish™) are a sound, effective therapeutic for the management of early caries lesions and relief of dentinal hypersensitivity.

While 5% NaF fluoride varnishes are most beneficial when used for preventing, arresting, and even reversing (in many cases) non-cavitated lesions, for cavitated lesions they are less effective [726,727]. So besides sealants or resin-infiltrants, is there a noninvasive option for managing dentin caries that removes the need for drilling? Yes! But, caution must be exercised. As depicted in **Figure 8.2**, 38% silver diamine fluoride (SDF) provides about 70% reduction in caries, and has been used outside the US for decades (particularly in Japan, Australia, and Mexico) [728]. The success of SDF is due to the combination of high fluoride content plus silver (which manifests its own antimicrobial properties), and is recommended as a surrogate for invasive restorative procedures in primary dentition [727-729]. In addition to early childhood caries (ECC), SDF may be recommended for elderly patients, as well as special-needs patients who present clinical challenges. In fact, SDF has been considered the best topical anticaries therapy for primary dentition and elderly populations [730]. Though lower concentration SDF is available, it seems 38% (~ 44,000 ppm fluoride) is most effective, with one treatment providing adequate but waning protection over a two-year period [729]. But while no drilling is required, there are limitations. Of primary concern is the relatively high amount of silver and fluoride delivered to the oral environment [728]. Therefore, SDF presents elevated risks for accidental ingestion by vulnerable populations, including children, the elderly, and special needs [727,729]. Also of concern is the jet-black residue from deposited silver that remains in the arrested cavitation, which unavoidably creates unappealing cosmetic effects, especially in the anterior teeth [727,731–733]. Other issues may include the metallic taste, soft tissue irritations, and parental perceptions on staining [732,733]. In turn, these limitations might be mitigated according to the skill and care of the clinician. Thus, the risk-benefit relationship for a given patient must be weighed carefully, and should include availability of other fluoride formats, access to professional dental care, and the economics of the dental situation [727,729]. And, with respect to preventing dental decay, SDF appears at least as good relative to other fluoridated formats [730,731].

Topical fluorides: Toothpastes

Next to water fluoridation, fluoride dentifrices provide arguably the most consistent exposure to fluoride on a worldwide basis [695,734]. Evolving from the original Crest® formulation with stannous fluoride, fluoride dentifrices in the US are regulated by the Food and Drug Administration [149], allowing for only stannous fluoride, sodium monofluorophosphate, or sodium fluoride [648,734]. Elsewhere, (in Europe, for instance), the list of approved fluoride compounds is longer [735]. Presently, the level of caries reduction appears to be about 24% for dentifrices comprising at least 1,000 ppm fluoride and up to about 1,250 ppm fluoride [736–738]; the caries reduction increases to about 36% for fluoride concentrations between 2,400 ppm and 2,800 ppm fluoride [738]; and, for fluoride levels 5,000 ppm fluoride (which are regarded professional-strength dentifrices in the US [676]) and above, the reduction in caries can reach, on average, 75% [737]. In this limit, these professional dentifrices are recommended for patients most at-risk for dental decay, including those with xerostomia, a history of dental decay, and even those wearing orthodontia. Relative to the other fluoride formats, approximate caries reduction benefits from dentifrices with levels near 1,000 ppm and 5,000 ppm fluoride are shown in **Figure 8.2**.

As fluoride toothpaste formulations evolve, some are designed to help promote additional benefits, including remineralization and/or relief from dentinal hypersensitivity. One example is the inclusion of calcium phosphate, of which there are several choices commercially available from various manufacturers. As such, it is helpful to touch on the benefits of such combination dentifrices since several are commercially available worldwide. But instead of reviewing several of these systems, as the inventor of an innovative form of calcium phosphate (the functionalized tricalcium phosphate system, which is discussed further in Chapter 9) incorporated into two fluoride dentifrices marketed by 3M Oral Care, I am intimately familiar with how these systems work and will limit the discussion to these. And, also being familiar with testing models and strategies for the evaluation of fluoride-containing dentifrices, in the next section I provide a narrative on the ability of these combination dentifrices to provide remineralization benefits. Moreover, evidence of both types of fluoride-based mineralization categorized in **Figure 8.1** (i.e., fluorapatite and calcium fluoride-like mineral) can be observed within the subsurface lesion.

> **NOTE:**
>
> As an inventor of the functionalized tricalcium phosphate systems, I claim vested interests in the dentifrices discussed in the next section. However, the data and information presented were not unduly influenced by these interests, and whenever possible independent studies are referenced. The two Clinpro™ dentifrice systems presented here manifest a unique remineralization approach (discussed in detail in Chapter 9), and because they are commercially available in many countries, including those in North America, South America, Europe, Asia, Middle East, and Africa, along with Australia & New Zealand, it makes sense to explore them a bit further.
>
> Importantly, the discussion that follows also allows the reader to visualize and explore the differences in fluoride-based mineralization (i.e., fluorapatite and calcium fluoride-like mineral from **Figure 8.1**) achieved within the subsurface lesion from two different fluoride-containing toothpastes; notably, such evidence within the subsurface lesion is often challenging to observe without sample destruction/distortion, so this is a great opportunity to provide an example.

Examples of the remineralization benefits of sodium fluoride plus calcium phosphate toothpaste: Clinpro™ toothpastes comprising functionalized tricalcium phosphate and either 950 ppm or 5,000 ppm fluoride.

Given the abundance of dentifrices to choose from, what helps distinguish one from another? While flavor [739] and appearance [740] surely factor into one's decision, therapeutic benefits [741] and the dentist's recommendations [739] are also important. Still recognized as the only clinically proven anticaries agent in the US, fluoride has established itself as a gold standard over the last 50 years.

But as discussed, efforts to extract further benefits from fluoride are ever-present, with most exploring novel ways to link calcium and phosphate to fluoride. While some of these will be revisited in Chapter 9, others are left to excellent reviews [734,742]. Here, I draw attention to two relatively new dentifrices introduced by 3M Oral Care that comprise a functionalized tricalcium phosphate ingredient: Clinpro™ Tooth Crème [743] and Clinpro™ 5000 [744]. Clinpro™ Tooth Crème and Clinpro™ 5000 are pH-neutral and contain 0.21% NaF (or, 950 ppm fluoride) and 1.1% NaF (or, 5,000 ppm fluoride), respectively. Also, the levels of functionalized tricalcium phosphate (referred to as 'fTCP' or 'TCP' for topical preparations marketed by 3M Oral Care) in each dentifrice are 0.05% (Clinpro™ Tooth Crème) and 0.08% (Clinpro™ 5000), respectively. These low levels of calcium and phosphate help meet low-supersaturation conditions for calcium-rich mineralization and will be discussed further in the next chapter. Clinpro™ Tooth Crème is designed to replace an existing daily dentifrice by providing safe and effective anticaries benefits at the tooth surface and subsurface. Due to the slightly lower fluoride level compared to normal over-the-counter (OTC) toothpaste (e.g., 1,100 ppm fluoride), this dentifrice is especially useful for those at low- to moderate-risk for tooth decay, as well as those seeking a lower-fluoride option. Ideal for those with elevated risks for tooth decay (e.g., for those with orthodontia, experiencing xerostomia, or exhibiting a history of tooth decay) or tooth sensitivity (e.g., from gingival recession), Clinpro™ 5000 is a professional-strength dentifrice designed for weekly or daily use, depending on the recommendation of the dental professional and/or the patient's needs. While sold globally, depending on the reader's geography, each of these is available from a dental professional, a pharmacy, or from an online marketplace (e.g., in the US, Clinpro™ Tooth Crème is available on Amazon.com).

Like the 3M varnish formulations, these Clinpro™ dentifrices comprise a customized form of β-tricalcium phosphate, where the functionalized form of the tricalcium phosphate is tailored to meet the design and intent of a topical fluoride format; for instance, the version of tricalcium phosphate in a dentifrice is different than that for a varnish [650,670,671,707]. For these dentifrices, β-tricalcium phosphate fused with low amounts of sodium lauryl sulfate (i.e., 2% sodium lauryl sulfate with 98% β-tricalcium phosphate) to create the functionalized material. The optimized combination of fluoride plus functionalized tricalcium phosphate builds on fluoride's clinically proven benefits without compromising fluoride bioavailability or requiring water-free or split-chamber compartments. Supported with multiple research grants from the US National Institute of Dental and Craniofacial Research and the State of Indiana [745], to date, this is the first and only form of calcium phosphate to have its solubility engineered to match the fit and function of the fluoride preparation (e.g., dentifrice or varnish)—all without compromising fluoride bioavailability.

Consistent with the presentation of fluorapatite and calcium fluoride formation (e.g., **Figure 8.1**), the morphology of incipient lesions (about 70 μm deep) treated with either Clinpro™ Tooth Crème or Clinpro™ 5000 bear out elements of these minerals as revealed by X-ray and scanning electron microscopy (SEM) studies in **Figure 8.3** [114]. The two graphs in **Figure 8.3** depict the long-range (wide-angle X-ray diffraction, WAXD, top graph) and short-range (small-angle X-ray diffraction, SAXS, bottom graph) order of the enamel structure. The corresponding SEM images correspond to depths about 30 μm into the enamel substrates.

Upon demineralization, loss of periodicity and crystallite volume resulted in lower WAXD intensity (as shown in the red curve); in contrast, as shown by the higher WAXD signals, both Clinpro™ Tooth Crème and Clinpro™ 5000 produced remineralization (the green and blue curves, respectively) that restored periodicity to levels approaching sound enamel (i.e., the black curve). Separately, the SAXS signal details the presence of high-surface area regions, such as that produced from voids or small crystallites [114,142,151,152]. Thus, relative to sound enamel (black curve), the lineshape corresponding to scattered signal from the incipient lesion (red curve) indicates the presence of voids and/or small crystallites. The SEM images for sound enamel and incipient lesions illustrate these differences, with sound enamel manifesting longer, densely-packed crystallites while shorter, disorganized, and loosely-packed crystallites comprise the enamel lesion.

When incipient lesions are treated with Clinpro™ Tooth Crème or Clinpro™ 5000, lesion structure and morphology were altered significantly. With respect to Clinpro™ Tooth Crème, the SAXS signal indicates a narrower lineshape (green curve) relative to the incipient lesion (red curve), and therefore, a fundamental change in the microstructure. Supported with microhardness measurements made on the same enamel cross-sections that were evaluated with X-ray diffraction and SEM, Clinpro™ Tooth Crème effected significantly harder (i.e., stronger) enamel relative to the incipient lesion [114]. Hence, the narrower lineshape represents the presence of new crystallites arranged in more or less the same orientation, and differs from the void structure that evolved during lesion formation. This observation is consistent with the micrograph for the lesion treated with Clinpro™ Tooth Crème, almost mirroring the crystallite length, size, and orientation in the micrograph for sound enamel.

So with respect to lesions remineralized with Clinpro™ Tooth Crème, petrographically, the newly formed crystallites appear enamel-like (i.e., apatite-like), while strengthening of the enamel lesion (determined from microhardness measurements [114]) suggests remineralization was likely produced through the formation of fluorapatite [34,578,643,649,650]: both of these characteristics are consistent with the FAP categorization in **Figure 8.1**. As discussed in Chapter 9, solubility product calculations reveal mineralization produced from Clinpro™ Tooth Crème largely include fluorapatite, hydroxyapatite, and some calcium fluoride; importantly, these calculations do not show evidence of other calcium phosphate phases. These data are supported with published laboratory and clinical research on this dentifrice system, which shows Clinpro™ Tooth Crème delivers fluoride [746–750], remineralizes incipient caries lesions [114,139,746–750], effects subsurface remineralization [114,751–756], and reduces dentinal hypersensitivity [757–759]. Importantly, despite being formulated with less fluoride compared to standard OTC toothpastes (e.g., 1100 ppm fluoride), the efficacy is at least as good as (and often better than) these systems, as well as others that may contain additional mineralizing agents: for example, on a per-gram-fluoride basis, the *in situ* remineralization effected by Clinpro™ Tooth Crème (which contains 0.21% NaF, and 0.05% functionalized tricalcium phosphate, TCP) was at least 5x better than other fluoride pastes, including one comprising 0.2% NaF and 10% casein phosphopeptide-amorphous calcium phosphate (CPP-ACP) [756]. Altogether, these results demonstrate Clinpro™ Tooth Crème delivers acid-resistant, enamel-like remineralization.

Given that high-fluoride dentifrices can effect, on average, 75% reduction in caries, it is important to understand how they function. With respect to lesions treated with the higher fluoride dentifrice (Clinpro™ 5000) the SAXS signal produced a dramatically intense and narrower lineshape (blue curve) relative to the less-intense signals from the incipient lesion (red curve) and the lesion treated with Clinpro™ Tooth Crème (green curve): these features indicate unique remineralization. Using microhardness measurements made on the same enamel cross-sections that were evaluated with X-ray diffraction and SEM, Clinpro™ 5000 produced significantly harder (i.e., stronger)

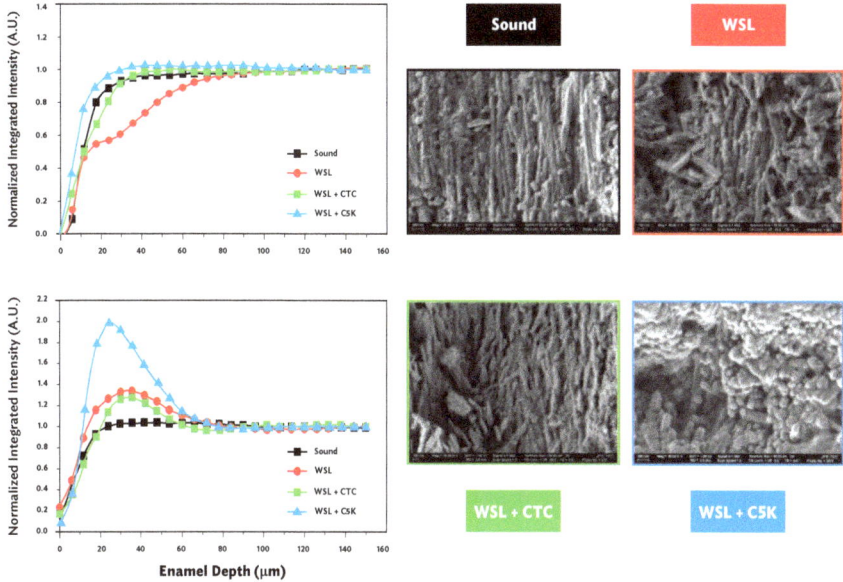

Figure 8.3. Microstructure examinations of enamel cross-sections using wide-angle X-ray diffraction (WAXD, top graph) and small-angle X-ray scattering (SAXS, bottom graph), and scanning electron microscopy (SEM) (from [114]). The X-ray diffraction data were collected from the outer surface of enamel down to 150 μm. The SEM images of enamel cross-sections (about 30 μm into the enamel substrates) were collected at 30,000x magnification (the white scale bars correspond to either 200 nm (for Sound and WSL + C5K) or 100 nm (for WSL and WSL + CTC). Four X-ray and SEM data sets are shown: Sound enamel (black line and symbol); white-spot lesion (WSL, red line and symbol) enamel; and WSL treated with either Clinpro™ Tooth Crème or Clinpro™ 5000 and cycled in a 10-day remineralization/demineralization pH cycling model with either Clinpro™ Tooth Crème (CTC, green line and symbol) or Clinpro™ 5000 (C5K, blue line and symbol). The demineralization was performed by immersion in a lactic acid-polymer solution partially saturated with hydroxyapatite (pH 5).

enamel relative to the incipient lesion, although it was comparable to that produced from Clinpro™ Tooth Crème and points to the inherent diffusive limitations in enamel from high-fluoride formats [114,700]. This is further observed as the center of the SAXS peak appears to be shifted to shallower depths by about 10 μm relative to that obtained from lesions treated with Clinpro™ Tooth Crème. Because the intense SAXS signal is very different relative to sound enamel, enamel lesions, and even lesions treated with Clinpro™ Tooth Crème, it likely arises from the formation of an abundance of high surface-area mineral. In viewing the micrograph, the enamel cross-section reveals the presence of globular minerals intermixed with crystallite laths, features that are not fully similar to the crystallite size, length, or orientations characteristic of sound enamel. These agglomerations bear the hallmarks of calcium fluoride (and calcium fluoride-like mineral), reflecting the categorization of fluoride minerals shown in **Figure 8.1**, and are consistent with expectations and results from high-fluoride formats [626,636,638–643,652–654].

In Chapter 9, calculations on the expected mineralized phases will show Clinpro™ 5000 encourages mostly calcium fluoride and fluorapatite (along with some hydroxyapatite). Consistent with those calculations, the morphology of the mineralization within the body of the incipient lesion demonstrates the ability of Clinpro™ 5000 to form calcium fluoride (and/or calcium fluoride-like minerals) reservoirs: as previously discussed, these reservoirs are thought to be important in sustaining fluoride exposure to the tooth [652–654]. Furthermore, in addition to the antimicrobial properties afforded by high-fluoride preparations [760–763], these mineralization data help explain the efficacy of this dentifrice. As shown in published laboratory and clinical studies, Clinpro™ 5000 is particularly effective in delivering fluoride to the teeth [746], producing strong, acid-resistant mineral at the enamel surface and subsurface [674,675,746,752,764], and reducing dentinal hypersensitivity [758,765,766] relative to conventional and high-fluoride preparations, including those with other nonfluoride therapeutic agents [674,675,746,764]. In particular, high-fluoride topical formats, while especially effective for those with impaired salivary function [761,767], generally do not penetrate deeply into the enamel lesion [674,675,746,768]. However, Clinpro™ 5000 overcomes this limitation by virtue of the functionalized tricalcium phosphate system to provide significantly better subsurface lesion penetration and strengthening relative to fluoride alone [671,674,675,746]. With respect to microbial control, twice daily use of Clinpro™ 5000 depressed levels of cariogenic bacteria (*Lactobacillus* and *S. mutans*) and reduced lactic acid production [769]. Finally, Clinpro™ 5000 improves salivary buffer capacity and promotes fluoride retention in plaque fluid [770], the latter of which is considered essential in the management of caries [771].

So how might these benefit an at-risk patient? Providing remineralization benefits at and below the tooth surface and promoting fluoride retention in the plaque and salivary fluids, both of these fluoridated dentifrices can be implemented in an oral hygiene plan for moderate-to-high risk patients, including those with:

✓ a history of caries;

✓ dental erosion;

✓ tooth wear;

✓ enamel hypoplasia;

✓ dry-mouth conditions;

✓ dentinal hypersensitivity;

✓ tender gingiva;

✓ exposed root surfaces; and,

✓ those fitted with orthodontia or other permanent and/or semipermanent intraoral devices.

For example, a patient manifesting several restorations and dry-mouth conditions resulting from daily medicines might brush her teeth with the high-fluoride dentifrice (Clinpro™ 5000) before bed, while the lower-fluoride option (Clinpro™ Tooth Crème) might be used in the morning and throughout the day. As such, these at-home fluoridated dentifrices promote remineralization, which is a key component to minimally invasive strategies [772], and is discussed in Chapter 10.

Action of fluoride in the oral environment: Dentition and microbes

Given the above exposition of various dental formats and the corresponding fluoride concentrations, it is important to explore the action of fluoride in the oral environment. As discussed in detail in this chapter, the fluoride concentrations vary widely depending on the topical format, but how much fluoride can accumulate in enamel? In general, regular exposure of fluoride in the oral environment leads to fluorine enrichment in the outer layers [699,700,773]. In fact, even in a low-fluoride environment, permanent dentition (erupted and unerupted) can accommodate five times as much fluoride in the outer enamel compared to the inner layers (i.e., near dentin) [773]. While fluorine may be present in low amounts throughout the enamel matrix during enamel formation, higher fluorine content accumulates into the outer enamel (up to ~ 0.1 mm) of unerupted and posterupted teeth, with permanent teeth generally having relatively higher fluorine content compared to primary dentition. In contrast to nonfluorosed enamel, mottled enamel typically has higher fluorine content throughout the enamel (not just in the outer layers) [699]. But regardless of the type or age of enamel (including primary, permanent, or mottled), there appears to be a ceiling of about 1% for fluorine accumulation [699].

Of course, establishing sustained levels of fluoride in the enamel, let alone the oral environment, influences the nature of the remineralization/demineralization balance [771]. Several ways to attain higher fluoride levels in the mouth include periodic applications of high-fluoride topicals (e.g., fluoride varnish and prescription-strength fluoride dentifrice) and/or continuous exposure to low-fluoride formats (e.g., water fluoridation and OTC fluoride toothpaste). But the reader may wonder: why are multiple treatments needed if the tooth can accommodate a limited amount of fluoride? The short answer is: clearance. Fluoride is cleared from the oral environment in several ways, including salivary flow, intake of food and drink (especially acidic foods and beverages), lack of proper daily oral hygiene, accumulation in the plaque and salivary fluids, and coordination/attachment to microbes.

For instance, within 30 minutes of a 4-minute acidulated phosphate fluoride gel (1.23% NaF) topical application, the cohort that rinsed with tap water over two 30-second periods exhibited significantly less enamel fluoride uptake (about 40% less) compared to the group that did not rinse [690]. Further, these two cohorts were tracked over the course of 3 weeks, and by day 3, the reductions in enamel fluoride uptake were 30% and 42% for the no-rinse and rinse groups, respectively [690]. These reductions continued so that by the end of three weeks, the reductions in enamel fluoride uptake were 48% and 57% for the no-rinse and rinse groups, respectively [690]. Thus, after the single gel treatment (which would be given, for instance, as an in-office preventive measure after a dental cleaning) and a return to daily oral hygiene (which presumably would involve exposure to fluoridated water and/or topical fluoride format such as an OTC toothpaste), about half of the deposited fluoride into enamel was lost. The leaching of fluoride may have been due to a number of factors including, quite simply, normal diet and salivary activity. In any case, this response echoes other studies [636,651], and demonstrates the dynamism of the oral environment and the transient relationship between fluoride and the dentition. It is for these reasons that continuous exposure to fluoride is recommended [34,652,653,771].

Most of this presentation on fluoride has emphasized its hard-tissue role but it's important to also address its role in the microbial environment, which includes the salivary and plaque fluids contacting the teeth. For instance, while accumulation of fluoride in enamel creates harder and less soluble mineral, fluoride also discourages microbial colonization and acidogenic processes as envisioned in **Figure 8.4**. The last two categories on the right (i.e., 'Strengthen Enamel' and 'Increase Enamel Acid-Resistance') correlate well with the fluoride level-caries reduction trends in **Figure 8.2**. In general, the greater the exposure of enamel to fluoride, the stronger and more acid-resistant the enamel becomes [626,630,647,648,737,746,771]. The remaining three categories, however, are related to the microbial aspects of fluoride and are also sensitive to the amount of fluoride present.

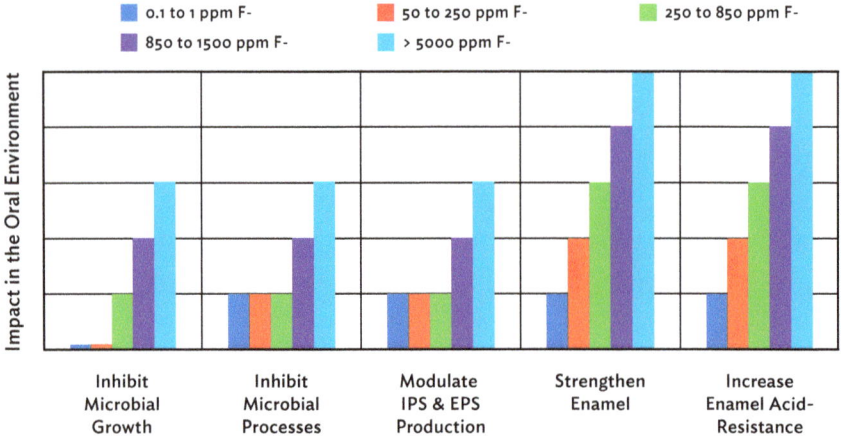

Figure 8.4. Impact of fluoride concentration on five selected categories in the oral environment (categorized from left to right): inhibition of microbial growth [50,762,763,775,776]; inhibition of microbial processes (e.g., fermentation of sugar) [50,760,762,763,775–780]; modulation of intracellular and extracellular polysaccharide (IPS and EPS, respectively) production [57,61,799]; strengthen enamel [630,648,737,746]; and, increase enamel acid-resistance [626,630,647,648].

As discussed in Chapters 2 and 7, the prospects of developing a caries vaccine are fraught with challenges, including the difficulty in identifying a particular process expressed by the microbe, such as adhesion or fermentation [83,518]. Most of the causative attention is directed to S.

mutans, but as discussed, this pathogen is not likely a dominant player in incipient enamel lesion formation; instead, it thrives in the organic-rich environment of dentin [38,39,43–45,47]. But if one were to focus on *S. mutans* (i.e., indicating active cavitations extending into dentin), the many dominant pathways manifested by *S. mutans* make vaccine development particularly elusive [518]. This would include cell division, cell synthesis, cell-signaling, transport, virulence factors, metabolic pathways for glucan production and/or carbohydrate synthesis, and adhesion [74]. But while the world waits for improvements in vaccine research, fortunately, there is an economic, abundant, and effective tool already at our disposable for managing microbial activity (including *S. mutans*): fluoride!

As mentioned earlier in this chapter, fluoride concentrations as low as 1 ppm are effective in reducing acid production from pathogenic species [50]. But does fluoride affect other properties, such as growth, lethality, and plaque formation? The answers are: yes, yes, and yes, but depend critically on fluoride source and concentration. For example, laboratory cell culture studies show stannous fluoride (SnF_2) and sodium fluoride (NaF) have different minimum concentrations for bacteriostatic or bactericidal action on *S. mutans* [774], while the minimum fluoride needed to inhibit growth was found to be about 250 ppm [50]. Following a dose-response relationship, fluoride can exert the following effects [50,762,763,775–778]:

✓ bactericidal;

✓ bacteriostatic (i.e., stunting microbial growth);

✓ depressed acid production;

✓ inhibition of glycolytic activity; or,

✓ inhibition of cation (e.g., K^+) and phosphate accumulation.

Additionally, microbial adenosine triphosphate (ATP) content appears to be sensitive to fluoride concentration [760,779], while the ability for microbes to maintain an acidic environment (i.e., by *S. mutans*) is also disrupted with fluoride [780]. Altogether, these effects provide the basis for the generalized fluoride sensitivity effect in the 'Inhibit Microbial Growth' and 'Inhibit Microbial Processes' categories of **Figure 8.4**.

Fluoride's ability to affect microbial activity becomes especially important, and heartening, for those prone to decay or deminer-alization (i.e., usually these populations have compromised saliva quality and/or quantity). For example, in a study on patients with carcinoma who received tumor-suppressing radiation that crippled their salivary glands and rendered them xerostomic, the use of a 1% NaF (5,000 ppm fluoride) gel over the course of 36 months resulted in significant reduction in caries incidence relative to those using a nonfluoride gel; importantly, these reductions were achieved without dietary restrictions [761].

At this stage it's important to address the possibility of microbes developing resistance to fluoride. This has long been a concern, and studies have been performed to figure out if and how microbes adapt to fluoride exposure. In one study involving children living in a community with water fluoridation, isolated cultured microbes obtained from plaque sampling struggled to grow even after subjected to a fluoride-free environment for 16 hours. Importantly, fluoride did not shift the ecology of the oral envi-ronment to favor cariogenic species and may have stimulated commensal species instead [781]. Separately, a laboratory study monitored the impact of fluoride on *S. mutans*: while its population growth was reduced, became stabilized, but was not eliminated, the glycolytic activity was dramatically reduced at the onset, and ceased to occur when consistently exposed to fluoride. Thus, any apparent tolerance to fluoride by *S. mutans* was muted by the lack of metabolic action [44,776]. And while fluoride-resistant strains may need higher fluoride levels to inhibit growth [762], viability does not appear to be affected [762], while glycolytic activity remains suppressed in the presence of fluoride [782]. The ability of oral microbes, especially *S. mutans*, to survive (albeit in a vegetative state) in the presence of fluoride is due to its abundance of ABC-type transporters [74], and has recently been traced to a bevy of fluoride-sensitive riboswitches that, when triggered, readily expel the ion [783,784]. However, fluoride does not seem to affect *S. mutans* plaque adherence [785], so physical removal remains important (i.e., brush your teeth!).

An interesting aspect influencing fluoride's impact on oral microbes is the role of divalent cations (e.g., Mg^{2+} and Ca^{2+}). Investigations show bidentate coordination of these cations with *S. mutans*, whereby calcium displays a stronger affinity relative to magnesium [786]; but in the presence of fluoride, one of these bidentate ligands becomes altered to accommodate fluoride, thus suggesting monodentate binding with the microbe, whereby the effect is again greater with calcium relative to magnesium [763,786]. Because the cellular walls and plaque matrix are rich in anions, particularly in carboxylate and phosphate groups, coordination with either calcium or magnesium ions can be expected. And when coupled with fluoride, it seems the dual coordination of the cation (e.g., Ca^{2+}) to both the microbial anions (e.g., carboxylate or phosphate groups) and fluoride would help produce cariostatic behavior, possibly through the establishment of fluoride reservoirs and the 'starving' of the microbe of important cations [786,787].

But while Mg^{2+} may be linked to glycolytic activity, the role of Ca^{2+} appears less clear. Indeed, Ca^{2+} has been shown to be linked to cellular membrane integrity and metabolic activity [787–789], but this certainly does not appear ubiquitous for prokaryotic systems [790]. For example, with respect to *S. mutans*, apparently low amounts of Ca^{2+} are required for viability; at higher Ca^{2+} concentrations, the culture count becomes depressed [790]. For low amounts of Mg^{2+} or Ca^{2+} in the presence of fluoride, when the fluoride concentration is increased from moderate to high, *S. mutans* viability actually improves, with Ca^{2+} bolstering colony counts better than Mg^{2+} [763]. Perhaps accounting for this range in behavior is the ability of *S. mutans* to shape-shift its cellular structure in response to external triggers (e.g., from neutral to acidic pH) [514]. After all, this microbe exhibited shape-changing properties unique enough to warrant its Latin naming by Clarke '*mutans*' [74,514].

Here's another consideration with respect to high or low calcium loading that can ultimately bear on the design of topical systems comprising fluoride and calcium (e.g., remineralization dentifrices, such as Clinpro™ Tooth Crème which has a low calcium loading, or GC America's Tooth Mousse (or MI Paste), which has high calcium loading): when large amounts of 'free' calcium are present, these cations may bind to the cellular walls preventing morphological flexibility and functionality that might otherwise lead to growth and other activity. But, in the low-calcium limit, there exists biochemical opportunity for membrane-dependent activity (e.g., division of cells, movement, flexibility, etc). So in a fluoride-free environment (which includes environments that have effectively low levels of fluoride due to undesirable calcium-fluoride interactions), high calcium loading might be a promising strategy from a microbial population control perspective, but this is insufficient in addressing other mechanisms of microbial control (e.g., glycolysis), and does not seem to promote improved clinical control of tooth decay relative to fluoride [791,792].

So long as fluoride is present and available, it can remain an effective anticaries agent. This condition is critical, and was the reason many early fluoride dentifrices failed to show a clinical caries reduction (i.e., the calcium abrasives were not stabilized sufficiently to prevent premature calcium-fluoride interactions prior to immediate use) [628], and why ultimately, a stabilized fluoridated toothpaste proved to be clinically effective [633]. This also contributes to the reason there now exists an anticaries drug monograph for fluoridated systems marketed in the US [149,734].

So with respect to high calcium loading, although microbial population growth might be limited, an abundance of Ca^{2+} risks neutralizing fluoride's availability and action in the oral environment. Additionally, high calcium loading may stimulate tartar and/or non-enamel-like mineral formation, as well as possible soft-tissue irritations that result from these mineral formations. Even further, calcium may actually trigger plaque formation from cariogenic bacteria [791]. To that end, fluoride preparations mirroring the calcium content of saliva (i.e., low saturation levels) may improve the quality of the remineralization while maintaining microbial efficacy. This concept is evaluated in Chapter 9 through solubility calculations, and pertains to the design of the functionalized tricalcium phosphate system described earlier in this chapter.

The last category of **Figure 8.4** to be discussed, 'Modulate IPS & EPS Production', is an extension of the 'Microbial Processes' and emphasizes the impact of fluoride on the intra- and extracellular polysaccharides (IPS and EPS, respectively) synthesized by cariogenic bacteria. In general, polysaccharides are critical to the survival of microbial colonies [56,794,795]: IPS serve as energy stores when pabulum is low or nonexistent, while the EPS is core to bacterial attachment, growth, recruitment (e.g., quorum-sensing), sustenance (again, when external sources are insufficient or absent), protection against host defenses, and enhanced resistance to antimicrobials [796,797]. As an example of plaque robustness, undisturbed dental plaque (over a 24-hour period) limited the penetration—and therefore the bactericidal activity—of chlorhexidine to the outer plaque material (~ 2 μm), leaving the bulk of the microbes, including those nearest to the tooth structure, untouched [53].

IPS and EPS are produced from carbohydrates, especially sucrose, a polysaccharide comprising one glucose ring and one fructose ring. Representing major constituents in dental plaque, dextrans and levans are generated from glucose and fructose, respectively, and are readily synthesized by cariogenic bacteria, including *Lactobacillus* and *Streptococcus* species [55,56,58,794,798]. Between the two types of polysaccharides, levans are readily hydrolyzed in an acidic environment as well as by saliva, thus rendering them particularly suitable for IPS storage [58,798]. In contrast, dextrans are poorly hydrolyzed by acids and saliva, and are resistant to attack from mixed microbial cultures [58,798]. So between the two polysaccharides, dextrans (or dextran-like polysaccharides) buttress the resilient cariogenic biofilms responsible for dental caries [58,794,798].

So if saliva, commensal bacteria, and antimicrobials exhibit limited action on counteracting dextrans (e.g., formation, adhesion, or solubility), and brushing and/or flossing may not reach all crevices or pores in the mouth that harbor biofilm formation (e.g., especially if one is fitted with orthodontic braces), what else might exert influence on IPS or EPS? Again, the answer is fluoride. Fluoride not only encumbers IPS accumulation [61] but also modulates EPS formation, whether it increases the fraction of soluble dextrans (or, dextran-like polysaccharides) [57] or alters EPS composition (at 70 ppm fluoride) to favor fructose catabolism (i.e., synthesis of levans or levan-like polysaccharides) [799]. This behavior is notable, since such behavior is dissimilar to cations, including magnesium, manganese, or calcium, all of which appear to stimulate dextran production [793]. Thus, another mode of action by fluoride is the inhibition, reduction, or compositional shift of polysaccharide synthesis by cariogenic bacteria, with the estimated impact in the oral environment as suggested in **Figure 8.4**.

While **Figure 8.4** emphasizes the effect of fluoride dose, one can also infer from these data that high frequency applications of low-fluoride concentrations can also exert an antidecay benefit [771].

In addition to the multiple modes previously listed, fluoride also bears on one more: rate of remineralization. Ordinarily, remineralization is driven by salivary constituents (i.e., calcium and phosphate) [90], but addition of fluoride to calcium phosphate solutions produces an extraordinary result: acceleration of remineralization [86,771,800–802]. For instance, under physiological conditions (including neutral pH), octacalcium phosphate (OCP) is likely to form as an intermediate phase in the progression to apatite [805]. But, the inclusion of low amounts of fluoride (e.g., 0.1 ppm fluoride) into supersaturated calcium phosphate solutions bypasses this transient phase in the nucleation of apatite-like seeds (i.e., homonucleation) [800,806], as well as in mineral growth onto preformed apatite seeds or enamel substrates (i.e., heteronucleation) [807]. While fluoride shortens the transition time to apatite formation, it also affects crystal seed and growth morphology from supersaturated calcium phosphate solutions [806]. These studies reveal mineralization processes are sensitive to fluoride, and the next chapter will take a closer look at some notable remineralization systems that strive to enhance remineralization through combinations of fluoride, calcium, and phosphate.

Summary

In this chapter, we have covered several mechanisms by which fluoride exerts its impact. In short, the benefits of regular (and safe) exposures of sustained fluoride are manifold:

1. Reduce enamel solubility

2. Modulate microbial action

3. Enhance remineralization

Thus, fluoride effects physical, chemical, and biological change that impacts tooth structure and the microbial environment, demonstrating there is no single mode of action [808]. In turn, the multipronged action of fluoride can provide excellent anticaries benefits at various stages of one's life and health, such as:

1. prior to eruption of primary dentition (i.e., less than 2 years of age);

2. prior to eruption of secondary dentition (i.e., up through ~ 21 years of age);

3. after invasive restorative, orthodontic, prosthodontic, and cosmetic procedures;

4. when saliva flow is minimal due to medical and/or health reasons; or

5. according to dynamics of hygiene, diet, behavior, and/or lifestyle.

But despite the multimodal effects of fluoride, it is appealing to identify a foremost mechanism because it simplifies understanding and communication from both patient and clinician perspectives. Ideally, clinicians would customize a patient's needs based on his or her dietary habits, predisposition to dental decay, access to and quality of dental care, and understanding of specific risk factors. Perhaps the multiaction benefits of fluoride are too expansive to aptly grasp, especially as research continues to evolve the role of fluoride, at least among academicians; in turn, it is human nature to settle into a 'favorite' mindset or school of thought (e.g., a sports team; managing one's financial outlook; daily routines or schedules; a job or career; where to live; what type of car to drive; food choice; education preference; and so on), where a given role might satisfy a clinician's understanding of fluoride, and may certainly be age- or education-related.

For example, while varnishes probably deliver safer levels of fluoride compared to gels, gels are the status quo in certain communities [809,810]. And there exists confusion among dental practitioners and researchers on the dominant mechanism of fluoride [809,810]. On one hand such questions might be construed inappropriate or misleading, since the action of fluoride can certainly depend on the status of one's life situation. For example, as discussed in Chapter 2, the oral flora appears unique for those experiencing dental decay. Thus, perhaps achieving low-level fluoride is challenging and/or insufficient in managing an at-risk patient with elevated risk factors. Although it is common that patients visit practitioners when health problems arise (e.g., [811]), the clinician needs to be more than a mechanic (i.e., detect and repair problems) and engage in positive approaches and caries prevention guidelines [692,809,812]. Likewise, the patient needs to become more involved and knowledgeable about his/her oral care. In either case, the clinician and the patient have a responsibility to be proactive, where open and honest discussions on general well-being, habits and behaviors, notable life events, and health goals can lead to better oral health [139]. As proactivity necessarily involves prevention, fluoride, the most well-researched and clinically proven agent, will naturally be a cornerstone of an effective oral hygiene plan [34,692–696]. These aspects will be covered in additional detail in Chapter 10 but it is important to recognize fluoride's place in the vanguard of decay prevention.

In closing, I covered some key aspects of fluoride, including its anticaries history, the multipronged mechanistic underpinnings, and features of some popular topical fluoride formats. But the benefits of fluoride would be limited in the absence of our natural remineralizing system: saliva. Efforts to bridge the efficacy of fluoride with the remineralizing force of saliva has, therefore, led to newer innovations that seek to combine these two to provide better oral health benefits. This important and ever-evolving field is the subject of the next chapter.

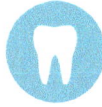

CHAPTER NINE

Remineralization

THE ABILITY OF SALIVA TO NATURALLY REHARDEN ENAMEL was presented in 1910 by Head and was based on probing enamel specimens with a lancet [209]. Head continued this line of research and presented in 1912 hardness measurements he made on softened enamel through the use of a mechanical device he constructed [87]. These measurements moved him to believe that enamel is not 'dead' (as was conventionally thought, since there was no conduit extending fluids from the body or blood to enamel) but, in fact, undergoes physical changes, even if the structure was weakened by acidic insults. As the nature of these physical changes necessarily involves various calcium phosphate (and/ or fluoride) phases, this chapter explores some of the principal calcium compounds that precipitate and/or integrate into tooth structure from supersaturated environments.

Indeed, there are many therapeutic formulations commercially available or in development but it is not the scope here to review all of these. Instead, identifying one or two key high-level differentiators will help improve the reader's understanding to enable him/her to make a more informed decision as to why a given formulation might or might not be used. Such distinctions can be accomplished through comparisons among several calcium phosphate systems on the basis of supersaturation and formation of possible mineral phases. In doing so, estimations of possible mineral phases from some commercially available formats can also be determined, and I have done just that based on published data for some toothpastes and varnishes.

And with support from independent scientific research published more than 40 years ago, I am not the first to show that the 'more is better' thesis need not apply to calcium in the remineralization of the teeth. In fact, the opposite can be very effective, where 'less is more' provides efficient remineralization from low supersaturation calcium phosphate systems.

This chapter is personal for me, where my passion to develop an improved remineralization system was born out of an exasperation of a long, personal history of dental decay that I attributed, in part, to a lack of effective preventive strategies. In fact, I was moved to apply my formal PhD-level training in the chemistry and physics of condensed materials (including ice) to researching prospective remineralizing agents for use in preventive dentistry. In the course of this research, it made sense to also understand the mineralizing characteristics of saliva, including the nature of minerals saliva can produce. As such, I believe this is a good place to start the discussion.

Calcium phosphates and the formation of hydroxyapatite

Consideration of the calcium phosphate content of the supersaturated biological fluids, saliva and plasma, leads to an interesting distinction: though bone and teeth comprise calcium phosphate mineral, the fluids supporting these structures (i.e., plasma and saliva, respectively) manifest different ratios of calcium to phosphate (Ca/P): approximately 0.3 and 2.2 for saliva and blood, respectively [91,159,813–818]. And in contrast to these Ca/P ratios, the major inorganic constituent of enamel and bone, which appears to be variations of carbonate hydroxyapatite, bears a Ca/P ratio of about 1.67 [21,819–823].

Before pressing forward too far, just a quick note about hydroxy-apatite (HAP): it is understood that the mineral in bone and teeth is not solely hydroxyapatite but rather a blend of various apatites (including calcium-deficient, carbonate, and substituted HAP) [823]. However, HAP still remains abundant in teeth and bone and so for sake of experimental simplicity and understanding, HAP is widely used as the *de facto* analogue. The following discussion then assumes HAP is the principal mineral in bone and teeth.

It is understood that the mineral in bone and teeth is not solely hydroxyapatite but rather a blend of various apatites.

So how might different Ca/P ratios affect mineralization? That HAP forms (with a Ca/P ratio of ~ 1.67) in the teeth and bone regardless of the supersaturation level (i.e., whether Ca/P is 0.3 or 2.2), demonstrates that the thermodynamics of both saliva and blood support formation of, or maintenance of, apatite-like mineral. In contrast, the kinetics of HAP formation is influenced by several factors, including the Ca/P ratio, and this ultimately affects the quantity and quality of apatite formation [824].

For instance, it has been reported that HAP formation is not observed from low supersaturation mediums in the absence of a seed or substrate [825]. Instead, other calcium phosphate phases nucleate first, and transition to HAP according to the stability of the phase (from least to most stable) [826], including dicalcium phosphate dihydrate (DCPD) and octacalcium phosphate (OCP) [660,804,825]; or, directly from amorphous calcium phosphate [200,827,828]. Since such succession necessarily requires time, the ripening to HAP is not fast and can last many hours, days, or even weeks [200,829]. The formation kinetics are sensitive to various factors, such as temperature, pH, additives (e.g., fluoride, collagen, chondroitin), seeds (or substrates, such as enamel or HAP discs), degree of supersaturation (i.e., constituent concentration such as Ca^{2+} and $PO_4{}^{3-}$), and Ca/P ratio of the supersaturated solution, so HAP formation can be accelerated [86,800,805,824,825,830–832]; in contrast, crystallization inhibitors (e.g., Zn^{2+}, Mg^{2+}, pyrophosphate— which may be too abrasive to gingiva and exposed root surfaces—and statherin) frustrate HAP formation [833–836].

As realized by surface rehardening measurements or precipitation reaction studies, other examples of accelerating mineralization include the elevation of the Ca/P ratio from 1 to 1.67 [86], or increased concentration of calcium and phosphate in the supersaturated solutions [825,837]. Agitation also promotes mineral formation from supersaturated solutions [826,838], and this might be realized, for instance, through stimulation of saliva (e.g., via mastication), swilling, mouthrinsing, and even toothbrushing.

Instead of adjusting the degree of supersaturation or Ca/P ratio, another approach involves seeds or substrates (usually crystalline) immersed in the supersaturated solution [826, 830,831,838–840], a scenario which mimics the teeth and saliva in the oral environment. Here, HAP crystals or enamel slabs or powder are used as the substrate and immersed in a calcium phosphate solution supersaturated with respect to HAP [830,831,839]. HAP readily deposits onto the substrate or newly formed crystallites [824] and, with proper experimental parameters, may do so without the generation of transient phases [831,840].

In reviewing these studies, the majority of HAP-formation research as it relates to dental enamel has emphasized Ca/P ratios having, at minimum, equal calcium and phosphate concentrations (i.e., Ca/P = 1), but mostly favoring Ca/P of about 1.67 (i.e., the molar ratio of calcium-to-phosphorous for HAP) [86,200,800,822,824,825,827,830–832,837]. However, notable exceptions include the transformation from ACP to HAP, where the Ca/P ratio was 0.7 [828], along with remineralization of etched enamel by calcifying solutions having a similar Ca/P ratio [841].

And, the bulk of HAP-formation research as it relates to dental enamel has also utilized highly supersaturated calcium phosphate solutions (e.g., [86,200,800,824,825,827,830–832,837,840,842]). However, exceptions to this include the low-supersaturation, HAP-seeded experiments [831,829], where calcium concentrations were 0.4 mM or 0.3 mM and the corresponding Ca/P ratios were 1.5 and 1.67, respectively. Incidentally, the formation of HAP in these independent studies (which were fluoride-free) took about the same time to form (~ 24 hours) relative to high supersaturated solutions, and underlines the influence that a seed or substrate [838] and water [200] have on mineralization phenomena. Even further, the nature of the transient phase is fundamentally distinct: instead of progressing through calcium phosphate phases such as DCPD, OCP, or even tricalcium phosphate (TCP), low supersaturated solutions may produce a calcium-rich phase (Ca/P ~ 1.9) that cures to HAP (i.e., Ca/P ~ 1.7) within a day at 25°C [831] (and, at biological temperatures near 37⁰C, this would occur much more quickly). Here we note that while tetracalcium phosphate (TTCP, Ca/P ~ 2) might be formed, it is not familiar in biological systems, and it is unstable in aqueous environments where it rapidly dissolves to precipitate HAP [843]. Still, with respect to the low supersaturated phase, perhaps a transient TTCP-like mineral phase might be initially created given the Ca/P ratio, a situation that may be especially poignant at pH less than 3.9, where calcium-deficient HAP is likely to exist (as opposed to DCPD) [843].

Accelerating remineralization

So adjusting Ca/P ratios and increasing the degree of supersaturation can accelerate HAP mineralization rate—but why might this be important?

Saliva, the natural biological remineralizing fluid, is phosphate-rich (having at least 3 mM) and modestly supersaturated with respect to calcium (Ca^{2+} ~ 1 mM) [91,564,844]. While saliva naturally remineralizes softened enamel [87,89,90,106,209,841], the effects can be limited [388,841,845]. Such limitations, however, can be overcome in the presence of fluoride (e.g., [160,633,635]), and reflects the initial observations that low-level fluoride (e.g., 1 ppm fluoride, or ~ 0.05 mM) leads to accelerated remineralization [86,800].

Therefore, in order to counter short hygienic events, poor salivary flow or quality, salivary clearance, diffusion into plaque biofilms, or simply to meet the demands created by demineralized teeth, the ability to quickly form HAP (or apatite-like mineral) is attractive in the defense against dental caries, and has driven most of the research into prospective topical treatments (e.g., [842]). This stems in part from the accelerated mineralizing benefits observed when fluoride supplements supersaturated calcium phosphate solutions [86,800].

In turn, academic and commercial strategies have sought to accelerate the formation of HAP (and, other minerals) by way of either increasing the degree of supersaturation (utilizing Ca/P ratios approaching 1.67) or including additives (e.g., F^-, Sr^{2+}, Zn^{2+}) with the aim of rapidly remineralizing (i.e., resupplying with calcium and phosphate, and fluoride, if present) weakened enamel.

How to remineralize the demineralized tooth

The properties of the demineralized tooth structure influences remineralization.

For instance, enamel lesions and eroded (or etched) enamel respond differently to remineralization, with the former limited by diffusive processes while the latter is sensitive to interface reactions [846]. This means that remineralization of enamel lesions (which then necessarily involves penetration into the enamel subsurface) will be slower, while the surface of etched enamel will respond more quickly to deposition processes.

From a clinical perspective, the benefits of multiple fluoride treatments administered over a short timescale lead to a point of diminishing returns at or near the enamel surface. For instance, thrice daily brushing with 1,100 ppm fluoride plus weekly 12,500 ppm fluoride acidulated phosphate fluoride (APF) gel treatments produced limited remineralization of caries-like lesions beginning as early as the first APF treatment [847]. Separately, in a 20-day laboratory model emulating incipient lesions observed clinically, the surface remineralization achieved from an enhanced 5,000 ppm fluoride dentifrice saturated after 10 days [746]. And another clinical study demonstrated that while remineralization of caries-like lesions is rapid after a single pH-neutral 1,000 ppm fluoride (NaF) treatment (i.e., after a month the remineralization rate increased from 16% to 26%), a second fluoride treatment produced limited to no effects compared to the control (i.e., no second fluoride treatment given) [848].

Therefore, while the surface of enamel lesions may respond quickly to remineralization, diffusion into the lesion subsurface will be the rate-limiting step and will, therefore, limit the rate of remineralization *in vivo* [771]. So strategies aimed at accelerating the clinically slow remineralization of lesions have led to the design of topical 'remineralization' systems, whereby pH, fluoride concentration, and/or calcium phosphate supersaturation are adjusted:

✓ low pH systems (e.g., APF, stannous fluoride gels or dentifrices);

✓ high fluoride concentration formats (e.g., 5% NaF varnish or 1.1% NaF dentifrices or gels); or,

✓ those with high calcium phosphate loading or supersaturation (e.g., bioglass (e.g., Novamin®), casein phosphopeptide-amorphous calcium phosphate (CPP-ACP), and amorphous calcium phosphate (ACP).

With respect to eroded enamel, the nature of the surface is again prone to rapid remineralization or deposition: for instance, eroded enamel responds very well to higher amounts of fluoride and/or frequency of applications [160,161,849,850]. The reactivity of the tooth surface is likely linked to the increase in porosity and surface areas created by erosive processes [851]. But due to the challenges of remineralizing eroded enamel [138], it is important that the etched surface is not bombarded with an abundance of precipitates or deposits that cannot integrate effectively with enamel [113,852].

Thus, creation of fluoride reservoirs (e.g., calcium fluoride or calcium fluoride-like deposits) and/or apatite-like mineral is preferable to the production of random, uncontrolled heterogeneity of precipitated or deposited minerals [824], which may otherwise potentially increase the risks for tartar-like formation, counter the efficacy of fluoride (through undesirable binding), or create an abundance of non-enamel-like mineral (a noninsignificant fraction of which might be cleared from the oral environment by saliva and, therefore, swallowed).

Systems for remineralization: Introduction

Armed with the knowledge that rapid remineralization of weakened teeth can be achieved through the addition of fluoride, high amounts of calcium and phosphate, and/or calcium-rich Ca/P ratios, it is possible to gain insight into putative minerals formed based on composition of the remineralizing system.

> **NOTE:**
>
> The following discussion takes a hard look at several commercially available calcium phosphate systems. As a researcher immersed in this space, I take a close look at the functionalized tricalcium phosphate system (i.e., the system I developed, also referred to as 'TCP' or 'fTCP'), which is a relatively low supersaturation system, along with a couple other calcium phosphate technologies that are relatively high supersaturation systems and have been around for at least 10 years in some variation (i.e., 'CPP-ACP' and 'ACP'); for others (e.g., Novamin® bioglass or calcium carbonate-arginine combination), I only comment where necessary for the sake of brevity. But this exposition is meant to help clarify differences among supersaturated systems based on science instead of artful (and often misleading) marketing or personal bias (which we all have, whether we admit it or not). The reader is encouraged to pry deeper into the references used in this section for further information as needed.

First, I have presented numerous examples in this chapter and the previous one explaining how and why fluoride should be foundational in the design of effective anticaries remineralizing systems [578]. Now, let's consider the use of nonfluoride agents, of which there are many [742]. First, in comparison with fluoride, none appear to provide superior benefits relative to fluoride over the long term, and this is magnified when several factors are considered.

For instance, a relatively newer approach is a dentifrice that comprises an insoluble calcium compound (such as calcium carbonate) plus arginine (which may elevate mouth pH [70,71]) plus fluoride (the source of which is sodium monofluorophosphate, NaMPF). This system relies on high supersaturation (i.e., high loading) of insoluble calcium carbonate, along with an amino acid (i.e., arginine) that may help elevate mouth pH (or at least help calcium carbonate adhere to the dentition). While this system may sound promising, especially for hypersensitivity relief [853], here are some key drawbacks with respect to remineralization:

✓ The approach of elevating mouth pH is not new (i.e., see Chapter 7) and has been suggested previously (e.g., hydrolysis of arginine by oral *Streptococcus* species have been studied since the 1920s [532,533]), but, as reported by Davies and King, for example, such systems fail to reduce caries increments [82]. Perhaps these past studies bear on recent ones, where clinical plaque diversity couldn't be achieved. And perhaps of some concern, the virulence of lactate-producing microbes increased after cessation of use [72].

✓ The insolubility of the calcium compound may be great for plugging openings or gaps (and may bode well as a dental hypersensitivity treatment, at least in the short-term [853]), but does not participate in remineralization processes, and therefore may not be effective in addressing erosive [854] or caries lesions [540] relative to existing fluoride therapies. Perhaps this contributes to its limited benefits for low- to moderate-risk populations [538], who may already harbor less-cariogenic bacteria [40].

✓ Due to potential bioavailability issues with the insoluble calcium compounds, the use of NaMFP is chosen; however, in dentifrice use, it has been reasoned that NaF is superior to NaMPF [855].

✓ Importantly, at a cost about 40% higher compared to standard dentifrices, the modest benefits achieved in low- to moderate-risk populations (in studies which were sponsored by the company with vested interests in the technology, Colgate-Palmolive) may not be economically or demographically motivating [540].

Similarly, another agent, Novamin®, is also proposed for remineralization [856]. However, instead of remineralization [857] and like the calcium carbonate-arginine combination above, this technology might be better suited to the relief of dental hypersensitivity [859,860], at least short-term [861]. This system relies on high supersaturation (i.e., high loading) of highly soluble forms of calcium and phosphate glass-like material. One reason this technology may be limiting is that it encourages deposition of glass-like particles whose morphology and composition are not apatitic [861]. Another is that it does not maintain sufficient stability when combined with fluoride in an aqueous environment [862]. Finally, fluoridated formulations using Novamin® have to utilize what some consider to be the less-preferable NaMFP (e.g., [855]) as a means of avoiding undesirable calcium-fluoride interactions (e.g., [863]) due to the highly soluble calcium species in the system. As fluoridated dentifrice guidelines are regulated in the US, it is noteworthy that the Sensodyne® Repair & Protect dentifrice replaces the Novamin® ingredient with stannous fluoride (e.g., [864]), despite recognition of the Novamin® ingredient for hypersensitivity benefits [865]. Altogether, these characteristics underline limitations in the remineralizing potential of Novamin® [857].

For purposes of clarity, I define dental remineralization as the ability to deliver mineralizing components to the tooth that leads to acid-resistant, apatite-like, or calcium fluoride-like mineralization at the tooth surface and within the subsurface [650]; notably, this view echoes independent views on remineralization [771].

As such, nonapatitic mineral phases deposited or formed *in situ* on the tooth surface may frustrate surface demineralization but may not necessarily promote subsurface remineralization. Though possibly serving as a sacrificial layer for the evolution of calcium and phosphate ions for reprecipitation purposes [667,866], instead, these ions may become cleared from the oral environment (i.e., due to saliva or dietary events) [91], may be utilized in ongoing mineral growth processes driven by saliva (i.e., which has implications for tartar formation) [104,654], or may bind with fluoride or plaque constituents, which, in turn, may limit the effect of fluoride on microbial growth and/or processes [763,786].

Predicting mineral phases from the concentration of mineralizing ions (e.g., calcium, phosphate, and fluoride) is one way to evaluate a given supersaturated system [867,868]. Solubility product calculations can, therefore, be used to probe the mechanisms contributing (or not) to remineralization from topically applied calcium phosphate (CaP) systems [125,817,844,869].

To compare three popular CaP systems noted above (i.e., TCP, ACP, and CPP-ACP), I have calculated the solubility products in both dentifrice and varnish formats. For reference purposes, I have also calculated the minerals that may form from saliva, as well as some fluoride-only systems. Instead of relying on performance/evaluation models (some of which may be especially sensitive to a given CaP system), this approach facilitates answers to the fundamental questions such as "how does this CaP system work?" or "what are the differences among these CaP systems?."

To get started, first we must consider the most likely minerals that may be produced from supersaturated remineralizing systems. As shown in **Table 9.1**, eight mineral phases are listed, along with the shorthand notation, chemical formula, and Ca/P ratio for each. This list is not inclusive, as several notable phases are missing, including amorphous calcium phosphate (ACP, which may appear as a transient and/or initial phase in the ripening to HAP) [827,828], tetracalcium phosphate (TTCP, a possible unlikely phase in biological systems) [843], and alpha-tricalcium phosphate (α-TCP, a high-temperature form of beta-tricalcium phosphate) [805]. However, as each of those minerals is a transient phase and not as stable under physiological conditions (much like DCPD [645], DCPA [645] or OCP [804]) for the sake of simplicity and probability (i.e., following Ostwald ripening), they are omitted as final solubility products. To that end, the relative ease of solubility of these calcium phosphate minerals at pH 7 can be expressed as follows [805]:

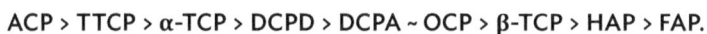

ACP > TTCP > α-TCP > DCPD > DCPA ~ OCP > β-TCP > HAP > FAP.

Because our comparative assessments will involve versions of ACP and beta-tricalcium phosphate (β-TCP) these warrant some commentary.

Systems for remineralization: ACP

This mineral phase is present in biological systems and also derives from prepared supersaturated calcium phosphate solutions. Contrary to synthetic ACP and thermodynamics observed in the laboratory, biological ACP is very stable, makes up an appreciable fraction of bone mineral (e.g., ~ 40% in human, bovine, and murine femur), and slowly converts to apatite-like mineral over the course of the subject's lifetime (e.g., the murine femur content of ACP decreased from 69% to 36% from an age of five days to over the course of 70 years) [819]. ACP does not have a rigidly defined chemical composition, but tends to have Ca/P ratios between 1.44 and 1.55, which, therefore, bears on tricalcium phosphates (i.e., Ca/P ~ 1.5) [819], and has been described as a Posner cluster, with formula $Ca_9(PO_4)_6$ [828]. Furthermore, due to the comparable Ca/P ratios, studies suggested synthetic ACP is likely nano-crystalline (or, at least noncrystalline) tricalcium phosphate (which would necessarily include phases corresponding to β-TCP) [819].

Due to its instability, synthetic ACP converts to apatite in aqueous environment. However, this conversion appears to be autocatalytic, depending critically on water [827], with the rate dependent on the quantity of apatitic crystals formed (or present) and not on the supersaturated nature of the solution [819]. As discussed earlier in this chapter, the rate of conversion to apatite is heavily influenced by additives [667,819], including fluoride, which seems to bypass the middleman OCP phase [807]. In fact, in the absence of water, the conversion will slow dramatically [819,827] and thus has major implications for those with low salivary flow, where those with dry-mouth conditions (e.g., including those with xerostomia, along with other factors such as sleep, medications, and overall health) may not realize the endpoint ripening benefits of apatite formation. Another low-hydration environment may also include certain regions in the enamel subsurface (barring large demineralized zones) or undisturbed plaque traps. Therefore, because the oral environment exhibits greater biological, chemical and physical properties compared to 'clean' laboratory evaluations of mineral formation and growth, it can, therefore, be expected that not all of the calcium phosphate delivered from the topical preparation will progress CaP phase ripening to apatite-like mineral.

Two dominant types of amorphous calcium phosphate utilized in topical dental preparations CPP-ACP (i.e., 'stabilized' ACP, also known as Recaldent™ and is found in GC America preparations such as Tooth Mousse, Tooth Mousse Plus, MI Paste, MI Paste Plus, and MI Varnish) and ACP (i.e., 'unstabilized' ACP, sometimes referred to as Enamelon™ or Liquid Calcium™ and is presently found in some Premier and Arm & Hammer dental preparations). The former is comprised of casein peptides that bind to amorphous calcium phosphate and prevent the ripening to apatite, while rapid precipitation is encouraged in the 'unstabilized' ACP [870]. Both the former and latter both rely on high calcium phosphate supersaturation in constructing the synthetic ACP phase, which can form in the matter of minutes [667,871]. As an example, the amount of calcium in ACP [663–666] or CPP-ACP [869] dental preparations can be at least 75x higher relative to normal saliva [91,844] (e.g., about 75 mM compared to 1 mM, respectively). Under physiological conditions (i.e., 37°C, pH 7.4) and in the absence of fluoride, the test-tube conversion period can take 90 minutes to reach the OCP phase, and then days until ripening to apatite is complete [827,871]. In the presence of fluoride, the reaction rate is increased (e.g., 3x faster in some laboratory experiments [802]) and transient phases may be bypassed [807]. But once ACP forms, the conversion to apatite will be influenced by the myriad constituents (some of which will inhibit mineralization) and/or level of hydration in the mouth.

Systems for remineralization: β-TCP, functionalized tricalcium phosphate, and calcium fluoride

This CaP mineral phase has limited solubility, is very stable under ambient conditions, but can readily transition to HAP [805,872,873]. β-TCP manifests unique properties (e.g., **Figure 9.1**), including the lack of phosphate moieties along with underbonded calcium oxide environments (i.e., CaO_3) [874], features which render this material the basis for the functionalized tricalcium phosphate systems [650,670–672]. The use of β-TCP, however, is not new [875]: recipes and applications for 'phosphate of lime' were outlined in the 1810 issue of Encyclopaedia

Brittanica (e.g., including for the remedy of rickets and soft bones) [876], advertisements for the relief of dentinal hypersensitivity appeared in 1873 (**Figure 9.2**), and it was also used as a biomaterial (referred to as 'triple calcium phosphate') in pioneering studies on the use of bioactive implants in bone repair [829]. In the US, β-TCP is recognized as a Class II medical device for bone remodeling [877], and there are a number of commercial versions used for such (e.g., Periophil; PremierTCP™; ChronOS™); but with respect for its use in topical dental applications, the functionalized form of β-TCP is the first and only version used in fluoridated preparations for remineralization of teeth (e.g., [702], [703], [743], and [744]).

The only nonphosphate mineral in **Table 9.1**, calcium fluoride (CaF_2), is also familiar. It remains practically insoluble at neutral pH, but is susceptible to dissolution under acidic conditions, a feature which makes it promising as a source of slow-release fluoride [652–654].

CALCIUM COMPOUND	SHORTHAND	FORMULA	Ca/P
Dicalcium phosphate anhydrous	DCPA	$CaHPO_4$	1
Dicalcium phosphate dihydrate	DCPD	$CaHPO_4 \cdot 2H_2O$	1
Octacalcium phosphate	OCP	$Ca_8H_2(PO_4)_6 \cdot 5H_2O$	1.33
Beta-tricalcium phosphate	β-TCP	$β\text{-}Ca_3(PO_4)_2$	1.5
Hydroxyapatite	HAP	$Ca_{10}(PO_4)_6(OH)_2$	1.67
Fluorapatite	FAP	$Ca_{10}(PO_4)_6F_2$	1.67
Calcium fluoride	CaF_2	CaF_2	----

Table 9.1 Some possible calcium compounds produced from saliva and/or dental treatments supersaturated with calcium, phosphate, and/or fluoride constituents. This list includes shorthand notation, stoichiometric formula, and calcium:phosphate ratio (Ca/P). For other calcium compounds, see [805].

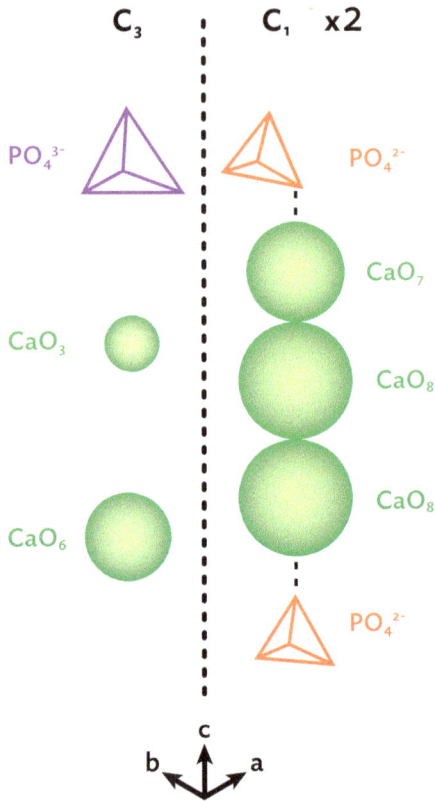

Figure 9.1. Schematic of the C_3 and C_1 symmetry sites of the β-TCP unit cell based on neutron diffraction data [671,874]. As noted in the figure, the C_3 symmetry site lacks a phosphate polyhedron and houses an underbonded CaO_3 cluster, thus providing a basis for functionalization [650,670–672].

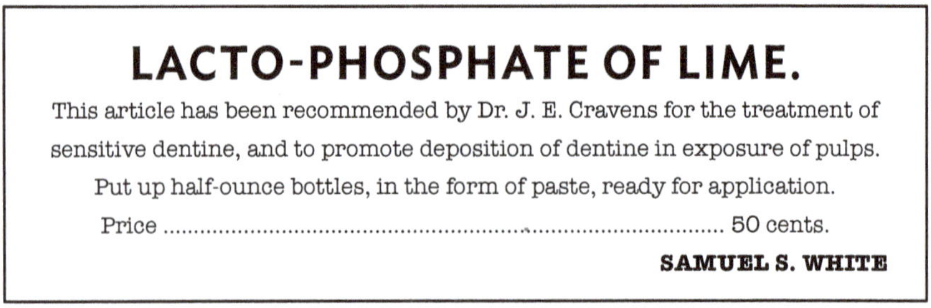

Figure 9.2. An 1873 advertisement by the S.S. White Company for the relief of dentinal hypersensitivity (from [875]).

Mineral phase calculations: Background

In biological systems there can exist more than one calcium phosphate (CaP) phase, as noted for the case of bone [819]. And given the heterogeneity of the oral environment (e.g., as noted by differences in salivary and biofilm fluoride levels [724], or supra- and subgingival plaque constituency [54]), which will affect rates of remineralization (i.e., the inhibition, retardation or acceleration of phase transformations to apatite-like mineral), it follows that more than one CaP phase can be expected to exist when supersaturated CaP systems are introduced.

To calculate potential solubility products, and therefore possible mineral phases, I utilized the Visual MINTEQ 3.1 chemical equilibrium model [878]. These assessments are based on thermodynamic tables established by collaborations between several US agencies beginning in the 1970s and continuing on into the 1990s. Although the dental research community has invoked such calculations to explore possible CaP phases (e.g., CPP-ACP [869], human saliva [844], and artificial salivas [817]), there have been few published cross-comparisons among different systems [879].

In calculating the possible CaP and fluoride mineral phases from various remineralizing systems, I have made four separate comparisons grouped according to topical modality (i.e., either paste or varnish):

✓ the first and second sets of calculations derive calcium mineral phases from calcium, phosphate, and/or fluoride content from commercially available calcium pastes/dentifrices based on theoretical and measured amounts, respectively; and,

✓ the third and fourth sets of calculations are based on measurements of calcium, phosphate, and fluoride eluted from several commercially available varnish systems under neutral and acidic conditions.

Mineral phase calculations: Dentifrices and pastes

In the <u>first</u> comparison, the following calcium compounds in pastes or dentifrices were used based on labeled (i.e., theoretical) content [666,879]:

1. Enamelon™ ACP: ACP is precipitated from two distinct salts that are introduced simultaneously during a brushing event: calcium sulfate (with 0.3% Ca^{2+}) and monoammonium orthophosphate (with ~ 0.9% $H_2PO_4^-$); also contains 1,130 ppm fluoride;

2. GC Tooth Mousse: loaded with 10% CPP-ACP;

3. GC Tooth Mousse Plus: loaded with 10% CPP-ACP plus 900 ppm fluoride;

4. 3M Clinpro™ Tooth Crème: loaded with 0.05% functionalized TCP plus 950 ppm fluoride. Note: for this dentifrice, only about 10% of the total functionalized TCP is soluble based on the design functionalization and the nature of β-TCP [671];

5. 3M Clinpro™ 5000: loaded with 0.08% functionalized TCP plus 5,000 ppm fluoride. Note: for this dentifrice, only about 10% of the labeled functionalized TCP is soluble based on the design functionalization and the nature of β-TCP [671]; and,

6. Saliva: used approximate calcium and phosphate concentrations of 58 ppm and 513 ppm, respectively [91,844], with 0 ppm fluoride; this group is used for reference purposes.

The results of the chemical equilibrium analysis for this <u>first</u> comparison are shown in **Figures 9.3** thru **9.6**.

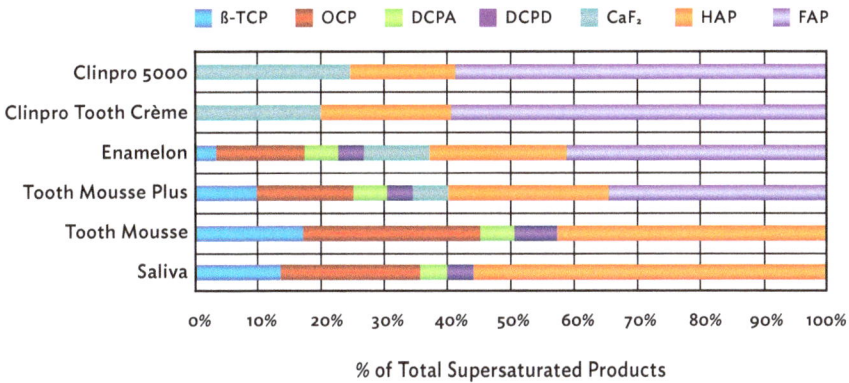

Figure 9.3. Distribution of solubility products estimated from chemical equilibrium calculations using Visual MINTEQ [878]. Data based on theoretical amounts (i.e., first comparison) for pastes [666,879] and saliva [91,844]. For the Clinpro™ dentifrices, the level of functionalized TCP were reduced to 10% to reflect the design of the low solubility characteristics of the functionalized TCP system [671].

From a remineralization perspective, it is desirable to produce HAP, FAP, and CaF_2 since these provide enamel-like mineralization, increased resistance to demineralization, and reservoirs of fluoride. With respect to the groups listed in **Figure 9.3**, the distributions (listed in descending order) are as follows:

1. Clinpro™ 5000: 100% are HAP, FAP, and/or CaF_2;

2. Clinpro™ Tooth Crème: 100% are HAP, FAP, and/or CaF_2;

3. Enamelon™ ACP: 75% are HAP, FAP, and/or CaF_2;

4. Tooth Mousse Plus: 65% are HAP, FAP, and/or CaF_2;

5. Saliva: 58% is HAP; and,

6. Tooth Mousse: 45% is HAP.

What explains these percentages?

These observations demonstrate the low supersaturation design of the functionalized tricalcium phosphate (i.e., TCP or fTCP) systems in the Clinpro™ dentifrices lead to 'quality' mineral formation (i.e., here, I'm referring to HAP, FAP, and CaF_2 as 'quality' mineral phases), while the high supersaturation formulas of Tooth Mousse and Enamelon™ groups can produce a heterogeneous blend of minerals, including those that are not HAP, FAP, or CaF_2 (i.e., β-TCP, OCP, DCPA, DCPD). As saliva is naturally inclined to facilitate remineralization, these calculations support this biological fluid in its basic ability to produce HAP. As fluoride improves the remineralization process, it inherently minimizes the amount of non-apatite-like or calcium fluoride-like phases; but when CaP supersaturation levels are very high or at least high enough that the fluoride concentration becomes marginalized or otherwise diminished, the generation of non-apatite-like or non-calcium-fluoride-like mineral becomes more pronounced.

As mentioned previously, high CaP supersaturation conditions produce nonapatitic mineral phases. But nonapatitic mineral may confer benefit if pronounced deposition of CaP mineral could be achieved at the tooth surface without being otherwise cleared from the oral cavity (e.g., swallowed). This mineral might be expected to provide mineralizing ions upon salivary action or exposure to acidic challenges (e.g., consuming a low-pH drink), that could reprecipitate mineral (apatitic and/or nonapatitic) on the tooth surface. In doing so, this may provide sufficient protection against subsurface demineralization due to limited diffusion processes [866]. However, the same diffusive limits at the tooth surface would also limit remineralization within subsurface lesions.

Regardless of the nature of the CaP remineralizing system, however, when immersed in the oral environment with saliva, remineralization will be modulated due to myriad intervening factors: after all, *in vivo* remineralization is not a rapid process [771]. And, if the environment is low in moisture, the progression rate of transitory CaP phases into apatite-like mineral will be reduced [827]. For these reasons, a CaP system (i.e., Clinpro™) with efficient calcium and phosphate loading that facilitates calcium fluoride (and/or calcium-fluoride-like) and/or direct (i.e., without undergoing CaP phase transitions [831,840]) apatite-like mineral formation may be especially appealing [650].

An analysis of the F^-, Ca^{2+}, and PO_4^{3-} components (shown in **Figures 9.4** thru **9.6**) helps explain this perspective. As F^- ions may readily participate in fluorapatite and/or CaF_2 formation, the abundance of 'free' F^- species (**Figure 9.4**) encourage production of enamel-like, acid-resistant mineral. Other species facilitating the formation of enamel-like or calcium fluoride-like mineral apparently include 'free' Ca^{2+}, along with CaF^+, HPO_4^{2-}, $H_2PO_4^-$ (from **Figures 9.5** and **9.6**), which are relatively abundant in the low supersaturation groups (i.e., Clinpro™ and saliva). In contrast, $CaPO_4^-$, $CaH_2PO_4^+$, and $CaHPO_4$(aq) (from **Figures 9.5** and **9.6**), which are components of DCPA, DCPD, and OCP, are relatively abundant among the highly supersaturated groups (i.e., Tooth Mousse, Tooth Mousse Plus, Enamelon™). Among

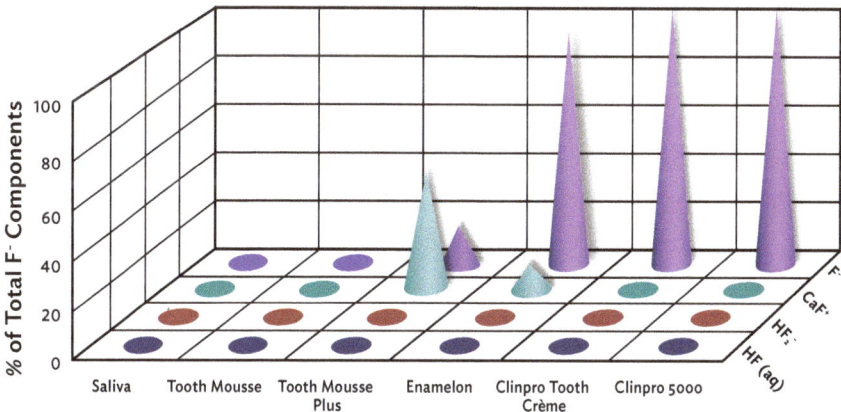

Figure 9.4. Distribution of fluoride (F^-) components (i.e., HF(aq), HF_2^-, CaF^+, F^-) determined from chemical equilibrium calculations using Visual MINTEQ [878] based on the first comparison groups in **Figure 9.3**.

the high supersaturation groups, that Enamelon™ produces about 10% more of the 'quality' remineralizing minerals (i.e., here 'quality' refers to HAP, FAP, or CaF_2) relative to Tooth Mousse Plus may be related to its relatively greater concentration of Ca^{2+} and $H_2PO_4^-$. The fact that saliva produces a fair amount of $CaHPO_4(aq)$ helps explain why HAP is not the only phase that can exist.

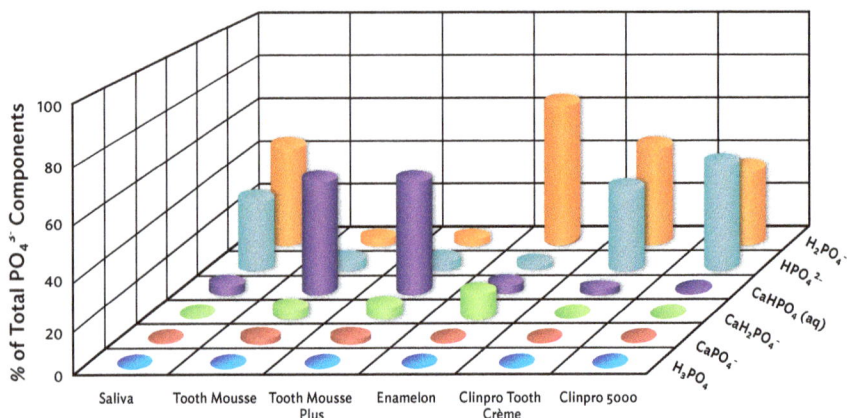

Figure 9.5. Distribution of orthophosphate (PO_4^{3-}) components (i.e., H_3PO_4, $CaPO_4^-$, $CaH_2PO_4^+$, $CaHPO_4(aq)$, HPO_4^{2-}, $H_2PO_4^-$) determined from chemical equilibrium calculations using Visual MINTEQ [878] based on the first comparison groups in **Figure 9.3**.

The <u>second</u> comparison is made based on measured calcium, phosphate, and fluoride contents from commercially available pastes/dentifrices (i.e., from Table 1 of [879]):

1. Placebo: same formulation as the Tooth Mousse and Tooth Mousse Plus, but lacks CPP-ACP and fluoride. The mean calcium and phosphate concentrations were measured to be 9.1 ppm and 1.4 ppm, respectively, with fluoride not detected (therefore, 0 ppm);

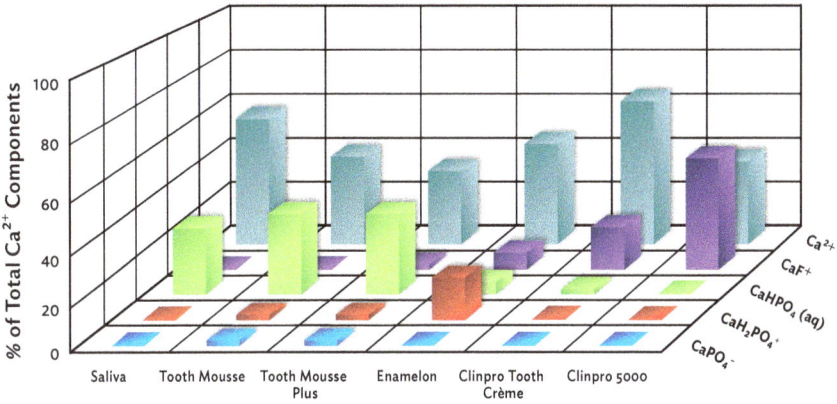

Figure 9.6. Distribution of calcium (Ca^{2+}) components (i.e., $CaPO_4^-$, $CaH_2PO_4^+$, $CaHPO_4$(aq), CaF^+, Ca^{2+}) determined from chemical equilibrium calculations using Visual MINTEQ [878] based on the first comparison groups in **Figure 9.3**.

2. GC Tooth Mousse (0 ppm fluoride): the mean calcium and phosphate concentrations were measured to be 338.1 ppm and 226.3 ppm, respectively, with fluoride not detected (therefore, 0 ppm);

3. GC Tooth Mousse Plus (900 ppm fluoride): the mean calcium, phosphate, and fluoride concentrations were measured to be 404.7 ppm, 253.2 ppm, and 48.4 ppm, respectively;

4. 3M Clinpro™ Tooth Crème (950 ppm fluoride): the mean calcium, phosphate, and fluoride concentrations were measured to be 8.9 ppm, 1.6 ppm, and 52.2 ppm, respectively;

5. Colgate (1,000 ppm fluoride): the mean calcium and fluoride contents were measured to be 5.7 ppm and 51.6 ppm, respectively; phosphate content was not detected (therefore, 0 ppm); and,

6. Neutrafluor 5000 (5,000 ppm fluoride): the mean calcium and fluoride contents were measured to be 45 ppm and 268.5 ppm, respectively; phosphate content was not detected (therefore, 0 ppm).

The results of the chemical equilibrium analysis for this second comparison are shown in **Figures 9.7** thru **9.10**.

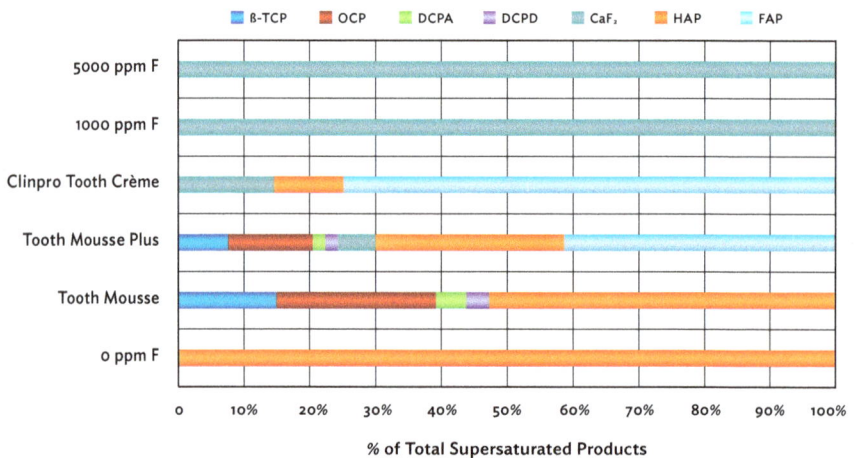

Figure 9.7. Distribution of solubility products estimated from chemical equilibrium calculations using Visual MINTEQ [878]. Data based on measured (i.e., second comparison) amounts for pastes/dentifrices [879].

As similarly assessed in the first comparison, the goal is to produce HAP, FAP, and CaF_2 since these produce enamel-like mineralization, increased resistance to demineralization, and reservoirs of fluoride; therefore, with respect to the groups listed in **Figure 9.7**, the distributions (listed in descending order) are as follows:

1. Placebo: 100% is HAP;

2. Colgate: 100% is CaF_2;

3. Neutrafluor 5000: 100% is CaF_2;

4. Clinpro™ Tooth Crème: <u>100%</u> are HAP, FAP, and/or CaF_2;

5. Tooth Mousse Plus: <u>75%</u> are HAP, FAP, and/or CaF_2; and,

6. Tooth Mousse: <u>55%</u> is HAP.

The discussion provided for in the <u>first</u> set of comparisons also applies here. These observations indicate the fluoride-only (i.e., Colgate and Neutrafluor) dentifrices only produce calcium fluoride, and the lack of detectable phosphate precludes other mineral possibilities. Similarly, the placebo paste lacked fluoride but contained low levels of calcium and phosphate to produce HAP and no other CaP mineral phase. This finding is consistent with low supersaturation mineral nucleation studies [831,839]. Consistent with the calculations for the <u>first</u> comparison, Clinpro™ yields only HAP, FAP, and/or CaF_2. As the calcium and phosphate contents were lower in this <u>second</u> comparison, the mineral phase amounts for Tooth Mousse Plus and Tooth Mousse are also lower, and are about 10% lower relative to those amounts from the <u>first</u> comparison. Underlining the sensitivity of the degree of supersaturation from highly supersaturated systems, these results echo the previous analysis in that a mixture of possible CaP mineral phases for Tooth Mousse and Tooth Mousse Plus exists that extend beyond HAP, FAP, or CaF_2 (i.e., β-TCP, OCP, DCPA, DCPD).

And in this study, the calculations demonstrate that the CaP system with low saturation (i.e., Clinpro™) facilitates calcium fluoride (and/or calcium-fluoride-like) and/or direct apatite-like mineralization [650].

Analyses of the F^-, Ca^{2+}, and PO_4^{3-} components (shown in **Figures 9.8** thru **9.10**) reveal similar information compared with the <u>first</u> set of comparisons. Notably, 'free' F^- ions are fairly abundant (**Figure 9.8**), with the lack of appreciable CaF^+ due to overall lower calcium levels relative to the <u>first</u> comparison.

The relatively fewer orthophosphate (**Figure 9.9**) and/or calcium (**Figure 9.10**) species is due to the overall lower calcium, phosphate, and fluoride contents used in this second comparison calculation. But consistent with the first comparison, the production of enamel-like, acid-resistant mineral seems to be dependent on 'free' Ca^{2+}, which practically all the groups can produce to some extent by virtue of the relatively low calcium and phosphate contents (i.e., relative to the first comparison). In **Figure 9.10**, the fluoride-only and Clinpro™ groups share a relative abundance of the CaF^+ moiety, suggesting the remineralization profiles are similar and likely constitute a combination of FAP and/or CaF_2, thus explaining the mineral phase possibilities shown in **Figure 9.7**.

And because all groups demonstrated the capacity to form 'quality' remineralizing mineral (i.e., again, here I use 'quality' to refer to HAP, FAP, or CaF_2 as these are comparatively less soluble than other CaP phases while promoting enamel-like mineralization), the prominence of HPO_4^{2-} and $H_2PO_4^-$ in all groups seems to correspond to the importance of these components in evolving CaP mineral that might effectively integrate with the tooth. In fact, observations suggest the presence of HPO_4^{2-} helps modulate the size and solubility of calcium fluoride-like minerals in the oral environment [652]. These observations appear to apply to the measured calcium, phosphate and/or fluoride concentrations from the pastes evaluated in these two sets of comparisons.

Notably, the number of orthophosphate species is expanded for Tooth Mousse and Tooth Mousse Plus (**Figure 9.9**) as $CaHPO_4(aq)$ is noticeably present in these two groups, and this likely gives rise to the possibility of nonapatitic CaP mineral precipitations, including OCP, DCPD, and DCPA. As the $CaHPO_4(aq)$ component was found in both the first and second comparisons and may be related to nonapatitic mineral, this finding warrants further commentary. The $CaHPO_4(aq)$ orthophosphate species has been implicated in the remineralization of lesions [206,869]. Our calculations reveal the evolution of nonapatitic

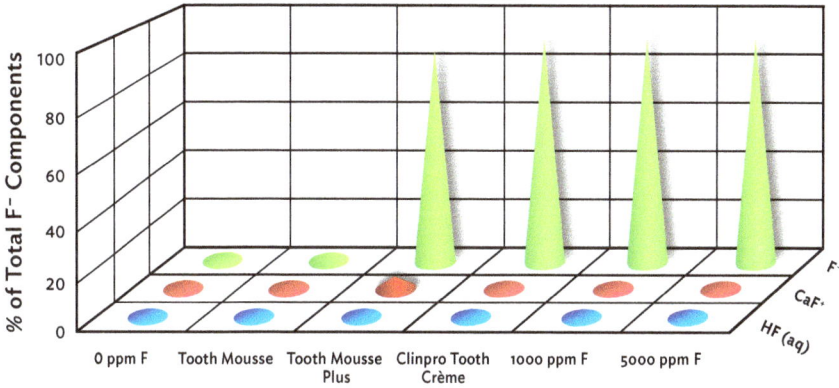

Figure 9.8. Distribution of fluoride (F^-) components (i.e., $HF(aq)$, HF_2^-, CaF^+, F^-) determined from chemical equilibrium calculations using Visual MINTEQ [878] based on the second comparison groups in **Figure 9.7.**

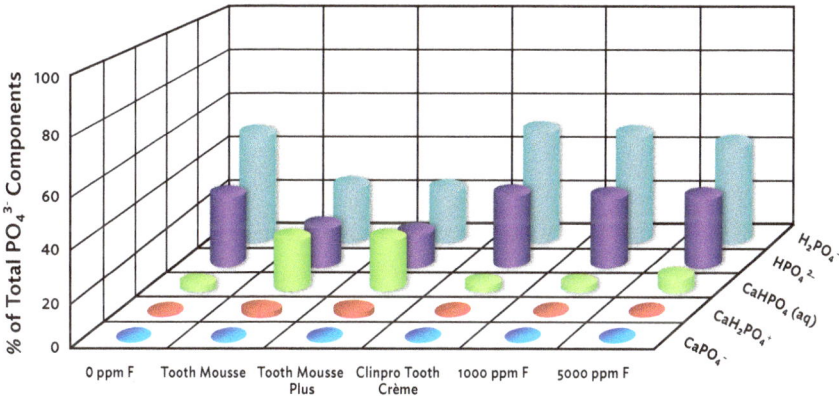

Figure 9.9. Distribution of orthophosphate (PO_4^{3-}) components (i.e., $CaPO_4^-$, $CaH_2PO_4^+$, $CaHPO_4(aq)$, HPO_4^{2-}, $H_2PO_4^-$) determined from chemical equilibrium calculations using Visual MINTEQ [878] based on the second comparison groups in **Figure 9.7.**

mineral includes this orthophosphate species. As such, it is possible this neutrally charged moiety may contribute to nonapatitic remineralization of weakened enamel structure, perhaps diffusing and/or precipitating as OCP or DCPD. While certainly contributing to deposition of mineral, this phase does not provide comparable acid-resistance relative to HAP, FAP, or CaF_2 (or calcium fluoride-like mineral) and may not transition to an apatite-like mineral once present in the oral environment (especially in low-moisture conditions).

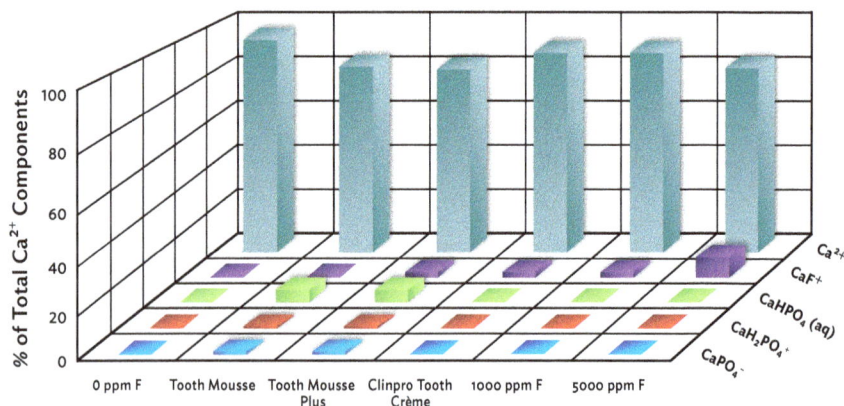

Figure 9.10. Distribution of calcium (Ca^{2+}) components (i.e., $CaPO_4^-$, $CaH_2PO_4^+$, $CaHPO_4(aq)$, CaF^+, Ca^{2+}) determined from chemical equilibrium calculations using Visual MINTEQ [878] based on the second comparison groups in **Figure 9.7**.

Mineral phase calculations: Varnishes. The last two comparisons (i.e., third and fourth comparisons) involve potential solubility products formed by fluoride varnishes. The third comparison involves calculations made on calcium, phosphate, and fluoride released from the following varnish systems over the period of 24 hours at 37°C at neutral pH [706]:

1. Duraphat: the mean calcium and fluoride concentrations were measured to be 2.5 μmol/g and 74.7 μmol/g, respectively, with phosphate not detected (therefore, 0 μmol/g);

2. MI Varnish: the mean calcium, phosphate, and fluoride concentrations were measured to be 18.2 μmol/g, 31.5 μmol/g, and 1,139.9 μmol/g, respectively;

3. Enamel Pro: the mean calcium, phosphate, and fluoride contents were measured to be 16.4 µmol/g, 199.2 µmol/g, and 687.5 µmol/g, respectively; and,

4. Clinpro™ Varnish: the mean calcium, phosphate, and fluoride concentrations were measured to be 3.2 µmol/g, 0.8 µmol/g, and 74 µmol/g, respectively.

The results of the chemical equilibrium analysis for this third comparison are shown in **Figures 9.11** thru **9.14**.

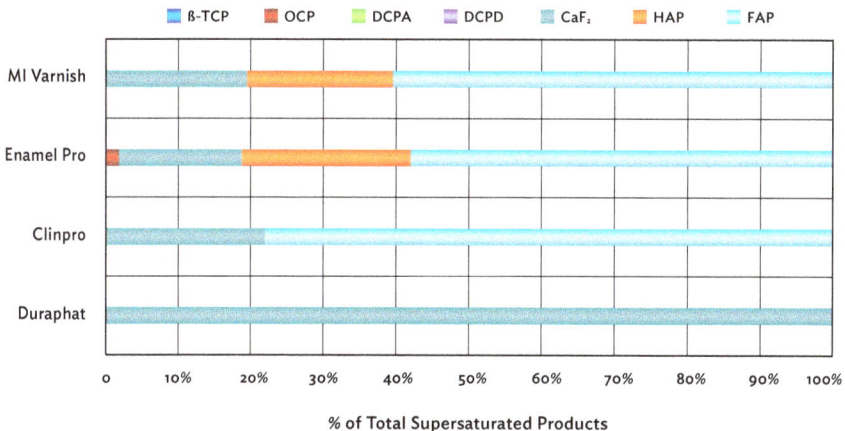

Figure 9.11. Distribution of solubility products estimated from chemical equilibrium calculations using Visual MINTEQ [878]. Data based on measured (i.e., third comparison) amounts for varnishes under neutral conditions [706].

While toothpastes are designed to frequently refresh the oral environment with remineralizing agents (most notably, fluoride), varnishes are applied relatively infrequently, have much higher fluoride content, and are meant to sustain delivery or deposition of fluoride into enamel [636,651,657,658] through the formation of fluorapatite, calcium fluoride, and/or calcium fluoride-like mineralization [652,656]. Therefore, mineralization characteristics from fluoridated toothpastes and fluoridated varnishes can be expected to be different, and this is where chemical equilibrium calculations can help identify possible mineral phases.

With respect to the groups listed in **Figure 9.11**, the distributions (listed in descending order) of FAP and/or CaF_2 are as follows:

1. Duraphat®: <u>100%</u> is CaF_2;

2. Clinpro™: <u>100%</u> are FAP and CaF_2;

3. MI Varnish: <u>78%</u> are FAP and CaF_2; and,

4. Enamel Pro: <u>73%</u> are FAP and CaF_2.

The purpose of a fluoride varnish is to prolong fluoride retention in and/or on the tooth surface, and all groups appear to deliver these benefits through formation of at least one type of fluoridated mineral. Fluorapatite is less soluble than hydroxyapatite and suggests immediate mineral integration with the tooth, while calcium fluoride reservoirs help sustain the action of fluoride in the oral environment. The dominant form of fluoride was the same for the four different varnishes (i.e., F^-) and corresponds well to the relatively large percentages of CaF_2 and FAP calculated for each system.

Notably, the mineral phases predicted by these solubility product calculations have been observed in or on tooth structure. For instance, with respect to the Clinpro™ system, these calculations are consistent with independent observations of the existence of both CaF_2 (scanning electron microscopy) and FAP (X-ray diffraction) [880–882]. Thus, chemical equilibrium calculations (like the one used here) provide support in the characterization of supersaturated remineralizing systems [817,844,869].

Although less resistant to acid attack, HAP may also be produced (e.g., MI Varnish and Enamel Pro) and contribute to enamel-like mineralization. For infrequent varnish applications, however, fluoridated mineral phases help deliver sustained benefits and may, therefore, be preferable relative to delivery of nonfluoridated phases. Frequent application of remineralization dentifrices and pastes can subsequently complement fluoride varnish treatment through the formation of fluoridated, apatitic, and perhaps nonapatitic mineral (e.g., like those calculated from the first and second comparison sets).

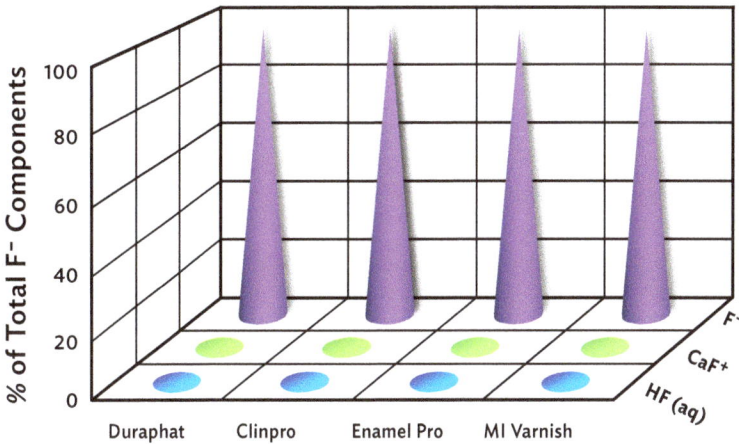

Figure 9.12. Distribution of fluoride (F^-) components (i.e., HF(aq), CaF^+, F^-) determined from chemical equilibrium calculations using Visual MINTEQ [878] based on the third comparison groups in **Figure 9.11**.

As HPO_4^{2-} appears to be influential in fluoride mineralization [652,655], the presence of this component bears importance for fluoride varnishes just as it did for fluoride dentifrices (i.e., the first and second comparisons). Under the neutral conditions used here, it is likely this moiety and its $H_2PO_4^-$ counterpart can readily form calcium fluoride-like mineral and may integrate with the tooth structure directly. In fact, it is likely the slightly higher amount of the $H_2PO_4^-$ moiety may contribute to the relatively greater likelihood of forming FAP from the Clinpro™ varnish. In any event, the importance of forming calcium fluoride-like mineral remains paramount from topical high-fluoride formats such as fluoride varnishes.

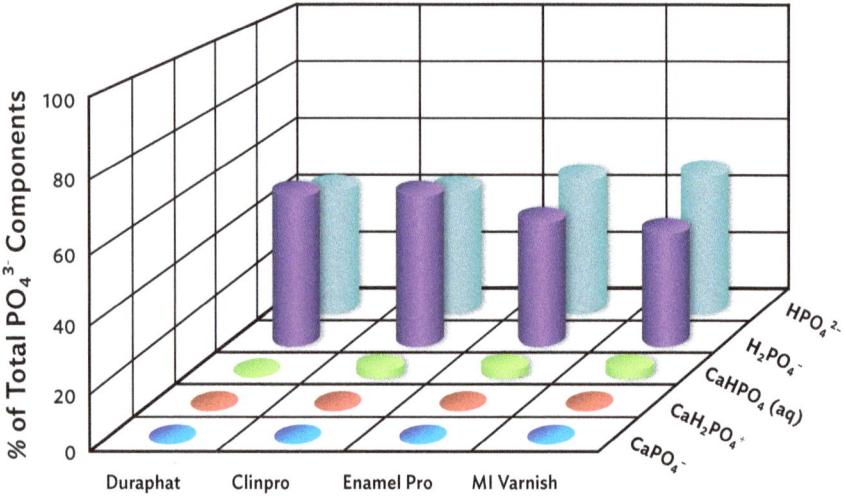

Figure 9.13. Distribution of orthophosphate (PO_4^{3-}) components (i.e., $CaPO_4^-$, $CaH_2PO_4^+$, $CaHPO_4$(aq), HPO_4^{2-}, $H_2PO_4^-$) determined from chemical equilibrium calculations using Visual MINTEQ [878] based on the third comparison groups in **Figure 9.11**.

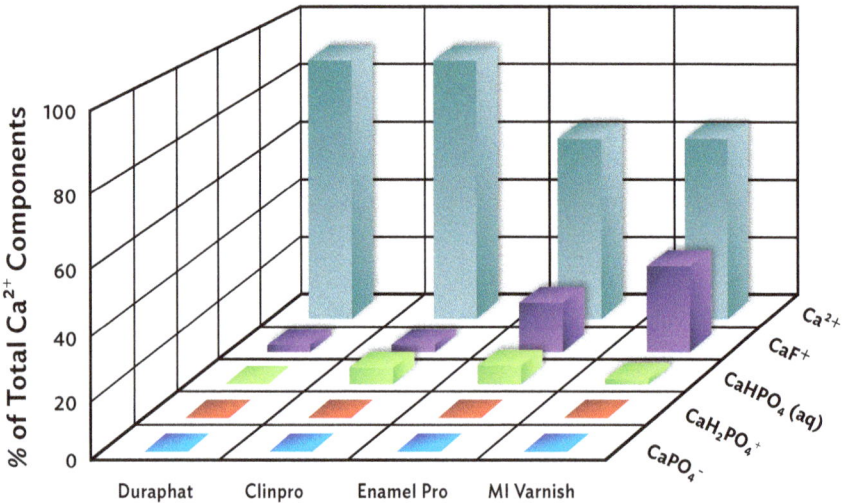

Figure 9.14. Distribution of calcium (Ca^{2+}) components (i.e., $CaPO_4^-$, $CaH_2PO_4^+$, $CaHPO_4$(aq), CaF^+, Ca^{2+}) determined from chemical equilibrium calculations using Visual MINTEQ [878] based on the third comparison groups in **Figure 9.11**.

With respect to the calcium components, Enamel Pro produces $CaHPO_4$(aq) in a relatively significant amount, which helps explain the formation of HAP (and to a lesser degree, OCP). The relatively high 'free' Ca^{2+} content produced from Duraphat® and Clinpro™ likely drives the relatively higher CaF_2 and FAP contents, respectively, and underlines the differences that exist in the interplay of ionic components among the CaP remineralizing systems. By avoiding the heterogeneity in the nucleation and growth of various mineral phases that evolves from highly supersaturated systems is one reason a low and/or sustained-release supersaturated CaP system (with fluoride, of course) may drive more efficient remineralization.

The final (i.e., <u>fourth</u>) comparison involves measurements made on calcium, phosphate, and fluoride released from the following varnish systems over the period of 24 hours at 37°C under acidic conditions (pH ~ 4.8) [883]:

1. Duraphat: the mean calcium, phosphate, and fluoride concentrations were measured to be 5.66 µmol/g, 3.32 µmol/g, and 56.3 µmol/g, respectively;

2. MI Varnish: the mean calcium, phosphate, and fluoride concentrations were measured to be 36.77 µmol/g, 44.75 µmol/g, and 1,149.31 µmol/g, respectively;

3. Enamel Pro: the mean calcium, phosphate, and fluoride contents were measured to be 11.49 µmol/g, 159.48 µmol/g, and 506.72 µmol/g, respectively; and,

4. Clinpro™ Varnish: the mean calcium, phosphate, and fluoride concentrations were measured to be 4.16 µmol/g, 2.02 µmol/g, and 175.87 µmol/g, respectively.

Results of the chemical equilibrium analysis for this fourth comparison are shown in **Figure 9.15**. The relatively low levels of calcium and phosphate release under these acidic conditions (pH ~ 4.8) apparently preclude formation of CaP mineral. Because the results reveal only the production of fluoridated minerals under these acidic conditions, further detail regarding the fluoride, calcium, and phosphate components are omitted for brevity. In essence, all varnishes are able to produce fluoridated mineral, including formation of FAP (~ 25%) for the MI Varnish group. This mineral may form due to the relatively high fluoride content evolved from its rapid dissolution properties (e.g., 'rapid-release'). Still, calcium fluoride (and/or calcium fluoride-like mineral), which was predicted to form for all the systems, is preferred for sustained benefits, since this mineral may act as a reservoir of calcium and fluoride for subsequent integration with weakened enamel structure [652–654]. But despite the large differences in measured fluoride released from the different varnish systems (contrasting by as much as 15x among varnishes), the formation of calcium fluoride-like mineral indicates each of these varnishes may inhibit demineralization, at least under the acidic conditions used in this laboratory study [883].

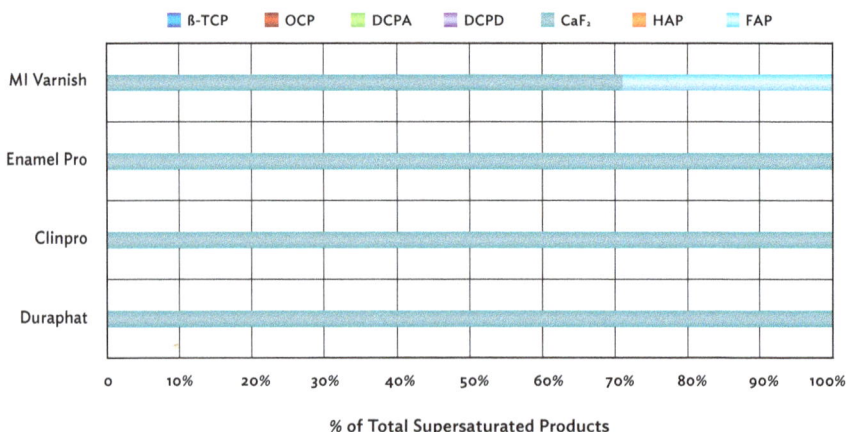

Figure 9.15. Distribution of solubility products estimated from chemical equilibrium calculations using Visual MINTEQ [878]. Data based on measured (i.e., fourth comparison) amounts for varnishes under acidic conditions [883].

Some final thoughts regarding remineralization from high and low CaP supersaturation

These four comparisons of both pastes/dentifrices and varnishes help shed light on the expected calcium-containing minerals that may be created from various remineralizing systems. Certain systems may favor the formation of HAP, FAP, and/or CaF_2, which can provide quality remineralization in terms of appearance, acid-resistance, and integration with existing tooth structure. But the mineral phase calculations also present clear possibilities for nonapatitic minerals, which may also be important, especially if reservoirs of calcium and phosphate are desired or if large deposits of minerals are needed to prevent demineralization [667,866].

Thus, highly supersaturated systems can provide benefits, as they may impart remineralization benefits provided sufficient amounts of 'free' fluoride are available (e.g., even 1 ppm fluoride is sufficient to accelerate remineralization [86,800,866]). After all, both amorphous and non-apatite-like minerals are known to exist in biological systems and remain stable [819,884–886].

Still, concerns exist for highly supersaturated systems, including the reduction in 'free' fluoride that interacts with the tooth, plaque, or saliva, increased chance of clearance from the oral cavity (i.e., through swallowing), delayed transitions to HAP, FAP, or CaF_2 mineral, the creation of non-enamel-like aggregates that may encumber remineralization of weakened tooth structure, and possible gingival irritations. Lastly, the transition from nonapatitic CaP phases to enamel-like phases (i.e., HAP or FAP) requires moisture (e.g., saliva) [827]. Such transitions would be severely limited (and possibly nonexistent then) for those with xerostomia, and also those experiencing nagging dry-mouth characteristics.

Based on the remineralization evidence (including clinical success), there also seems to be economic inefficiencies, especially in comparison to the success of low supersaturated systems: for instance, although Tooth Mousse Plus contains more than 200x more calcium than Clinpro™ Tooth Crème, this rather large differential has not been observed clinically in independent studies [756,887]: for example, salivary levels of calcium were found to be significantly *higher* for Clinpro™ Tooth Crème (which is formulated with 0.05% TCP + 950 ppm fluoride) compared to a GC Tooth Mousse Plus (which comprises 10% CPP-ACP plus 900 ppm fluoride) in a randomized, double-blind clinical trial [887]. And on a per-gram-fluoride basis, Clinpro™ Tooth Crème provided at least 5x better remineralization than other fluoride pastes, including the combination of a fluoride paste (1,000 ppm fluoride) and GC Tooth Mousse Plus (10% CPP-ACP plus 900 ppm fluoride). Similarly, on a per-CaP-load basis, this remineraliza-tion benefit swells to about 200x *in favor of* Clinpro™ [756]. And with the cost of the TCP products less than those with CPP-ACP (e.g., on average at least 20% less based on reputable vendors as listed on the Internet and dental supply houses), the economic benefits to the patient should not be ignored.

Although the 'stabilized' CPP-ACP technology reports clinical success and has many studies [870,888], there are also clinical studies demonstrating its limitations, especially in comparison with fluoride-only therapies, where little to no additional remineralization effects are observed (e.g., [756,791,889–891]). Currently, multiple independent assessments render this technology as promising for the short-term (at best) [892], but withhold recommendations for long-term use [791,893–896], especially when CPP-ACP is combined with fluoride [895,896], due in part to nonsignificant clinical benefits, questionable study design or quality, and/or potential for high risk of bias regarding the majority of the data amassed thus far [893,895].

With respect to 'unstabilized' ACP, there is evidence for clinical success, especially for the relief of dentinal hypersensitivity [897]. This promising technology stems from a first-generation approach at combining fluoride with high amounts of calcium and phosphate (i.e., 'ACP') to effect mineral depositions [667]. Since the original research (e.g., [663]), the 'ACP' approach has experienced a few transitions throughout its history (including a business reorganization, having started out as Enamelon™ in the late 1990s before a bankruptcy shifted progress). Although considered promising [870], the lack of independent (i.e., similar to the Novamin® and CPP-ACP studies, company reports or sponsored studies pose ever-present risks for bias) or clinical comparison studies remains a concern [666,668,870].

Thus, differences in the degree of supersaturation help distinguish functionalized tricalcium phosphate from other CaP systems. In contrast to most formulations (e.g., those with ACP, CPP-ACP, bioglass), the functionalized tricalcium phosphate is a low supersaturation system due to low loading (e.g., 0.08% TCP in Clinpro™ 5000) and tailored solubility (e.g., < 1.5 mM soluble calcium in Clinpro™ 5000). This results in a formulation that emulates salivary calcium content (~ 1 mM) and contrasts those exhibiting high supersaturation (e.g., at least 75 mM for ACP or CPP-ACP).

As independent data continue to emerge, the clinical data amassed on the fluoride plus functionalized tricalcium phosphate systems (e.g., including those demonstrating superior benefits relative to fluoride alone and at least as good a performance relative to high supersaturation systems [139,160,161,673,675,708,711,724,725,751,756,759,766,769,770]) continue to validate the potential of low supersaturation approaches [831,839] and also underlines the innovative design of functionalized tricalcium phosphate.

Proper dosing helps reduce potential undesirable side-effects (which practically always exist in an effective medicament) while maintaining health and economic balance. The medical industry is well-versed in prescribing the proper dose of therapeutics to effectively rectify or manage a specific condition. In doing so, this highlights the power of the active drug ingredient and the efficiency of the medium from which it is delivered. In doing so, the amount of therapeutic agent needed to attain an outcome or manage a given situation constitutes an effective dose. This reasoning was a major consideration in the development of the functionalized tricalcium phosphate systems.

For instance, the use of 5,000 ppm fluoride dentifrices can achieve 75% reduction in caries incidence relative to standard 1,000 ppm fluoride dentifrices [737]. So is there a similar, unequivocal clinical benefit of having 5% or 10% CaP relative to 1%, or even sub-1% (e.g., 0.08% functionalized tricalcium phosphate in Clinpro™ 5000)? Presently, I am unaware that any such data exists.

In specialized cases (e.g., special-needs populations) more than one remineralization topical might be needed to counter the patient's oral health risk. However, as a primary mode of protection, a fluoride-only or fluoride plus low-CaP supersaturation remineralization treatment should be used on the basis of efficient remineralization. Then, if high-CaP supersaturation treatments are used, they should be used as an adjunct to progress the remineralization initiated by the low-CaP supersaturation system (i.e., which serves as the initial 'seeding' treatment).

As an example, consider a xerostomic patient where salivary flow is cripplingly absent and the clinician recommends the use of Clinpro™ Tooth Crème and GC Tooth Mousse. Clinpro™ Tooth Crème encourages acid-resistant, enamel-like mineral integration from fewer, better-matched calcium and fluoridated phases relative to Tooth Mousse, which precipitates heterogeneous calcium phosphate phases (e.g., HAP, FAP, and CaF_2 as shown in **Figures 9.3** and **9.7**). In the event Clinpro™ Tooth Crème might not meet the patient's needs for remineralization, follow-on applications of Tooth Mousse might provide supplemental reservoirs of calcium and phosphate.

But in contrast to the two-step remineralization example described above, a single high-fluoride modality comprising a low supersaturation CaP system may be used instead. For example, relative to lower-fluoride treatments, Clinpro™ 5000 (a 1.1% NaF dentifrice) provides enhanced remineralization and hypersensitivity benefits while suppressing activity from microbial pathogens. These low supersaturation dentifrices may be especially helpful for those with dry-mouth conditions, since the minerals formed do not rely on moisture to deliver the mineralizing benefit. Importantly, compared to multistep procedures, a single preparation can help encourage patient compliance while limiting additional expenditures. This comment becomes magnified when one considers whether the economic cost meets or exceeds the actual benefits [540,756].

Of course, some situations may warrant the use of more than one topical. For instance, if maintaining a moist environment is troublesome, other modalities may be necessary (e.g., lozenge, sprays, gels, etc.). In the end, the clinical outcome desired for a given patient matters most, and should dictate the choice and use of the remineralization system(s) [139], along with any economic factors [540]. In other words, if one remineralization system doesn't present economic and/or functional benefits, perhaps another one will.

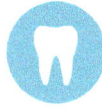

CHAPTER TEN

Put It to Practice

THUS FAR, DEMINERALIZATION AND REMINERALIZATION FACTORS in the spirit of preventive dentistry have been explored. When the remineralization agents (including fluoride and saliva) cannot compete with microbial mayhem and acid insults, inflammation of the soft tissue and/or weakening of the hard tissue ensue. But the scope of this book is not intended to address irreparable tooth destruction, where substantial modification (i.e., loss) of tooth structure occurs due to disease progression or through corrective, stabilizing procedures by the clinician. Instead, the material in the preceding chapters has provided the framework to better understand how minimally invasive strategies can be effective in clinical practice. While some of the strategies are discussed here, interested readers are strongly encouraged to explore the excellent references used in this chapter to glean more information.

Minimally invasive dentistry

Today, minimally invasive dentistry (MID) is a cornerstone of preventive dentistry, aiming to preserve, recover, and/or stabilize the tooth structure using nonoperative methodologies, resorting to restorative intervention only when no other options are viable [297,692,772,898].

Notably, the concept of preventive dentistry is not new but has evolved over time, with views of what actually constitutes 'preventive dentistry' and the attendant strategies sometimes differing considerably over the years. For example, preventive dentistry strategies published in 1895 revealed that filling the tooth was a hallmark of good preventive efforts. In one instance, Dr. G. Newkirk stated *"The fissures and pits which cannot always be kept clean by the patient, should be filled upon the first indications of decay. Here is preventive dentistry in a nutshell."* [899]. But while 'filling' a tooth usually involved invasive procedures along with a metallic restoration [900], it might also involve simple cleaning and cementing of the frank lesion without excavation as recommended in 1895 [901]: *"The writer advises against any excavation—syringe thoroughly with warm water, dehydrate with alcohol, dry thoroughly, and fill with cement, placing the dry powder over the filling and pressing firmly with the finger. . . . This will preserve the teeth through the early grade of immaturity, preserving all of the tooth structure, retaining the natural color, and without inflicting pain."*

> *Today, minimal intervention in preventive dentistry emphasizes saving tooth structure, which is predicated on managing the decay process.*

Today, minimal intervention in preventive dentistry emphasizes saving tooth structure, which is predicated on managing the decay process [902]. Such strategies seek to either avoid the start of or delay the need for restorative procedures, which otherwise trigger the tooth's 'death spiral', whereby tooth structure gradually becomes diminished over the course of repeated restorative procedures. For instance, the average functional lifetime of posterior composite restorations is less than 10 years [903].

The theme here is cleanliness and is the same 100+ years ago [899] as it is today [297]: if the tooth is not clean, decay can ensue. Consistent with calls for managing carious lesions, those carious lesions that are cleansable (i.e., not cavitated), should be managed through biofilm removal (i.e., plaque), remineralization (e.g., fluoride), and/or sealing (e.g., sealants) [297].

Arguably the most critical part of oral hygiene is the frequent disruption of plaque. Commonly observed in those wearing orthodontic brackets [107–109], inadequate removal allows for adhesion, cohesion, and proliferation of microbial species. As noted in those abstaining from oral hygiene procedures for 10 days, the composition of supragingival plaque shifts to favor pathogens and may exert some irreversible behavior even if oral hygiene is reinstituted [904]. Diversity shifts have also been observed after cessation of arginine toothpaste [72]. These observations underline the robustness of plaque constituents and underline the importance of clean tooth surfaces [899]. To that end, studies with children and adults demonstrate that proper oral hygiene procedures can drastically reduce gingivitis, periodontitis, and caries experience [905].

As discussed in Chapter 8, the revolutionary anticaries agent, fluoride, catalyzes remineralization processes and helps thwart microbial pathogenic activity. Fluoride is thus a 'must-have' in the MID tool chest. While the oral environment naturally fosters remineralization [106], fluoride enhances this process [86,800] while also managing microbial activity [50,775]. But for this powerful remineralization agent to work most effectively, it is important that both clinicians and patients understand how it works and what topical formats are available. Unfortunately, these criteria are often lacking [809–812]. Recognizing that preexisting decay (e.g., secondary caries) is notoriously challenging to manage [906], clinicians must consider the possibility of using higher fluoride treatments and/or more aggressive remineralization approaches in order to achieve a desired oral health outcome [139,906].

Another aspect of minimally invasive intervention utilizes sealants or resin infiltrants for lesions that cannot be remineralized and need to be arrested. Sealants can be placed in those regions harboring plaque and/or food debris; in particular, sealants and/or resins can be applied to cavitations as a means of effectively arresting disease progression [262,263,297,907]. This may be especially appealing for primary dentition, where the lifetime of the protective sealant/resin outlasts the residency of the tooth. With respect to permanent dentition, sealing may help extend the point at which more aggressive intervention becomes inevitable: such stopgap measures may be favored in instances where health-related concerns outweigh risks of invasive dental procedures, or if patients decline aggressive treatment as a matter of preference. For even greater benefits, periodic applications of fluoride varnish to the sealed region are also recommended [262].

The use of air abrasion on questionably carious teeth to arrest potential progression has been considered as a minimal intervention option [908,909]. In principle, this would accomplish minimal removal of enamel tissue, which would, in turn, minimize the size of the ensuing restoration. But this conservative yet invasive procedure has fallen out of favor due in part to the following reasons: it does not necessarily stave off subsequent caries progression, still requires acid etching, has limited restorative applications, can introduce iatrogenic factors, initiates the restorative cycle (regardless how minimal the restoration might be), and importantly, may be unnecessary if less-invasive remineralization therapies can be used [910]. In contrast, and corresponding with the latter point, MID advocates improved plaque removal techniques along with remineralization therapies to heal accessible (or, cleansable), noncavitated decay.

If decay has progressed into dentin (especially for primary dentition), MID recommends an additional level of care involving sealants or resin infiltrants [297]. But if the decay is not manageable (i.e., cannot be readily cleaned, stabilized, or remineralized) and/or the decay has progressed to deep within the tooth structure, then excavations may be necessary [297]. Presently, emerging evidence strongly supports the use of stepwise excavation in permanent teeth in order to remove as little dentin as possible [253,297].

In short, MID plans work, provided both the clinicians and patients are in accord, and the patients understand their options and are motivated to take ownership of their oral health [898,911]. Otherwise, risks related to the expertise of the clinician, the patient's understanding, and the communication between the two interested parties can arise that can reduce the likelihood of success and limit the overall health outcome. These aspects are discussed in the next section.

Clinicians, patients, and the clinician-patient relationship

While aspects of conservative dentistry have been expressed above, the degree of success remains dependent on the characteristics of the clinician and of the patient. Oral hygiene or caries management plans can fail for reasons including limited or insufficient resources (e.g., funding or outreach mechanisms), clinician-patient misunderstandings, poor clinical plan design, poor compliance to the customized plan, and apathy.

As discussed previously, some limitations pertain to clinicians' general knowledge of fluoride and the various topical fluoride formats; but there are other factors to consider. Understandably, clinician optimism can devolve when the patient (or the patient's family or caregivers) declines to or is unable to accept stewardship of his/her oral health [811]. But perhaps hitting closer to home, many clinicians may feel overwhelmed by the lack of financial incentives for preventive programs (e.g., lack of support from government agencies or insurance companies [811,902]), along with inadequate understanding, training, or promotion of preventive guidelines [811]. In fact, these factors may be contributing to noncompliance of dental practices with established guidelines [912]. Moreover, among clinicians there is often variability in models and terminology, as well as gaps between research and clinical practice [811,902,913,914]. For example, there are at least four systems assessing caries activity (i.e., ICDAS, CAMBRA, Nyvad, and CMS [902]) or tooth wear (i.e., Eccles Index, Tooth Wear Index, Lussi Index, and Basic Erosive Wear Examination [915]), respectively.

Acknowledging these obstacles [811,812], the onus still remains with the clinician to create a genuine, trusting clinician-patient relationship. Though this may be challenging, improved health outcomes can be achieved when the patient feels or believes there is trust, rapport, understanding, satisfaction, involvement, motivation, and safety [916].

Among the features of a healthy clinician-patient relationship, patient fears present a challenge that the clinician may not have fully anticipated, or even contributed to previously. While few are likely to be enthusiastic about a medical visit (e.g., even a routine physical exam needed for a sporting activity), a trip to the dentist can be even more foreboding, especially by one who has a history of tooth decay, pain, or sensitivity. For instance, among 15 various fears listed in the Children's Fear Survey Schedule—Dental Subscale (CFSS-DS), the actions of injections, choking, having a stranger touch them, and drilling were most feared among Japanese children (in contrast, the practitioner's attire or having instruments in the mouth were not as feared) [917]. Additionally, children visiting private practices displayed greater fears relative to those visiting the university clinic (Pediatric Dental Clinic at Okayama University Dental Hospital). Notably, these fears are not unique to Japanese culture, as other cultures (e.g., Netherlands, China, Finland) reported injections, choking, and drilling as the top fears [917]. This means that having one invasive procedure (e.g., a restoration) could meet all four of these primary fears, while preventive treatments including fluoride gels can elicit perhaps two. These results support the finding that by the time the child turns 18 years of age, an acquired fear of the dentist has been attained by those with caries experience [918]. Even into adulthood, the dislike of the sound of the dental drill remains strong [919].

Thus, patients with a history of caries often have reservations, including fear and doubt. A clinical approach or plan that is too limiting, nagging, indicting, unsustainable, and/or simply doesn't seem to apply to 'real' humans (e.g., "I mean, who doesn't enjoy a dessert or treat?!") may therefore diminish, or even lose, the ability to build clinician-patient trust through meaningful, proactive, healthy, and reasonable discussions.

One way of constructing a solid clinician-patient relationship is achieved through effective, two-way communication [916]. This necessarily involves the patient and can help motivate the patient toward a better oral health outcome. In designing the patient's customized plan, it is essential the patient understands the clinician's recommendations and possible alternatives. For instance, as stated in the American Dental Association's Principles of Ethics and Code of Professional Conduct regarding Patient Autonomy, *"the dentist has a duty to respect the patient's rights to self-determination and confidentiality."* [920]. Furthermore:

"This principle expresses the concept that professionals have a duty to treat the patient according to the patient's desires, within the bounds of accepted treatment, and to protect the patient's confidentiality. Under this principle, the dentist's primary obligations include involving patients in treatment decisions in a meaningful way, with due consideration being given to the patient's needs, desires, and abilities, and safeguarding the patient's privacy."

The above statement underlines the importance of effective communication with the patient, so prior to managing a dental situation, effective communication is key (i.e., the patient understands the options and recommendations of the clinician). This is probably one of the biggest hurdles facing the clinician: ensuring the patient has more than one option, understanding the patient's unique situation, and then respecting the patient's ultimate decision, even if the decision may not be commensurate with the clinician's professional opinion.

This may seem obvious, but does the patient actually understand and/or agree with the clinician's recommendations? While the expectations, goals, and plans to address oral maladies and achieve optimum oral health may seem clear and aligned during the clinician-patient conversation, in actuality there is strong evidence there is a disconnect in the take-home message. For example, Misra et al. found that dentists recalled providing much more information and agreement on actions than patients remembered [921]. In fact, this disparity was found to be significantly different (p < 0.05) for the 26 consultations, with the dentists recalling almost twice as much dental advice than what the patients recalled. Separately, another study underlined that patient recognition of oral health terminology does not imply understanding [922].

These studies demonstrate that gaps in understanding exist and are relevant to 'real world' scenarios. Therefore, if the patient (including adults, children, parents, guardians, caregivers, etc.) may not fully understand the recommendations and instructions from the expert, might this not contribute to situations of poor patient compliance where the patient (whether it's a child or adult) does not recall—and therefore cannot perform—the recommendations? Also, what if the patient is unable or unwilling to follow the clinician's advice? Already bombarded with information overload in today's societies, along with myriad other details that life naturally presents, compliance with therapeutic instructions can be elusive. Strategies to improve compliance may include written instructions and/or periodic phone or e-mail follow-ups given shortly after and before the subsequent dental visit. Such approaches are part of a patient-centered approach where communication and oversight can help improve overall patient outcome [297,139,921,923].

Call to action: Advocating minimal intervention

Clinicians must remain mindful of the dreaded restorative 'death spiral' [903]. As documented in the 19th century, it was common for some dentists (especially early-career dentists) to trumpet their skills in filling the tooth and fixing the problem, regarding their restoration as superior relative to nature's original structure [924]. But is this valid today? Recently, a meta-analysis study evaluated over 18,000 practitioners and found that more than 21% would opt for the invasive 'drill-and-fill' option for enamel-only lesions compared to less-invasive approaches [925]. Separately, Gordan et al. reported that among 197 small, large, and public health dental practices in the Dental Practice-based Research Network (in the United States, Denmark, Norway, and Sweden), 75% (or 7,073) restorations were replaced compared to 25% (or 2,411) that were repaired [926]. Among all three dental practice types, secondary caries was the major reason (i.e., 43%) for justifying replacement or repair, while larger and/or public health practices were more likely to repair than replace restorations compared to small group practices. But among all three practice types and indicating perhaps a change in philosophy favoring minimal intervention, younger graduates from dental schools and those having been the original dentist who made the restoration conferred a significantly greater tendency to make repairs compared to replacements [926].

Regarding restorative options, the patient's attitude might be very clear (especially in today's 'on-demand' society): "just fix it now so I don't have to bother with it." Despite personality or philosophical differences, patients must be informed of less-invasive but perhaps more patient-dependent (i.e., 'more involved') options, including sealants, high-fluoride therapies, better hygiene practices, and/or shifts in dietary choices.

As an example, if the clinician observes an enamel lesion that appears to be progressing rapidly, a wait-and-see approach utilizing a high-fluoride dentifrice [737] requires minimal clinical intervention and minimal change to patient behavior. Importantly, this can directly be substituted for an existing dentifrice, rendering additional hygienic steps potentially unnecessary. So instead of restoring the tooth (and thus engaging the restoration death spiral clock), effective communication (i.e., mutual understanding of action, with follow-up conversations as necessary) with the patient about the noninvasive treatment, including frequency of use and goals expected, along with any other recommendations (e.g., dietary or behavioral), empowers the patient and assigns responsibility; then, at the follow-up visit, assessments and next-step decisions of the suspect tooth will be made. In this hypothetical scenario, responsibility, communication, and trust are under evaluation, and while this may ultimately result in some additional intervention, the experience (for better or worse, with the hope for the former!) will shape the clinician-patient relationship.

> **NOTE:**
>
> I have a history of dental decay and never enjoyed going to the dentist. This was magnified, as my brother, who lived with me in the same family/household, never had issues with tooth decay. This led to much confusion as to why, between the two of us, it was only I who experienced tooth decay, despite our similar diets (i.e., we ate carbohydrates regularly and happily) and hygienic behavior (twice a day brushing with an OTC fluoride toothpaste was 'sufficient'), coupled with limited dental understanding (i.e., besides 'sugar is bad for you'). Eventually, a visit to the dentist was something that seemed more bothersome and defeating, since at each visit (by multiple practitioners in different states and towns), there always seemed to be the discovery of some 'new' form of decay. Nevertheless, my view of practitioners has evolved in response to my improved understanding of dentistry and efforts to create better remineralization therapies that affect not just me but anyone with a history of tooth decay.

Interestingly, while professional cleanings can certainly help thwart disease risk factors, the tradition of infrequent visits to the dentist is not based on clinical evidence: originating from estimations of tooth failure and/or convenience of travel, especially through inclement weather and temperamental modes of transportation, six-month intervals have survived since the middle 19th century [903], while initial work with clinically applied topical fluoride solutions were given thrice annually (about every four months) [632]. Compared to the 19th and early 20th centuries, one muses that more frequent visits to the dental clinician in these modern times might be apropos (at least for patients with moderate or high risk for caries) given the relatively improved accessibility to a clinician; of course, this only works if the patient is willing to pay for these costs, even if insurance (or another third party payer) is unable or unwilling to do so.

Keeping in mind that preventive, restorative, and surgical treatment decisions often extend beyond the clinician and patient, when third-party payers (i.e., insurance) are thrown into the mix, this can certainly generate additional challenges [927]. One reason restorative intervention remains popular has to do with third-party financial incentives [902,903]. While discussions regarding insurance are outside the scope of this book, there is a tremendous unmet need to shift reimbursements and/or coverages from restorative or surgical intervention to assessments, diagnosis, prevention, and etiology [902]. Such shifts, such as the use of fluoride varnish in lieu of restorations for primary dentition, can help implement minimal intervention strategies, limit the pain and discomfort of the child, and thwart the restorative 'death spiral'—all while reducing the cost of government-sponsored expenditures [698]! As discussed in this chapter and elsewhere in this book, removal of plaque is critical to an effective minimal intervention approach. Thus, more frequent prophylaxis cleanings (i.e., more than twice annually), covered by a third-party payer, would be one example where third-party payers can help foster a healthy patient outcome through exercising preventive strategies. In fact, prevention of dental disease is a core tenet of the successful Apple Tree Dental nonprofit model that targets high-risk, high-need populations [928]. But, for minimal intervention systems to succeed on a massive scale, all stakeholders (i.e., clinician, patient, and third-party payer) need to be aligned.

Call to action: Nutritional knowledge

Dietary assessments can help the clinician shape a management plan for patients with moderate to high risks for caries and erosion. As discussed in detail in Chapter 6, the carbohydrates and acids in various foodstuffs can present demineralization risks—since digestion begins in the mouth, dental clinicians, therefore, have a vested interest in nutrition. However, nutritional expertise can help craft creative dietary strategies while maintaining a patient's philosophical preference. For example, one simple strategy for patients with higher risks for decay is implementing the use of sugar alternatives such as xylitol or erythritol in postmeal or postsnack mints or gums. This example demonstrates the importance of remineralization, a hallmark of minimal intervention strategies [772], which may help offset negative effects that can ensue from certain dietary selections. Additionally, familiarity with dietary selections that contain calcium can also provide benefits, while understanding that sour-flavored selections inherently pose greater risk for tooth demineralization.

While nutritional knowledge may be outside the limitations of dental clinicians (e.g., due to time and/or interest constraints), one solution would be to employ nutritional experts as part of the dental clinic team; or, since dental therapists can help improve access to oral care and are recommended for dental clinics [929], perhaps some might specialize in nutritional knowledge. In doing so, the dental experience is elevated and the 'dental home' can be better positioned to deliver a better oral care experience for the patient. Similarly, just as physicians can employ medical auxiliaries (e.g, physician's assistant, nurse practitioner), the addition of dental auxiliaries to a physician's clinic provides cross-expertise to help deliver overall care to the patient, thereby strengthening the 'medical home': for example, five part-time hygienists to a pediatric clinic provided care for over 2,000 children over 27 months [930]. Regardless of personnel, however, constructive conversations regarding foods and beverages should meet amenable thresholds of a patient's quality, capabilities, and pace of life.

And while soft drinks are known to be damaging to teeth (mainly due to low pH) [338], there is growing evidence that those formulated with high fructose corn syrup or artificial sweeteners pose significant health threats: distinct brain responses, increased triglyceride and fat contents, weight gain, reduced fertility, type 2 diabetes, poor cardiovascular health, and potentially higher mortality rates [327–329,931,932]. Notably, sucrose was more benign [327,329], so although it is condemned from a dental caries perspective [275,276], when compared with nonnutritive alternatives, it appears to confer less stress on systemic health [329]. And while sucrose is recognized as a casual factor in dental decay [275,276], it is challenging to remove it completely from one's diet [933]; moreover, unlike high fructose corn syrup (HFCS) [327,329] and zero-calorie sweeteners [931,932] and aside from obvious glycemic concerns for those with type 1 diabetes, there is little evidence connecting normal sucrose intake to metabolic syndrome and other risk factors for healthy adults [934,935]: for example, insulin sensitivity remained unchanged even with 25% substitution of sucrose for starch [935]. Therefore, while not beneficial for teeth, sucrose appears to be a better systemic alternative to HFCS and nonnutritive sweeteners in human nutrition. Of course, moderation of sugar intake and frequency, along with strategic dietary and behavioral choices (e.g., sequence of foods consumed, sugar substitutes, or chewing sugarless gum after a meal) can help effect favorable changes in oral pH and thwart the decay process. But if sucrose (at least 'added sucrose') is to be limited, to satisfy a 'sweet-tooth' for example, choosing plant-derived carbohydrates (which are comprised of starches or polysaccharides) in the form of fruits, vegetables, and cereals may be an excellent option [936]. Still, demineralization (e.g., due to erosion by food acids) can still occur, so plans to counter an unhealthy oral pH must be implemented from this perspective.

Call to action: Age-related health and perceptions

While systemic diseases typically predominate after maturity (e.g., baselines for high blood pressure, which is a leading global risk factor, usually begin around the age of 30 [937]), the risk for dental decay begins prior to the eruption of the first baby tooth [696]. From then on, managing oral hygiene becomes a lasting challenge, therefore necessarily becoming a habit.

Socioeconomic conditions certainly matter. Beginning in relatively young dentition (less than 18 years), the quality of oral hygiene can vary dramatically depending on socioeconomic factors: in one study, about 86% of 273 private-schooled 12- and 15-year-old children exhibited good oral health status compared to none of 331 same-aged government-schooled kids; in both instances, the girls had better oral health scores [938]. Clearly, this has implications for initiation of the restoration 'death spiral'.

The appearance of our teeth also matters. As noted in a study involving 138 soldiers (between ages of 18 and 21), the appearance of one's teeth matters considerably: while malocclusion affected about 47% of the soldiers, 72% reported being teased about their teeth, while 80% avoided smiling due to appearance of the teeth [939]. While malocclusion produces plaque traps that may be challenging to keep clean even if one is feeling self-confident, poor confidence in one's appearance may lead to extreme behavior: either neglect to properly care for the teeth due to a self-defeating, apathetic attitude or overaggressive therapy that may damage the gingiva or dentition (e.g., aggressive whitening procedures or toothbrushing). As it is said beauty resides in the eye of the beholder, this holds true for clinicians, orthodontists, and laypeople, with the latter often being most judgmental: in a separate study involving the evaluation of 41 sets of different teeth by 5 laypeople, 5 orthodontists, and 5 clinicians, laypeople were most critical and had concerns regarding tooth size, appearance, and color; orthodontists favored little gingiva display (and preferred fuller lips), while clinicians were mostly focused on tooth color [940]. Together, these data demonstrate physical aesthetics impact psychological wellness, which is an important characteristic of every human being, impacting a person's self-esteem, overall wellness, and interaction in society.

And as one progresses through life, disease risks correspondingly increase, and may become interconnected. Dental diseases, like periodontitis and caries, have been postulated as predictors for systemic diseases [941]. While this view remains debatable, ongoing research demonstrates a patient's behavior, nutrition, and overall systemic health is related to his or her oral environment [942–944]. As an example, for high-risk elderly populations living in nursing homes, a healthy oral environment appears to reduce the incidence of respiratory illnesses [944]. In general, due to the many confounders in oral and systemic diseases, any interrelationship, even if statistically significant, is relatively small [945]. Nevertheless, even without large epidemiological studies, casual factors can exist, with the relationship between periodontitis and cardiovascular disease (CVD) serving as an example: in a study with more than 9,000 American adults, those with periodontitis exhibited a 25% increase in coronary heart disease relative to those without periodontal disease [946]. And tobacco use, which affects practically all organs of the body, is known to exacerbate periodontal problems, and therefore serves to elevate CVD risk factors [947]. Finally and more recently, a review surmised the number of missing teeth appears to be linked, at least casually due to the common confounding risk factors, to increased CVD events; importantly, loss of teeth due to infection does not necessarily stave off CVD risk [948].

Final thoughts

In closing, although the dental clinician bears a tremendous and challenging responsibility, there remain opportunities to create meaningful change in the course of assessing and addressing oral health maladies during routine preventive or emergency-based appointments.

The abundance of research—both past and present—relating to dental science and amassed by dedicated and inspiring researchers around the globe is truly impressive and continues to build, shedding new information or ways of thinking with respect to assessing, probing, understanding, and managing oral health from a variety of perspectives and from experts in various fields of study, as catalogued in this book.

From factors involved in demineralization to the powerful effects of remineralization, one purpose of this book is to explore and bridge elements of preventive dentistry that can ultimately serve to support and empower the clinician and nonclinical researcher to deliver improved patient care. The body of work captured in this book supports minimally invasive strategies to manage stubborn oral health conditions, while also highlighting potential avenues of prevention-focused research and outreach. For those intrepid readers, the references in this book may be particularly useful.

Finally, the fact that dental caries continues to be a global problem confirms the challenges in managing a preventable disease. Therefore, because tooth decay, tooth erosion, hypersensitivity, and poor oral hygiene are still problematic, new approaches are needed. The perspectives shared in this book were constructed with the purpose of educating, awakening new ideas, and/or stimulating passions about a sensitive topic. As referenced throughout this book, these views are formed using scientific underpinnings and reflect my understanding, position, and personal involvement in preventive dentistry and oral health wellness.

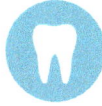

Bibliography

1. Selwitz RH, Ismail AI, Pitts NB. Dental Caries. *Lancet.* 2007; 369: 51–59.

2. Department of Health and Human Services, Office of Inspector General. Most Children with Medicaid in Four States Are Not Receiving Required Dental Services. January 2016. Report No: OEI-02-14-00490. Available from: https://oig.hhs.gov/oei/reports/oei-02-14-00490.pdf

3. The Kaiser Family Foundation. Children and Oral Health: Assessing Needs, Coverage, and Access. June 2012. Available from: http://kff.org/disparities-policy/issue-brief/children-and-oral-health-assessing-needs-coverage/

4. The Pew Charitable Trusts. A Costly Dental Destination: Hospital Care Means States Pay Dearly. February 28, 2012. Available from: http://www.pewtrusts.org/~/media/assets/2012/01/16/a-costly-dental-destination.pdf

5. American Academy of Pediatric Dentistry, Clinical Affairs Committee. Policy on Early Childhood Caries (ECC): Classifications, Consequences, and Preventive Strategies. 2016; 38(6): 52–54.

6. American Academy of Pediatric Dentistry, Clinical Affairs Committee. Guideline on Periodicity of Examination, Preventive Dental Services, Anticipatory Guidance/Counseling, and Oral Treatment for Infants, Children, and Adolescents. 2013; 37(6): 123–130.

7. Agency for Healthcare Research and Quality. Children's Dental Care: Advice and Checkups, Ages 2–17, 2008, Medical Expenditure Panel Survey. Available at: "https://meps.ahrq.gov/data_files/publications/st326/stat326.pdf" Accessed February 28, 2017.

8. Dye BA, Tan S, Smith V, Lewis BG, Barker LK, Thornton-Evans G, et al. Trends in oral health status: United States, 1988–1994 and 1999–2004. National Center for Health Statistics. *Vital Health Statistics*. 2007; 11(248): 1–92.

9. Peretz B, Ram D, Azo E, Efrat Y. Preschool caries as an indicator of future caries: a longitudinal study. *Pediatric Dentistry*. 2003; 25: 114–118.

10. McCarthy D, Radley DC, Hayes SL. Results from a Scorecard on State Health System Performance, 2015. The Commonwealth Fund. December 2015. Available from: http://www.commonwealthfund. org/publications/fund-reports/2015/dec/aiming-higher-2015

11. Miller WD. *Micro-Organisms of the Human Mouth*. Philadelphia: S.S. White Dental Mfg. Co., 1890.

12. Grine FE, Gwinnett AJ, Oaks JH. Early hominid dental pathology: interproximal caries in 1.5 million-year-old *Paranthropus Robustus* from Swartkrans. *Archives of Oral Biology*. 1990; 35(5): 381–386.

13. Shao J, Han Y, He W, Dai J, Duan Q. Dental caries in 104 skulls about 2,200 years ago from the site of the emperor Qinshihuang's mausoleum in China. *The Open Anthropology Journal*. 2010; 3: 20–24.

14. Walker MJ, Zapata J, Lombardi AV, Trinkaus E. New evidence of dental pathology in 40,000-year-old Neandertals. *Journal of Dental Research.* 2011; 90(4): 428–432.

15. Derise NL, Ritchey SJ, Furr AK. Mineral composition of normal human enamel and dentin and the relation of composition to dental caries. I. Macrominerals and comparison of methods of analyses. *Journal of Dental Research.* 1974; 53(4): 847–852.

16. Burnett FW, Zenewitz JA. Studies of the composition of teeth. VIII. The composition of human teeth. *Journal of Dental Research.* 1958; 37(4): 590–600.

17. Kolmas J, Slósarczyk A, Wojitowicz A, Kolodziejski W. Estimation of the specific surface area of apatites in human mineralized tissues using 31P MAS NMR. *Solid State Nuclear Magnetic Resonance.* 2007; 32(2): 53–58.

18. Roy S, Basu B. Mechanical and tribological characterization of human tooth. *Materials Characterization.* 2008; 59(6): 747–756.

19. Goldberg M, Kulkarni AB, Young M, Boskey A. Dentin: structure, composition and mineralization. The role of dentin ECM in dentin formation and mineralization. *Frontiers in Bioscience* (Elite Edition). 2011; 3: 711–735.

20. Palmer LC, Newcomb CJ, Kaltz SR, Spoerke ED, Stupp SI. Biomimetic systems for hydroxyapatite mineralization inspired by bone and enamel. *Chemical Reviews.* 2008; 108(11): 4754–4783.

21. Karlinsey RL, Mackey EC, Walker ER, Frederick KE. Spectroscopic evaluation of native, milled, and functionalized β-TCP seeding into dental enamel lesions. *Journal of Materials Science.* 2009; 44(18): 5013–5016.

22. LeGeros RZ. Calcium phosphates in demineralization/remineralization processes. *Journal of Clinical Dentistry.* 1999; 10: 65–73.

23. Robinson C, Shore RC, Brookes SJ, Strafford S, Wood SR, Kirkham J. The chemistry of enamel caries. *Critical Reviews in Oral Biology & Medicine.* 2000; 11(4): 481–495.

24. Bell T. "Chemical Composition of the Teeth." In: *The Anatomy, Physiology and Diseases of the Teeth.* Philadelphia: Carey and Lea, 1830.

25. Haverty D, Tofail SAM, Stanton KT, McMonagle JB. Structure and stability of hydroxyapatite: density functional calculation and Rietveld analysis. *Physical Review B.* 2005; 71(9): 9410301–941039.

26. Featherstone JDB, Goodman P, McLean JD. Electron microscope study of defect zones in dental enamel. *Journal of Ultrastructure Research.* 1979; 67(2): 117–123.

27. Yanagisawa T, Miake Y. High-resolution electron microscopy of enamel-crystal demineralization and remineralization in carious lesions. *Journal of Electron Microscopy.* 2003; 52(6): 605–613.

28. Arends J, Jongebloed WL. Ultrastructural studies of synthetic apatites. *Journal of Dental Research.* 1979; 58(Spec Iss B): 837–843.

29. Kerebel B, Daculsi G, Kerebel M. Ultrastructural studies of enamel crystallites. *Journal of Dental Research.* 1979; 58(Spec Iss B): 844–850.

30. Rönnholm E. An electron microscopic study of the amelogenesis in human teeth. I. The fine structure of the ameloblasts. *Journal of Ultrastructure Research.* 1962; 6(5): 2229–248.

31. Jongebloed WL, Molenaar I, Arends J. Morphology and size-distribution of sound and acid-treated enamel crystallites. *Calcified Tissue International.* 1975; 19(1): 109–123.

32. Applebaum E. Concerning the permeability of human enamel. *Journal of Dental Research.* 1931; 11(4): 611–620.

33. Voegel JC, Frank RM. Stages in the dissolution of human enamel crystals in dental caries. *Calcified Tissue Research.* 1977; 24(1): 19–27.

34. Featherstone JDB. Prevention and reversal of dental caries: role of low level fluoride. *Community Dentistry & Oral Epidemiology.* 1999; 27(1): 31–40.

35. Li K, Bihan M, Yoosph S, Methe BA. Analyses of the microbial diversity across the human microbiome. *PLoS ONE.* 2012; 7(6): e32118. http://journals.plos.org/plosone/article?id=10.1371/journal.pone.0032118

36. Bouslimani A, Porto C, Rath CM, Wang M, Guo Y, Gonzalez A, et al. Molecular cartography of the human skin surface in 3D. *Proceedings of the National Academy of Sciences.* 2015; 112(17): E2120-E2129.

37. Becker MR, Paster, BJ, Leys EJ, Moeschberger ML, Kenyon SG, Galvin JL, Boches SK, Dewhirst FE, Griffen AL. Molecular analysis of bacterial species associated with childhood caries. *Journal of Clinical Microbiology.* 2002; 40(3): 1047–1417.

38. Aas JA, Griffen AL, Dardis SR, Lee AM, Olsen I, Dewhirst FE, Leys EJ, Paster BJ. Bacteria of dental caries in primary and permanent teeth in children and young adults. *Journal of Clinical Microbiology.* 2008; 46(4): 1047–1417.

39. Simón-Soro A, Belda-Ferre P, Cabrera-Rubio R, Alcaraz LD, Mira A. A tissue-dependent hypothesis of dental caries. *Caries Research.* 2013; 47(6): 591–600.

40. Peterson SN, Snesrud E, Liu J, Ong AC, Kilian M, Schork NJ, Bretz W. The dental plaque microbiome in health and disease. *PLoS ONE.* 2013; 8(3): e58487. http://journals.plos.org/plosone/article?id=10.1371/journal.pone.0058487

41. Zaura E, Keijser BJF, Huse SM, Crielaard W. Defining the healthy "core microbiome" of oral microbial communities. *BMC Microbiology.* 2009; 9: 259. https://bmcmicrobiol.biomedcentral.com/articles/10.1186/1471-2180-9-259

42. Simón-Soro A, Tomás I, Cabrera-Rubio R, Catalan MD, Nyvad B, Mira A. Microbial geography of the oral cavity. *Journal of Dental Research*. 2013; 92(7): 616–621.

43. Johansson I, Witkowska E, Kaveh B, Holgerson PL, Tanner ACR. The microbiome in populations with a low and high prevalence of caries. *Journal of Dental Research*. 2013; 95(1): 80–86.

44. Loesche WJ. Role of *Streptococcus mutans* in human dental decay. *Microbiological Reviews*. 1986; 50(4): 535–380.

45. Takahashi N. Oral microbiome metabolism: from "Who are they?" to "What are they doing?." *Journal of Dental Research*. 2016; 94(12); 1628–1637.

46. Wang B-Y, Wu J, Lamont RJ, Lin X, Xie H. Negative correlation of distributions of *Streptococcus cristatus* and *Porphyromonas gingivalis* in subgingival plaque. *Journal of Clinical Microbiology*. 2009; 47(12): 3902–3906.

47. Wang Q, Luo Y, Shao Q, Kinlock BL, Wang C, Hildreth JEK, Xie H, Liu B. Heat-stable molecule derived from *Streptococcus cristatus* induces APOBEC3 expression and inhibits HIV-1 replication. *PLoS ONE*. 2014; 9(8): e106078. http://journals.plos.org/plosone/article/authors?id=10.1371/journal.pone.0106078

48. Pasteur L, Faulkner F, Robb DC. "The Physiological Theory of Fermentation." In: *Studies on Fermentation: The Diseases of Beer, Their Causes, and the Means of Preventing Them*. London: MacMillan & Co., 1879.

49. Leeuwenhoek, A. Microscopical observations, about Animals in the scurf of the Teeth, the Substance call'd Worms in the Nose, the Cuticula consisting of Scales. *Philosophical Transactions*. 1684; 14: 568–577.

50. Bibby BG, Van Kesteren M. The effect of fluorine on mouth bacteria. *Journal of Dental Research*. 1940; 19(4): 391–402.

51. Takahashi N, Nyvad B. The role of bacteria in the caries process: ecological perspectives. *Journal of Dental Research.* 2011; 90(3): 294–303.

52. Wood WR, Kirkham J, Marsh PD, Shore RC, Nattress B, Robinson C. Architecture of intact natural human plaque biofilms studied by confocal laser scanning microscopy. *Journal of Dental Research.* 2000; 79(1): 21–27.

53. Zaura-Arite E, van Marle J, ten Cate JM. Confocal microscopy study of undisturbed and chlorhexidine-treated dental biofilm. *Journal of Dental Research.* 2001; 80(5): 1436–1440.

54. Zijnge V, van Leeuwen BM, Degener JE, Abbas F, Thurnheer T, Gmür R, Harmsen HJM. Oral biofilm architecture on natural teeth. *PLoS ONE.* 2010; 5(2): e9321. doi: http://journals.plos.org/plosone/article?id=10.1371/journal.pone.0009321

55. Niven CF, Smiley KL, Sherman JM. The production of large amounts of a polysaccharid by *Streptococcus salivarius. Journal of Bacteriology.* 1941; 41(4): 479–484.

56. Wood JM, Critchley P. The extracellular polysaccharide produced from sucrose by a cariogenic *Streptococcus. Archives of Oral Biology.* 1966; 11(10): 1039–1042.

57. Treasure P. Effects of fluoride, lithium and strontium on extracellular polysaccharide production by *Steptococcus mutans* and *Actinomyces viscosus. Journal of Dental Research.* 1981; 60(3): 1601–1610.

58. Gibbons RJ. Formation and significant of bacterial polysaccharides in caries etiology. *Caries Research.* 1968; 2(2): 164–171.

59. Marsh PD, Keevil CW, Ellwood DC. Relationship of bioenergetics processes to the pathogenic properties of oral bacteria. *Journal of Dental Research.* 1984; 63(3): 401–406.

60. Luoma H, Tuompo H. The relationship between sugar metabolism and potassium translocation by the caries-inducing Streptococci and the inhibitory role of fluoride. *Archives of Oral Biology.* 1975; 20(11): 947–755.

61. Wegman MR, Eisenberg AD, Curzon MEJ, Handelman SL. Effects of fluoride, lithium and strontium on intracellular poly-saccharide accumulation in *S. mutans* and *A. viscosus. Journal of Dental Research.* 1984; 63(9): 1126–1129.

62. Meckel AH. The nature and importance of organic deposits on dental enamel. *Caries Research.* 1968; 2(2): 104–114.

63. Hannig M, Fiebiger M, Güntzer M, Döbert A, Zimehl R, Nekrashevych Y. Protective effect of the *in situ* formed short-term salivary pellicle. *Archives of Oral Biology.* 2004; 49(11): 903–910.

64. Mays TD, Holdeman LV, Moore WEC, Rogosa M, Johnson JL. Taxonomy of the genus *Veillonella* Prévot. *International Journal of Systematic Bacteriology.* 1982; 32(1): 28–36.

65. Arif N, Sheehy EC, Do T, Beighton D. Diversity of *Veillonella* spp. from sound and carious sites in children. *Journal of Dental Research.* 2008; 87(3): 278–282.

66. Kleinberg I. A mixed-bacteria ecological approach to understanding the role of the oral bacteria in dental caries causation: an alternative to *Streptococcus mutans* and the specific-plaque hypothesis. *Critical Reviews in Oral Biology & Medicine.* 2002; 13(2): 108–125.

67. Marsh PD. Dental plaque as a biofilm and a microbial community—implications for health and disease. *BMC Oral Health.* 2006; 6(Suppl 1): S14. https://www.ncbi.nlm.nih.gov/pmc/articles/PMC2147593/

68. Li T, Bratt P, Jonsson AP, Ryberg M, Johansson I, Griffiths WJ, Bergman T, Strömberg N. Possible release of an ArgGlyArgProGln pentapeptide with innate immunity properties from acidic

proline-rich proteins by proteolytic activity in commensal *Streptococcus* and *Actinomyces* species. *Infection and Immunity*. 2000; 68(9): 5425–5429.

69. Jurtshuk P Jr. 'Chapter 4: Bacterial Metabolism.' In: Baron S, editor. *Medical Microbiology. 4th Edition*. Galveston (Texas): University of Texas Medical Branch at Galveston; 1996. Available from: https://www.ncbi.nlm.nih.gov/books/NBK7919/.

70. Huang X, Schulte RM, Burne RA, Nascimento MM. Characterization of the arginolytic microflora provides insights into pH homeostasis in human oral biofilms. *Caries Research*. 2015; 49(2): 165–176.

71. Nascimento MM, Liu y, Kalra R, Perry S, Adewumi A, Xu X, Primosch RE, Burne RA. Oral arginine metabolism may decrease the risk for dental caries in children. *Journal of Dental Research*. 2013; 92(7): 604–608.

72. Koopman, JE, Hoogenkamp MA, Buijs MJ, Brandt BW, Keijser BJF, Crielaard W, ten Cate JM, Zaura E. Changes in the oral ecosystem induced by the use of 8% arginine toothpaste. *Archives of Oral Biology*. 2017; 73: 79–87.

73. Ruan Y, Shen L, Zou Y, Qi Z, Yin J, Jiang J, Guo L, He L, Chen Z, Tang Z, Qin S. Comparative genome analysis of *Prevotella intermedia* strain isolated from infected root canal reveals features related to pathogenicity and adaptation. *BMC Genomics*. 2015; 16(1): 122. https://bmcgenomics.biomedcentral.com/articles/10.1186/s12864-015-1272-3

74. Ajdić D, McShan WM, McLaughlin RE, Savić G, Chang J, Carson MB, Primeaux C, Tian R, Kenton S, Jia H, Lin s, Qian Y, Li S, Zhu H, Naja R, Lai H, White J, Roe BA, Ferretti JJ. Genome sequence of Streptococcus mutans UA159, a cariogenic dental pathogen. *Proceedings of the National Academy of Sciences*. 2002; 99(2): 14434–14439. http://www.pnas.org/content/99/22/14434.long

75. Griswold AR, Chen Y-YM, Burne RA. Analysis of an agmatine deiminase gene cluster in *Streptococcus mutans* UA159. *Journal of Bacteriology*. 2004; 186(6): 1902–1904.

76. Youngburg GE. Salivary ammonia and its relation to dental caries. *Journal of Dental Research*. 1935; 15(5): 247–263.

77. Grove CT, Grove CJ. The biochemical aspect of dental caries. *Dental Cosmos*. 1934; 76(10): 1029–1036.

78. Henschel CJ. "Dentifrice." US Patent 2,542,518. Issued February 20, 1951.

79. Wach EC. "Dentifrice." US Patent 2,542,886. Issued February 20, 1951.

80. Kesel RB. "Ammoniated Dentifrice." US Patent 2,622,058. Issued December 16, 1952.

81. Chernausek DS, Mitchel DF. Ammoniated dentifrices and hamster caries: II. The effectiveness of brushing the teeth with a control and an ammoniated dentifrice. *Journal of Dental Research*. 1951; 30(3): 393–398.

82. Davies GN, King RM. The effectiveness of an ammonium ion toothpowder in the control of dental caries. *Journal of Dental Research*. 1951; 30(5): 645–655.

83. Smith DJ. Prospects in caries vaccine development. *Journal of Dental Research*. 2012; 91(3): 225–226.

84. Vratsanos SM, Mandel ID. Comparative plaque acidogenesis of caries-resistant vs. caries-susceptible adults. *Journal of Dental Research*. 1982; 61(3): 465–468.

85. Abelson DC, Mandel ID. The effect of saliva on plaque pH in vivo. *Journal of Dental Research*. 1981; 60(9): 1634–1638.

86. Koulourides T, Cueto H, Pigman W. Rehardening of softened enamel surfaces of human teeth by solutions of calcium phosphates. *Nature*. 1961; 189: 226–227.

87. Head J. A study of saliva and its action on tooth enamel in reference to its hardening and softening. *Journal of the American Medical Association*. 1912; 59(24): 2118–2122.

88. Mandel I. The functions of saliva. *Journal of Dental Research*. 1987; 66 (Spec Iss): 623–627.

89. Amaechi BT, Higham SM. In vitro remineralisation of eroded enamel lesions by saliva. *Journal of Dentistry*. 2001; 29(5): 371–376.

90. Stookey GK. The effect of saliva on dental caries. *Journal of the American Dental Association*. 2008; 139(5 suppl): 11S-17S.

91. M Edgar, C Dawes, & D O'Mullane (Eds.). In: *Saliva and Oral Health, 3rd Edition*. London: British Dental Association, 2004.

92. Ekström J, Khosravani N, Castagnola M, Messana I. "Saliva and the Control of Its Secretion." O Ekberg (Ed.), In: *Dysphagia: Diagnosis and Treatment*. Berlin: Springer-Verlag, 2012, 19–47.

93. Brown LR, Dreizen S, Handler S, Johnston DA. Effects of xerostomia on oral microbes. *Journal of Dental Research*. 1975; 54(4): 740–750.

94. Ship JA. "Xerostomia: aetiology, diagnosis, management and clinical implications." M Edgar, C Dawes, & D O'Mullane (Eds.), In: *Saliva and Oral Health, 3rd Edition*. London: British Dental Association, 2004, 50–69.

95. Ben-Aryeh H, Roll N, Lahav M, Dlin R, Hanne-Paparo N, Szargel R, Shein-Orr C, Laufer D. Effect of exercise on salivary composition and cortisol in serum and saliva in man. *Journal of Dental Research*. 1989; 68(11): 1495–1497.

96. Dawes C. The effects of exercise on protein and electrolyte secretion in parotid saliva. *Journal of Physiology*. 1981; 320: 139–148.

97. Ligtenberg AJM, Liem EHS, Brand HS, Veerman ECI. The effect of exercise on salivary viscosity. *Diagnostics*. 2016; 6(4): 40.

98. Blannin AK, Robson PJ, Walsh NP, Clark AM, Glennon L, Gleeson M. The effect of exercising to exhaustion at different intensities on saliva immunoglobulin A, protein and electrolyte secretion. *International Journal of Sports Medicine*. 1998; 19(8): 547–552.

99. Gleeson M, Pyne DB. Exercise effects on mucosal immunity. *Immunology and Cell Biology*. 2000; 78: 536–544.

100. Cowman RA, Baron SS, Glassman AH, Davis ME, Strosberg AM. Changes in protein composition of saliva from radiation-induced xerostomia patients and its effect on growth of oral Streptococci. *Journal of Dental Research*. 1983; 62(3): 336–340.

101. Tenovuo J. "Protective functions of saliva." M Edgar, C Dawes, & D O'Mullane (Eds.), In: *Saliva and Oral Health*, 3rd Edition. London: British Dental Association, 2004, 103–119.

102. Applebaum E. The radiopaque surface layer of enamel and caries. *Journal of Dental Research*. 1940; 19(1): 42–46.

103. Whelton H. "Introduction: anatomy and physiology of salivary glands." M Edgar, C Dawes, & D O'Mullane (Eds.), In: *Saliva and Oral Health*, 3rd Edition. London: British Dental Association, 2004, 1–13.

104. Ten Cate JM. "The role of saliva in mineral equilibria—caries, erosion and calculus formation." M Edgar, C Dawes, & D O'Mullane (Eds.), In: *Saliva and Oral Health*, 3rd Edition. London: British Dental Association, 2004, 120–135.

105. Anderson BG. Clinical study of arresting dental caries. *Journal of Dental Research*. 1938; 17(6): 443–452.

106. Backer Dirks O. Posteruptive changes in dental enamel. *Journal of Dental Research*. 1966; 45(3): 503–511.

107. Moussa SA, Gobran HG, Salem MA, Barkat IF. Dental biofilm and saliva biochemical composition changes in your orthodontic patients. *Journal of Dentistry, Oral Disorders & Therapy*. 2017; 5(1): 1–5.

108. O'Reilly MM, Featherstone JDB. Demineralization and reminer-alization around orthodontic appliances: an in vivo study. *American Journal of Orthodontics & Dentofacial Orthopedics.* 1987; 92(1): 33–40.

109. Enaia M, Bock N, Ruf S. White-spot lesions during multibracket appliance treatment: A challenge for clinical excellence. *American Journal of Orthodontics and Dentofacial Orthopedics.* 2011; 140(1): e17-e24.

110. Haikel Y, Frank RM, Voegel JC. Scanning electron microscopy of the human enamel surface layer of incipient carious lesions. *Caries Research.* 1983; 17(1): 1–13.

111. Goulet D, Brudevold F, Tehrani A, Attarzadeh F. Sugar clearance from saliva and intra-oral spaces. *Journal of Dental Research.* 1985; 64(3): 411–415.

112. Zachrisson BJ, Nyøygaard L, Mobarak K. Dental health assessed more than 10 years after interproximal enamel reduction of mandibular anterior teeth. *American Journal of Orthodontics & Dentofacial Orthopedics.* 2007; 131(2): 162–169.

113. Siddiqui S, Anderson P, Al-Jawad M. Recovery of crystallographic texture in remineralized dental enamel. *PLoS ONE.* 2014; 9(10): e108879. http://journals.plos.org/plosone/article?id=10.1371/journal.pone.0108879

114. Asaizumi M, Yagi N, Aoyama K, Kato T, Kuga T, Oode N, Oda T, Sakurada T, Nagase S, Tabara T, Karlinsey RL. Observations of enamel microstructure in incipient lesions remineralized by NaF dentifrices. *Dental Research Management.* 2017; 2(1): 20–30. doi: http://edelweisspublications.com/edelweiss/article/Observations-Enamel-Microstructure-Incipient-Lesions-Remineralized-NaF-Dentifrices.pdf

115. Bottenberg P, Jacquet W, Behrens C, Stachniss V, Jablonski-Momeni A. Comparison of occlusal caries detection using the

ICDAS criteria on extracted teeth or their photographs. *BMC Oral Health.* 2016; 16(1): 93. https://bmcoralhealth.biomedcentral.com/articles/10.1186/s12903-016-0291-z

116. Hu J C-C, Hu Y, Smith CE, McKee MD, Wright JT, Yamakoshi Y, Papagerakis P, Hunter GK, Feng JQ, Yamakoshi F, Simmer JP. Enamel defects and ameloblast-specific expression in *enam* knock-out/*lacZ* knock-in mice. *Journal of Biological Chemistry.* 2008; 283(16): 10858–10871.

117. Shellis RP. Relationship between human enamel structure and the formation of caries-like lesions *in vitro*. *Archives of Oral Biology.* 1984; 29(12): 975–981.

118. Hamilton WJ, Judd G, Ansell GS. Ultrastructure of human enamel specimens prepared by ion micromilling. *Journal of Dental Research.* 1973; 52(4): 703–709.

119. Daculsi G, Kerebel B. High-resolution electron microscope study of human enamel crystallites: size, shape, and growth. *Journal of Ultrastructure Research.* 1978; 65(2): 163–172.

120. Orams HJ, Zybert JJ, Phakey PP, Rachinger WA. Ultrastructural study of human dental enamel using selected-area argon-ion-beam thinning. *Archives of Oral Biology.* 1976; 21(11): 663–675.

121. Orams HJ, Phakey PP, Rachinger WA, Zybert JJ. Ultrastructural changes in the translucent and dark zones of early enamel caries. *Journal of Oral Pathology.* 1980; 9(1): 54–61.

122. Rönnholm E. The amelogenesis of human teeth as revealed by electron microscopy. II. The development of enamel crystallites. *Journal of Ultrastructure Research.* 1962; 6(3–4): 249–303.

123. Hallsworth AS, Robinson C, Weatherell JA. Mineral and magnesium distribution within the approximal carious lesion of dental enamel. *Caries Research.* 1972; 6(2): 156–168.

124. Dibdin GH. The internal surface and pore structure of enamel. *Journal of Dental Research.* 1969; 48(Suppl 5): 771–776.

125. Shellis RP. A scanning electron-microscopic study of solubility variations in human enamel and dentin. *Archives of Oral Biology.* 1996; 41(5): 473–484.

126. Arends J, Dijkman T, Christoffersen J. Average mineral loss in dental enamel during demineralization. *Caries Research.* 1987; 21(3): 249–254.

127. Little MF, Casciani FS. The nature of water in sound human enamel. A preliminary study. *Archives of Oral Biology.* 1966; 11(6): 565–571.

128. Zahradnik RT, Moreno EC. Structural features of human dental enamel as revealed by isothermal water vapour sorption. *Archives of Oral Biology.* 1975; 20(5–6): 317–325.

129. Darling AI, Mortimer KV, Poole DFG, Ollis WD. Molecular sieve behaviour of normal and carious human dental enamel. *Archives of Oral Biology.* 1961; 5(12): 251–273.

130. Moreno EC, Zahradnik RT. The pore structure of human dental enamel. *Archives of Oral Biology.* 1973; 18(8): 1063–1068.

131. Dibdin GH, Poole DFG. Surface area and pore size analysis for human enamel and dentin by water vapour sorption. *Archives of Oral Biology.* 1982; 27(3): 235–241.

132. Dibdin GH. The water in human dental enamel and its diffusional exchange measured by clearance of tritiated water from enamel slabs of varying thickness. *Caries Research.* 1993; 27(2): 81–86.

133. Weatherell JA, Weidmann SM, Eyre DR. Histological appearance and chemical composition of enamel protein from mature human molars. *Caries Research.* 1968; 2(4): 281–293.

134. Burnett FW, Zenewitz JA. Studies of the composition of teeth. VII. The moisture content of calcified tooth tissues. *Journal of Dental Research.* 1958; 37(4): 581–589.

135. Dibdin GH. The stability of water in human dental enamel studied by proton nuclear magnetic resonance. *Archives of Oral Biology.* 1972; 17(3): 433–437.

136. Peigney A, Laurent C, Dumortier O, Rousset A. Carbon nanotubes-Fe-alumina nanocomposites. Part I: influence of the Fe content on the synthesis of powders. *Journal of the European Ceramic Society.* 1998; 18(14): 1995–2004.

137. Ludwig TG, Bibby BG. Acid production from different carbohydrate foods in plaque and saliva. *Journal of Dental Research.* 1957; 36(1): 56–60.

138. Lussi A, Carvalho TS. "Erosive tooth wear: a multifactorial condition of growing concern and increasing knowledge." A Lussi & C Ganss (Eds.), In: *Erosive Tooth Wear: A Phenomenon of Clinical Significance.* Basel: Karger Publishers, 2014, Vol 25, 1–15.

139. Thaper R, Karlinsey RL. Clinical observations on the remineralization of Stage 1 enamel caries lesions using a tray-based protocol: a case report. *International Journal of Dentistry and Oral Health.* 2015; 2(1): 1–4. doi: https://www.sciforschenonline.org/journals/dentistry/article-data/IJDOH-1-151/IJDOH-1-151.pdf

140. Applebaum E, Hollander R, Bödecker CF. Normal and pathological variations in calcifications of teeth as shown by the use of soft X-rays. *Dental Cosmos.* 1933; 75(11): 1097–1105.

141. Gomez J. Detection and diagnosis of the early caries lesion. *BMC Oral Health.* 2015; 15(Suppl 1): S3. doi: http://bmcoralhealth.biomedcentral.com/articles/10.1186/1472-6831-15-S1-S3

142. Crabb HSM. Structural patterns in human dental enamel revealed by the use of microradiography in conjunction with two dimensional microdensitometry. *Caries Research.* 1968; 2(3): 235–252.

143. Ripa LW. The histology of the early carious lesion in primary teeth with special reference to a "prismless" outer layer of primary enamel. *Journal of Dental Research.* 1966; 45(1): 5–11.

144. White DJ. Use of synthetic polymer gels for artificial carious lesion preparation. *Caries Research.* 1987; 21(3): 228–242.

145. Pearce EIF. A microradiographic and chemical comparison of in vitro systems for the simulation of incipient caries in abraded bovine enamel. *Journal of Dental Research.* 1983; 62(9): 969–974.

146. White DJ. Reactivity of fluoride dentifrices with artificial caries. I. Effects on early lesions: F uptake, surface hardening and remineralization. *Caries Research.* 1987; 21(2): 126–140.

147. White DJ. Reactivity of fluoride dentifrices with artificial caries. II. Effects on subsurface lesions: F uptake, surface hardening and remineralization. *Caries Research.* 1987; 22(1): 27–36.

148. White DJ. The application of in vitro models to research on demineralization and remineralization of the teeth. *Advances in Dental Research.* 1995; 9(3): 175–193.

149. Food and Drug Administration. Anticaries drug products for over-the-counter human use; final monograph. *Federal Register.* 1995; 60(194): 52474–52510.

150. Xue J, Zhang L, Zou L, Liao Y, Li J, Xiao L, Li W. High-resolution X-ray microdiffraction analysis of natural teeth. *Journal of Synchrotron Radiation.* 2008; 15(3): 235–238.

151. Yagi N, Ohta N, Matsuo T, Tanaka T, Terada Y, Kamasaka H, To-o K, Kometani T, Kuriki T. Evaluation of enamel crystallites in subsurface lesion by microbeam X-ray diffraction. *Journal of Synchrotron Radiation.* 2009; 16(3); 398–404.

152. Tanaka T, Yagi N, Ohta, T, Matsuo Y, Terada H, Kamasaka K, To-o K, Kometani T, Kuriki T. Evaluation of the distribution

and orientation of remineralized enamel crystallites in subsurface lesions by X-ray diffraction. *Caries Research.* 2010; 44(3): 253–259.

153. Ciccariello S, Goodisman J, Brumberger H. On the Porod law. *Journal of Applied Crystallography.* 1988; 21(2): 117–128.

154. Ciccariello S, Sobry R. Small-angle scattering intensity behaviours of cylindrical, spherical and planar lamellae. *Journal of Applied Crystallography.* 1999; 32(5): 892–901.

155. Fischer S, Diesner T, Rieger B, Marti O. Simulating the evaluating small-angle X-ray scattering of micro-voids in polypropylene during mechanical deformation. *Journal of Applied Crystallography.* 2010; 43(3): 603–610.

156. Featherstone JDB, ten Cate JM, Shariati M, Arends J. Comparison of artificial caries-like lesions by quantitative microradiography and microhardness profiles. *Caries Research.* 1983; 17(5): 385–391.

157. Kielbassa AM, Wrbas K-T, Schulte-Mönting J, Hellwig E. Correlation of transversal microradiography and microhardness on *in situ*-induced demineralization in irradiated and nonirradiated human dental enamel. *Archives of Oral Biology.* 1999; 44(3): 243–251.

158. Magalhães AC, Rios D, Moino AL, Wiegand A, Attin T, Buzalaf MAR. Effect of difference concentrations of fluoride in dentifrices on dentin erosion subjected or not to abrasion *in situ/ex vivo. Caries Research.* 2008; 42(2): 112–116.

159. Karlinsey RL, Mackey AC, Blanken DD, Schwandt CS. Remineralization of eroded enamel lesions by simulated saliva *in vitro. The Open Dentistry Journal.* 2012; 6(1): 170–176. doi: https://benthamopen.com/FULLTEXT/TODENTJ-6-170

160. Amaechi BT, Karthikeyan R, Mensinkai PK, Najibfard K, Mackey AC, Karlinsey, RL. Remineralization of eroded enamel by a NaF rinse contain a novel calcium phosphate agent in an *in situ* model:

a pilot study. *Clinical, Cosmetic and Investigational Dentistry.* 2010; 2: 93–100. doi: https://www.dovepress.com/remineralization-of-eroded-enamel-by-a-naf-rinse-containing-a-novel-ca-peer-reviewed-article-CCIDE

161. Mathews MS, Amaechi BT, Ramalingam K, Ccahuana-Vasquez RA, Chedjieu IP, Mackey AC, Karlinsey RL. *In situ* remineralisation of eroded enamel lesions by NaF rinses. *Archives of Oral Biology.* 2012; 57(5): 525–530.

162. Meurman JH, Frank RM. Progression and surface ultrastructure of in vitro caused erosive lesions in human and bovine enamel. *Caries Research.* 1991; 25(2): 81–87.

163. Humphrey LT, De Groote I, Morales J, Barton N, Collcutt S, Ramsey CB, Bouzouggar A. Earliest evidence for caries and exploitation of starchy plant foods in Pleistocene hunter-gatherers from Morocco. *Proceedings of the National Academy of Sciences.* 2014; 111(3): 954–959.

164. Lussi A, Jaeggi T, Zero D. The role of diet in the aetiology of dental erosion. *Caries Research.* 2004; 38(Suppl 1): 34–44.

165. Bartlett DW. The role of erosion in tooth wear: aetiology, prevention and management. *International Dental Journal.* 2005; 55(4): 277–284.

166. Uhlen M-M, Tveit AB, Stenhagen KR, Mulic A. Self-induced vomiting and dental erosion—a clinical study. *BMC Oral Health.* 2014: 14(1): 92. doi: https://bmcoralhealth.biomedcentral.com/articles/10.1186/1472-6831-14-92

167. Saeves R, Espelid I, Storhaug K, Sandvik L, Nordgarden H. Severe tooth wear in Prader-Willi syndrome. A case-control study. *BMC Oral Health.* 2012; 21(1): 12. doi: https://bmcoralhealth.biomedcentral.com/articles/10.1186/1472-6831-12-12

168. Geurtsen W. Rapid general dental erosion by gas-chlorinated swimming pool water. Review of the literature and case report. *American Journal of Dentistry.* 2000; 13(6): 291–293.

169. Mulic A, Tveit AB, Songe D, Sivertsen H, Skaare AB. Dental erosive wear and salivary flow rate in physically active young adults. *BMC Oral Health.* 2012; 12(1): 8. doi: https://bmcoralhealth. biomedcentral.com/articles/10.1186/1472-6831-12-8

170. Carvalho TS, Baumann T, Lussi A. Does erosion progress differently on teeth already presenting clinical signs of erosive tooth wear than on sound teeth? An in vitro pilot trial. *BMC Oral Health.* 2017; 17(1): 14. doi: https://bmcoralhealth.biomedcentral.com/ articles/10.1186/s12903-016-0231-y

171. Kopychka-Kedzierawski DT, Meyerowitz C, Litaker MS, Chonowski S, Heft MW, Gordan VV, Yardic RL, Madden TE, Reyes SC, Gilbert GH, and National Dental PBRN Collaborative Group. Management of dentin hypersensitivity by National Dental Practice-Based Research Network practitioners: results from a questionnaire administered prior to initiation of a clinical study on this topic. *BMC Oral Health.* 2017; 17(1): 41. doi: https://bmcoralhealth.biomedcentral.com/articles/10.1186/ s12903-017-0334-0

172. West N, Seong J, Davies M. "Dentine hypersensitivity." A Lussi & C Ganss (Eds.), In: *Erosive Tooth Wear: A Phenomenon of Clinical Significance.* Basel: Karger Publishers, 2014, Vol 25, 108–122.

173. Addy M, Smith SR. Dentin Hypersensitivity: An overview on which to base tubule occlusion as a management concept. *Journal of Clinical Dentistry.* 2010; 21(Spec Iss): 25–30.

174. Gillam DG, Mordan NJ, Newman HN. The dentin disc surface: A plausible model for dentin physiology and dentin sensitivity evaluation. *Advances in Dental Research.* 1997; 11(4): 487–501.

175. Pashley DH. Dynamics of the pulpo-dentin complex. *Critical Reviews in Oral Biology and Medicine.* 1996; 7(2): 104–133.

176. West NX, Lussi A, Seong J, Hellwig E. Dentin hypersensitivity: pain mechanisms and aetiology of exposed cervical dentin. *Clinical Oral Investigations.* 2013; 17(Suppl 1): S9-S19.

177. Goldberg M, Kulkarni AB, Young M, Boskey A. Dentin: Structure, Composition and Mineralization. *Frontiers in Bioscience.* 2011; 1(3): 711–735.

178. Pashley DH. Dentin permeability, dentin sensitivity, and treatment through tubule occlusion. *Journal of Endodontics.* 1986; 12(10): 465–474.

179. Brännström M, Lindén LÅ, Åström A. They hydrodynamics of the dental tubule and of pulp fluid. A discussion of its significance in relation to dentinal sensitivity. *Caries Research.* 1967; 1(4): 310–317.

180. Pashley DH, Tay FR, Haywood VB, Collins MA, Drisko CL. Dentin hypersensitivity: Consensus-based recommendations for the diagnosis and management of dentin hypersensitivity. *Inside Dentistry.* 2008; 4(9): 1–40.

181. Asaizumi M, Kato T, Kuga T, Oode N, Oda T, Sakurada T, Thomson K, Tabara T, Karlinsey RL. Submicron X-ray computed tomography of human dentin treated with topical fluoride modalities. *EC Dental Science.* 2016; 5(2): 992–1017. doi: https://www.ecronicon.com/ecde/pdf/ECDE-05-0000147.pdf

182. Asaizumi A. "BL47XU Spring-8 Synchrotron Radiation X-ray Submicron CT 1.1." 2015, https://youtu.be/8w-HjM616fI.

183. Karlinsey RL, Mackey AC, Schwandt CS. Effects on dentin treated with eluted multi-mineral varnish *in vitro. The Open Dentistry Journal.* 2012; 6(1): 157–163. doi: https://benthamopen.com/FULLTEXT/TODENTJ-6-157.

DEMIN/REMIN IN PREVENTIVE DENTISTRY

184. Lefèvre R, Frank RM, Voegel JC. The study of human dentine with secondary ion microscopy and electron diffraction. *Calcified Tissue International.* 1976; 19(1): 251–261.

185. Mjör IA, Nordahl I. The density and branching of dentinal tubules in human teeth. *Archives of Oral Biology.* 1996; 41(5): 401–412.

186. Willmott NS, Wong FSL, Davis GR. An X-ray microtomography study on the mineral concentration of carious dentine removed during cavity preparation in deciduous molars. *Caries Research.* 2007; 41(2): 129–134.

187. Ahmed M, Davis GR, Wong FSL. An X-ray microtomography study to evaluate the efficacies of caries removal in primary molars by hand excavation and chemo-mechanical technique. *Caries Research.* 2012; 46(6): 561–567.

188. Gysi A. An attempt to explain the sensitiveness of dentine. *British Journal of Dental Science.* 1900; 785(43): 865–868.

189. Theuns HM, Van Dijk JWE, Jongebloed WL, Groeneveld A. The mineral content of human enamel studied by polarizing microscopy, microradiography and scanning electron microscopy. *Archives of Oral Biology.* 1983; 28(9): 797–803.

190. Burke EJ, Moreno EC. Diffusion fluxes of tritiated water across human enamel membranes. *Archives of Oral Biology.* 1975; 20(5–6): 327–332.

191. Arends J, Jongebloed WL, Schuthof J. Crystallite diameters of enamel near the anatomical surface. *Caries Research.* 1983; 17(2): 97–105.

192. Shellis RP. Variations in growth of the enamel crown in human teeth and a possible relationship between growth and enamel structure. *Archives of Oral Biology.* 1984; 29(9): 697–705.

193. Palamara J, Phakey PP, Rachinger WA, Orams HJ. Electron microscopy of surface enamel of human unerupted and erupted teeth. *Archives of Oral Biology*. 1980; 25(11–12): 715–725.

194. Sakae T. Variations in dental enamel crystallites and microstructure. *Journal of Oral Biosciences*. 2006; 48(2): 85–93.

195. Hallsworth AS, Weatherell JA, Robinson C. Loss of carbonate during the first stages of enamel caries. *Caries Research*. 1972; 7(4): 345–348.

196. Vieira AR, Gibson CW, Deeley K, Xue H, Li Y. Weaker dental enamel explains dental decay. *PLoS ONE*. 2015; 10(4): http://journals.plos.org/plosone/article?id=10.1371/journal.pone.0124236

197. Eisenburger M, Shellis RP, Addy M. Scanning electron microscopy of softened enamel. *Caries Research*. 2004; 38(1): 67–74.

198. Dawes C. Salivary flow patterns and the health of hard and soft oral tissues. *Journal of the American Dental Association*. 2008; 139: 18S-24S.

199. Hara AT, Zero DT. "The potential of saliva in protecting against dental erosion." A Lussi & C Ganss (Eds.), In: *Erosive Tooth Wear: A Phenomenon of Clinical Significance*. Basel: Karger Publishers, 2014, Vol 25, 197–205.

200. Eanes ED, Gillessen IH, Posner AS. Intermediate states in the precipitation of hydroxyapatite. *Nature*. 1965; 208(5008): 365–367.

201. Zhang TH, Liu XY. Nucleation: what happens at the initial stage? *Angewandte Chemie International Edition*. 2009; 48(7): 1308–1312.

202. Koulourides TA, Buonocore MG. Effect of organic ions on solubility of enamel and dentin in acid buffers. *Journal of Dental Research*. 1961; 40(3): 578–593.

203. Sperber GH, Buonocore MG. Effect of different acids on character of demineralization of enamel surfaces. *Journal of Dental Research.* 1963; 42(2): 707–723.

204. Gray JA. Kinetics of the dissolution of human dental enamel in acid. *Journal of Dental Research.* 1962; 41(3): 633–645.

205. Gray JA. Kinetics of enamel dissolution during formation of incipient caries-like lesions. *Archives of Oral Biology.* 1966; 11(4): 397–421.

206. Featherstone JDB, Duncan JF, Cutress TW. A mechanism for dental caries based on chemical processes and diffusion phenomena during in vitro caries simulation on human tooth enamel. *Archives of Oral Biology.* 1979; 24 (2): 101–112.

207. Featherstone JDB, Rodgers BE. Effect of acetic, lactic and other organic acids on the formation of artificial carious lesions. *Caries Research.* 1981; 15(5): 377–385.

208. Geddes DAM, Weetman, Featherstone JDB. Preferential loss of acetic acid from plaque fermentation in the presence of enamel. *Caries Research.* 1984; 18(5): 430–433.

209. Head J. Enamel softening and rehardening as a factor in erosion. *Dental Cosmos.* 1910; 52(1): 46–48.

210. *CRC Handbook of Chemistry and Physics, 84th ed.* DR Lide (Ed.). Boca Raton: CRC Press LLC, 2003.

211. Housecroft CE, Sharpe AG. *Inorganic Chemistry, 2nd edition.* London: Pearson, 2005.

212. Greenwald I. The dissociation of some calcium salts. *Journal of Biological Chemistry.* 1938; 124(2): 437–452.

213. Daniele PG, Foti C, Gianguzza A, Prenesti E, Sammartano S. Weak alkali and alkaline earth metal complexes of low molecular weight ligands in aqueous solution. *Coordination Chemistry Reviews.* 2008; 252 (10): 1093–1107.

214. Budz JA, Lo Re M, Nancollas GH. The influence of high- and low-molecular-weight inhibitors on dissolution kinetics of hydroxyapatite and human enamel in lactate buffers: a constant composition study. *Journal of Dental Research.* 1988; 67(12): 1493–1298.

215. Bunting JW, Thong KM. Stability constants for some 1:1 metal-carboxylate complexes. *Canadian Journal of Chemistry.* 1970; 48(11): 1654–1656.

216. Featherstone JDB, Lussi A. "Understanding the chemistry of dental erosion." A Lussi (Ed.), In: *Dental Erosion.* Basel: Karger Publishers, 2006, Vol 20, 66–76.

217. Dojindo metal chelates chart. Available from: https://www.dojindo. com/Images/Product%20Photo/Chelate_Table_of_Stability_ Constants.pdf.

218. Geddes DAM. Acids produced by human dental plaque metabolism *in situ. Caries Research.* 1975; 9(2): 98–109.

219. Vanysek P. Ionic conductivity and diffusion at infinite dilution. *CRC Handbook of Chemistry and Physics.* Boca Raton: CRC Press LLC, 2000; 83.

220. Weng YH, Wei HJ, Tsai TY, Chen WH, Wei TY, Hwang WS, Wang CP, Huang CP. Separation of acetic acid from xylose by nanofiltration. *Separation and Purification Technology.* 2009; 67(1): 95–102.

221. Dey P, Linnanen L, Pal P. Separation of lactic acid from fermentation broth by cross flow nanofiltration: membrane characterization and transport modelling. *Desalination.* 2012; 288: 47–57.

222. Zare HR, Nasirizadeh N, Ardakani MM. Electrochemical properties of a tetrabromo-p-benzoquinone modified carbons paste electrode. Application to the simultaneous determination of ascorbic acid, dopamine and uric acid. *Journal of Electroanalytical Chemistry.* 2005; 577(1): 25–33.

223. Lyons MEG, Breen W. Ascorbic acid oxidation at polypyr-role-coated electrodes. *Journal of the Chemical Society, Faraday Transactions.* 1991; 87(1): 115–123.

224. Teixeira JA, Mota M, Venâncio A. Model identification and diffusion coefficients determination of glucose and malic acid in calcium alginate membranes. *The Chemical Engineering Journal.* 1994; 56(1): B9-B14.

225. Ryan PR, Delhaize E, Randall PJ. Malate efflux from root apices and tolerances to aluminium are highly correlated in wheat. *Functional Plant Biology.* 1995; 22(4): 531–536.

226. Khalifah RG. Carbon dioxide hydration activity of carbonic anhydrase: paradoxical consequences of the unusually rapid catalysis. *Proceedings of the National Academy of Sciences.* 1973; 70(7): 1986–1989.

227. Gros G, Moll W. Facilitated diffusion of CO_2 across albumin solutions. *The Journal of General Physiology.* 1974; 64(3): 356–371.

228. Delgado JMPQ. Molecular diffusion coefficients of organic compounds in water at different temperatures. *Journal of Phase Equilibria and Diffusion.* 2007; 28(5): 427–432.

229. Spiess AC, Zavrel M, Ansorge-Schumacher MB, Janzen C, Michalik C, Schmidt TW, Schwendt T, Büchs J, Poprawe R, Marquardt W. Model discrimination for the propionic acid diffusion into hydrogel beads using lifetime confocal laser scanning microscopy. *Chemical Engineering Science.* 2008; 63(13): 3457–3465.

230. Hunt JN, Knox MT. The slowing of gastric emptying by four strong acids and three weak acids. *The Journal of Physiology.* 1972; 222(1): 187–208.

231. Apelblat A. *Citric Acid.* Switzerland: Springer, 2014.

232. Handgraaf J-W, van Erp TS, Meijer EJ. *Ab initio* molecular dynamics study of liquid methanol. *Chemical Physics Letters.* 2003; 367(5): 617–624.

233. Krom MD, Berner RA. The diffusion coefficients of sulfate, ammonium, and phosphate ions in anoxic marine sediments. *Limnology and Oceanography.* 1980; 25(2): 327–337

234. Hui L, Leaist DG. Thermal diffusion of weak electrolytes: aqueous phosphoric and iodic acids. *Canadian Journal of Chemistry.* 1990; 68(8): 1317–1322.

235. Raju UK, Sethuram B, Rao TN. Conductometric study of ion-ion and ion-solvent interactions. III. Conductances of silver acetate in acetonitrile-water mixtures at 25°C. *Bulletin of the Chemical Society of Japan.* 1982; 55(1): 293–296.

236. Kovacs H, Mark AE, van Gunsteren WF. Solvent structure at a hydrophobic protein surface. *Proteins-Structure Function and Genetics.* 1997; 27(3): 395–404.

237. Li G, Kikuchi E, Matsukata M. Separation of water-acetic acid mixtures by pervaporation using a thin mordenite membrane. *Separate and Purification Technology.* 2003; 32(1): 199–206.

238. Araki T, Ito M, Oscarsson O. Anion permeability of the synaptic and non-synaptic motoneuron membrane. *The Journal of Physiology.* 1961; 159(3): 410–435.

239. Ito M, Kostyuk PG, Oshima T. Further study on anion permeability of inhibitory post-synaptic membrane of cat motoneurones. *The Journal of Physiology.* 1962; 164(1): 150–156.

240. Volkov AG, Paula S, Deamer DW. Two mechanisms of permeation of small neutral molecules and hydrated ions across phospholipid bilayers. *Bioelectrochemistry and Bioenergetics.* 1997; 42(2): 153–160.

241. Kielland J. Individual activity coefficients of ions in aqueous solutions. *Journal of the American Chemical Society.* 1937; 69(9): 1675–1678.

242. Collins KD. Sticky ions in biological systems. *Proceedings of the National Academy of Sciences.* 1995; 21(12): 5553–5557.

243. Striolo A, Chialvo AA, Cummings PT, Gubbins KE. Water adsorption in carbon-slit nanopores. *Langmuir.* 2003; 19(20): 8583–8591.

244. Kahlenberg L. *The Action of Solutions On The Sense Of Taste.* Madison: University of Wisconsin, 1898.

245. Sowalsky RA, Noble AC. Comparison of the effects of concentration, pH and anion species on astringency and sourness of organic acids. *Chemical Senses.* 1998; 23(3): 343–349.

246. Rönnholm E. III. The structure of the organic stroma of human enamel during amelogenesis. *Journal of Ultrastructure Research.* 1962; 6(3–4): 368–389.

247. Hagerman AE, Butler LG. The specificity of proanthocyanidin-protein interactions. *Journal of Biological Chemistry.* 1981; 256(9): 4494–4497.

248. Arends J, Schuthof J. Microhardness and lesion depth studies of artificial caries lesions: a comparison of gelatin and HEC based systems. *Journal de Biologie Buccale.* 1980; 8(2): 175–181.

249. Galil KA, Wright GZ. Acid etching patterns on buccal surfaces of permanent teeth. *Pediatric Dentistry.* 1979; 1(4): 230–234.

250. Hughes JA, West NX, Parker DM, van den Braak MH, Addy M. Effects of pH and concentration of citric, malic and lactic acids on enamel, in vitro. *Journal of Dentistry.* 2000; 28(2): 147–152.

251. Hosein I, Sherriff M, Ireland AJ. Enamel loss during bonding, debonding, and cleanup with the use of a self-etching primer. *American Journal of Orthodontics and Dentofacial Orthopedics.* 2004; 126(6): 717–724.

252. Hevinga MA, Opdam NJ, Frencken JE, Truin, GJ, Huysmans MCDNJM. Does incomplete caries removal reduce strength of restored teeth? *Journal of Dental Research.* 2010; 89(11): 1270–1275.

253. Franzon R, Guimarães LF, Magalhães CE, Haas AN, Araujo FB. Outcomes of one-step incomplete and complete excavation in primary teeth: A 24-month randomized controlled trial. *Caries Research.* 2014; 48(5): 376–383.

254. Meyer-Lueckel H, Paris S, Kielbassa AM. Surface layer erosion of natural caries lesions with phosphoric and hydrochloric acid gels in preparation for resin infiltration. *Caries Research.* 2007; 41(3): 223–230.

255. Croll TP. Enamel microabrasion for removal of superficial dis-coloration. *Journal of Esthetic and Restorative Dentistry.* 1989; 1(1): 14–20.

256. Tong LSM, Pang MKM, Mok NYC, King NM, Wei SHY. The effects of etching, micro-abrasion, and bleaching on surface enamel. *Journal of Dental Research.* 1993; 72(1): 67–71.

257. Meyer-Lueckel H, Paris S. Improved resin infiltration of natural caries lesions. *Journal of Dental Research.* 2008; 87(12): 1112–1116.

258. Kielbassa AM, Müller J, Gernhardt CR. Closing the gap between oral hygiene and minimally invasive dentistry: A review on the resin infiltration technique of incipient (proximal) enamel lesions. *Quintessence International.* 2009; 40(8): 663–681.

259. Omar SI. Using resin infiltration to treat developmental defects of enamel: Three case reports. Journal of Restorative Dentistry. 2013; 1(1): 31–35. Available from: http://www.jresdent.org/article. asp?issn=2321-4619;year=2013;volume=1;issue=1;spage=31;epage =35;aulast=Omar

260. Paris S, Meyer-Lueckel H. Inhibition of caries progression by resin infiltration *in situ*. *Caries Research.* 2010; 44(1): 47–54.

261. Martignon S, Ekstrand KR, Ellwood R. Efficacy of sealing proximal early active lesions: An 18-month clinical study evaluated by conventional and subtraction radiography. *Caries Research.* 2006; 40(5): 382–388.

262. Ekstrand KR, Bakhshandeh A, Martignon S. Treatment of proximal superficial caries lesions on primary molar teeth with resin infiltration and fluoride varnish versus fluoride varnish only: efficacy after 1 year. *Caries Research.* 2010; 44(1): 41–46.

263. Martignon S, Ekstrand KR, Gomez J, Lara JS, Cortes A. Infiltrating/sealing proximal caries lesions: A 3-year randomized clinical trial. *Journal of Dental Research.* 2012; 91(3): 288–292.

264. de Sousa SMG, Silva TL. Demineralization effect of EDTA, EGTA, CDTA and citric acid on root dentin: A comparative study. *Brazilian Oral Research.* 2005; 19(3): 188–192.

265. Chande KP, Manwar NU, Chandak MG, Lokade J, Chandak SR. Effect of chelating agents and irrigants on mineral content of root canal dentin: An *in vitro* study. *International Journal of Clinical Preventive Dentistry.* 2014; 10(3): 135–138.

266. Pérez-Heredia M, Ferrer-Luque CM, González-Rodríguez MP, Martín-Peinado FJ, González-López S. Decalcifying effect of 15% EDTA, 15% citric acid, 5% phosphoric acid and 2.5% sodium hypochlorite on root canal dentine. *International Endodontic Journal.* 2008; 41(5): 418–423.

267. González-López S, Camejo-Aguilar D, Sanchez-Sanchez P, Bolaños-Carmona V. Effect of CHX on the decalcifying effect of 10% citric acid, 20% citric acid, or 17% EDTA. *Journal of Endodontics.* 2006; 32(8): 781–784.

268. Miranda CB, Pagani C, Benetti AR, Matuda FDS. Evaluation of the bleached human enamel by scanning electö microscopy. *Journal of Applied Oral Science.* 2005; 13(2): 204–211.

269. de Oliveira R, Paes Leme AF, Giannini M. Effect of a carbamide peroxide bleaching gel containing calcium or fluoride on human enamel surface microhardness. *Brazilian Dental Journal*. 2005; 16(2): 103–106.

270. Efeoglu N, Wood D, Efeoglu C. Microcomputerised tomography evaluation of 10% carbamide peroxide applied to enamel. *Journal of Dentistry*. 2005; 33(7): 561–567.

271. Peutzfeldt A, Nielsen LA. Bond strength of a sealant to primary and permanent enamel: Phosphoric acid versus self-etching adhesive. *Pediatric Dentistry*. 2004; 26(3): 240–244.

272. Giannini M, Makishi P, Ayers APA, Vermelho PM, Fronza BM, Nikaido T, Tagami J. Self-etch adhesive systems: A literature review. *Brazilian Dental Journal*. 2015; 26(1): 3–10.

273. Jensen ME, Schachtele CF. The acidogenic potential of reference foods and snacks at interproximal sites in the human dentition. *Journal of Dental Research*. 1983; 62(8): 889–892.

274. Geddes DAM. Diet patterns and caries. *Advances in Dental Research*. 8(2): 221–224.

275. Zero DT. Sugars—the arch criminal? *Caries Research*. 2004; 38(3): 277–285.

276. Sheiham A, James WPT. Diet and dental caries: the pivotal role of free sugars reemphasized. *Journal of Dental Research*. 2015; 94(1): 1341–1347.

277. Zero DT, Lussi A. Erosion—chemical and biological factors of importance to the dental practitioner. *International Dental Journal*. 2005; 55(S4): 285–290.

278. Beighton D, Brailsford SR, Lynch E, Chen HY, Clark DT. The influence of specific foods and oral hygiene on the microflora of fissures and smooth surfaces of molar teeth: a 5-day study. *Caries Research*. 1999; 33(5): 349–356.

279. Rampersaud GC, Pereira MA, Girard BL, Adams J, Metzl JD. Breakfast habits, nutritional status, body weight, and academic performance in children and adolescents. *Journal of the American Dietetic Association*. 2015; 105(5): 743–760.

280. Petrie HJ, Stover EA, Horswill CA. Nutritional concerns for the child and adolescent competitor. Nutrition. 2004; 20(7): 620–631.

281. Gambon DL, Brand HS, Bots CP, Roos L, Veerman ECI. "Straw use in young children and the potential relation to tooth wear." Gambon DL (Ed.), In: *Dental erosion in children: risk factors in daily life in the 21st century*. Rotterdam: Optima Grafische Communicatie, 2011, 77–85.

282. Søvik JB, Skudutyte-Rysstad R, Tveit AB, Sandvik L, Mulic A. Sour sweets and acidic beverage consumption are risk indicators for dental erosion. *Caries Research*. 2015; 49(3): 243–250.

283. Foster GD, Wyatt HR, Hill JO, Makris AP, Rosenbaum DL, Brill C, Stein RI, Mohammed S, Miller B, Rader DJ, Zemel B, Wadden TA, Tenhave T, Newcomb CW, Klein S. Weight and metabolic outcomes after 2 years on a low-carbohydrate versus low-fat diet. *Annals of Internal Medicine*. 2010; 153(3): 147–157. https://www.ncbi.nlm.nih.gov/pmc/articles/PMC2949959/

284. World Health Organization. "Guideline: sugars intake for adults and children." Geneva: World Health Organization, 2015.

285. McCrory C, Vanderlee L, White CM, Reid JL, Hammond D. Knowledge of recommended calorie intake and influence of calories on food selection among Canadians. *Journal of Nutrition Education and Behavior*. 2016; 48(3): 199–207.

286. Borra S. Consumer perspectives on food labels. *American Journal of Clinical Nutrition*. 2006; 83(Suppl): 1235S.

287. Patterson NJ, Sadler MJ, Cooper JM. Consumer understanding of sugars claims on food and drink products. *Nutrition Bulletin.* 2012; 37(2): 121–130.

288. Gomez P, Werle COC, Corneille O. The pitfall of nutrition facts label fluency: easier-to-process nutrition information enhances purchase intentions for unhealthy food products. *Marketing Letters.* 2017; 28(1): 15–27.

289. Krebs JD, Elley CR, Parry-Strong A, Lunt H, Drury PL, Bell DA, Robinson E, Moyes SA, Mann JI. The Diabetes Excess Weight Loss (DEWL) Trial: a randomised controlled trial of high-protein versus high-carbohydrate diets over 2 years in type 2 diabetes. *Diabetologia.* 2012; 55(4): 905–914.

290. Dupuis L, Oudart H, René F, de Aguilar J-LG, Loeffler J-P. Evidence for defective energy homeostasis in amyotrophic lateral sclerosis: Benefit of a high-energy diet in a transgenic mouse model. *Proceedings of the National Academy of Sciences.* 2004; 101(30): 11159–11164.

291. Brinkworth GD, Noakes M, Clifton PM, Bird AR. Comparative effects of very low-carbohydrate, high-fat and high-carbohydrate, low-fat weight-loss diets on bowel habit and faecal short-chain fatty acids and bacterial populations. *British Journal of Nutrition.* 2009; 101(10): 1493–1502.

292. Crossner C-G, Hase JC, Birkhed D. Oral sugar clearance in children compared with adults. *Caries Research.* 1991; 25(3): 201–206.

293. Lagerlöf F, Oliveby A, Weetman DA, Geddes DAM. Intra- and inter-individual differences in salivary sucrose clearance over time. *Caries Research.* 1994; 28(5): 348–352.

294. Slare F. Concerning a person who had a new set of teeth after 80 years of age; with some observations upon the virtues and

properties of sugar. *Philosophical Transactions.* 1712; 28(337): 273–274.

295. Lingström P, Birkhed D, Granfeldt Y, Björck I. pH measurements of human dental plaque after consumption of starchy foods using the microtouch and the sampling method. *Caries Research.* 1993; 27(5): 394–401.

296. Bibby BG, Mundorff SA. Enamel demineralization by snack foods. *Journal of Dental Research.* 1975; 54(3): 461–470.

297. Schwendicke F, Frencken JE, Bjørndal L, Maltz, M, Manton DJ, Ricketts D, Van Landuyt K, Banerjee A, Campus G, Doméjean S, Fontana M, Leal S, Lo E, Machiulskiene V, Schulte A, Splieth C, Zandona AF, Innes NPT. Managing carious lesions: Consensus recommendations on carious tissue removal. *Advances in Dental Research.* 2016; 28(2): 58–67.

298. Guerini V. *A History of Dentistry: From the Most Ancient of Times Until the End of the Eighteenth Century.* New York: Lea & Febiger, 1909.

299. Bashir E, Gustavsson A, Lagerlöf F. Site specificity of citric acid retention after an oral rinse. *Caries Research.* 1995; 29(6): 467–469.

300. Amaechi BT, Higham SM, Edgar WM, Milosevic A. Thickness of acquired salivary pellicle as a determinant of the sites of dental erosion. *Journal of Dental Research.* 1999; 78(12): 1821–1828.

301. Zero DT. Etiology of dental erosion—extrinsic factors. *European Journal of Oral Sciences.* 1996; 104(2): 162–177.

302. Al-Dlaigan YH, Shaw L, Smith A. Dental erosion in a group of British 14-year-old school children. Part II: Influence of dietary intake. *British Dental Journal.* 2001; 190(5): 258–261.

303. Linkosalo E, Markkanen H. Dental erosions in relation to lac-tovegetarian diet. *European Journal of Oral Sciences*. 1985; 93(5): 436–441.

304. Järvinen VK, Rytömaa II, Heinonen OP. Risk factors in dental erosion. *Journal of Dental Research*. 1991; 70(6): 942–947.

305. Ganss C, Schlechtriemen M, Klimek J. Dental erosions in sub-jects living on a raw food diet. *Caries Research*. 1999; 33(1): 74–80.

306. Stephan RM, Miller BF. A quantitative method for evaluating physical and chemical agents which modify production of acids in bacterial plaques on human teeth. *Journal of Dental Research*. 1943; 22(1): 45–51.

307. U.S. Food & Drug Administration, Center for Food Safety & Applied Nutrition. "Appendix 3: Factors that affect microbial growth in food." In: *Bad Bug Book: Foodborne Pathogenic Microorganisms and Natural Toxins Handbook, 2nd Edition*. International Medical Publishing, 2012. Available from: https://www.fda.gov/food/foodborneillnesscontaminants/causesofillnessbadbugbook/

308. Klampfl CW, Buchberger W, Haddad PR. Determination of organic acids in food samples by capillary zone electrophoresis. *Journal of Chromatography A*. 2000; 881(1): 357–364.

309. Velioğlu YS. "Food Acids: Organic Acids, Volatile Organic Acids, and Phenolic Acids." F Yildiz (Ed.), In: *Advances in Food Biochemistry*. Boca Raton: CRC Press 2010, 313–339.

310. Grigor JMV, Johnson WS, Salminen S. "Food additives for special dietary purposes." AL Branen, PM Davidson, S Salminen, JH Thorngate III (Eds.), In: *Food Additives, 2nd Edition, Revised and Expanded*. New York: Marcel Dekker Inc., 2002, 339–348.

311. Jenab M, Sabaté N, Ferrari P, Mazuir M, Casagrande C, Deharveng G, Tjønneland A, Olsen A, Overvad K, Boutron-Ruault M-C, Clavel-Chapelon F, Boeing H, Weikert C, Linseisen J, Rohrmann

S, Trichopoulou A, Naska A, Palli D, Sacerdote c, Tumino R, Mattiello A, Pala V, Bueno-de-Mesquita HB, Ocké MC, Peeters PH, Engeset D, Skeie G, Jakszyn P, Ardanaz E, Quirós JR, Chirlaque MD, Martinez C, Amiano P, Berglund G, Palmqvist R, van Guelpen B, Bingham S, Key T, Riboli E. Consumption and portion sizes of tree nuts, peanuts and seeds in the European Prospective Investigation into Cancer and Nutrition (EPIC) cohorts from 10 European countries. *British Journal of Nutrition.* 2006; 96(Suppl 2): S12-S23.

312. Suliburska J, Krejpcio Z. Evaluation of the content and bioaccessibility of iron, zinc, calcium and magnesium from groats, rice, leguminous grains and nuts. *Journal of Food Science and Technology.* 2014; 51(3): 589–594.

313. Bolling BW, Chen C-Yo, McKay DL, Blumberg JB. Tree nut phytochemicals: composition, antioxidant capacity, bioactivity, impact factors. A systematic review of almonds, Brazils, cashews, hazelnuts, macadamias, pecans, pine nuts, pistachios and walnuts. *Nutrition Research Reviews.* 2011; 24(2): 244–275.

314. Pellegrini N, Serafini M, Salvatore S, Del Rio D, Bianchi M, Brighenti F. Total antioxidant capacity of spices, dried fruits, nuts, pulses, cereals and sweets consumed in Italy assessed by three different *in vitro* assays. *Molecular Nutrition & Food Research.* 2006; 50(11): 1030–1038.

315. Drewnowski A, Fulgoni III V. Nutrient profiling of foods: creating a nutrient-rich food index. *Nutrition Reviews.* 2008; 66(1): 23–39.

316. Açar ÖÇ, Gökmen V, Pellegrini N, Fogliano V. Direct evaluation of the total antioxidant capacity of raw and roasted pulses, nuts and seeds. *European Food Research and Technology.* 2009; 229(6): 961–969.

317. Schlörmann W, Birringer M, Böhm V, Löber K, Jahreis G, Lorkowski S, Müller AK, Schöne F, Glei M. Influence of roasting

conditions on health-related compounds in different nuts. *Food Chemistry.* 2015. 180(1 August): 77–85.

318. Garasky S, Mbwana K, Romualdo A, Tenaglio A, Roy M. Foods typically purchased by supplemental nutritional assistance program (SNAP) households. Prepared by IMPAQ International, LLC for United States Department of Agriculture, Food and Nutrition Service, November 2016. Available from: https://nopren.org/wp-content/uploads/2016/12/SNAPFoodsTypicallyPurchased.pdf

319. Berdmore T. *A Treatise on the Disorders and Deformities of the Teeth and Gums.* Dublin: John Exshaw, 1769.

320. Sánchez-Mata MC, Cabrera Loera RD, Morales P, Fernández-Ruiz V, Cámara M, Díez Marqués C, Pardo-de-Santayana M, Tardío J. Wild vegetable of the Mediterranean area as valuable sources of bioactive compounds. *Genetic Resources and Crop Evolution.* 2012; 59(3): 431–443.

321. Food and Nutrition Board, Institute of Medicine. *Dietary reference intakes for vitamin C, vitamin E, selenium, and carotenoids.* Washington D.C.: National Academy Press, 2000.

322. Gillooly M, Bothwell TH, Torrance JD, MacPhail AP, Derman DP, Bezwoda WR, Mills W, Charlton RW, Mayet F. The effects of organic acids, phytates and polyphenols on the absorption of iron from vegetables. *British Journal of Nutrition.* 1983; 49(3): 331–342.

323. Pérez AG, Olías R, Espada J, Olías JM, Sanz C. Rapid determination of sugars, non-volatile acids, and ascorbic acid in strawberry and other fruits. *Journal of Agricultural and Food Chemistry.* 1997; 45(9): 3545–3549.

324. Nour V, Trandafir I, Ionica ME. HPLC organic acid analysis in different citrus juices under reversed phase conditions. *Notulae Botanicae Horti Agrobotanici Cluj-Napoca.* 2010; 38(1): 44–48.

325. Viljakainen S, Visit A, Laakso S. Concentrations of organic acids and soluble sugars in juices from Nordic berries. *Acta Agriculturae Scandinavica, Section B, Soil and Plant Science.* 2002; 52(2): 101–109.

326. Sinki GS, Gordon RJ. "Flavoring Agents." AL Branen, PM Davidson, S Salminen, JH Thorngate III (Eds.), In: *Food Additives, 2nd Edition, Revised and Expanded.* New York: Marcel Dekker Inc., 2002, 341–408.

327. Bocarsly ME, Powell ES, Avena NM, Hoebel BG. High-fructose corn syrup causes characteristics of obesity in rats: Increased body weight, body fat and triglyceride levels. *Pharmacology Biochemistry and Behavior.* 2010; 97(1): 101–106.

328. Parker H. A sweet problem: Princeton researchers find that high-fructose corn syrup prompts considerably more weight gain. March 22, 2010. Available from: https://www.princeton.edu/news/2010/03/22/sweet-problem-princeton-researchers-find-high-fructose-corn-syrup-prompts

329. Ruff JS, Hugentobler SA, Suchy AK, Sosa MM, Tanner RE, Hite ME, Morrison LC, Gieng SH, Shigenaga MK, Potts WK. Compared to sucrose, previous consumption of fructose and glucose monosaccharides reduces survival and fitness of female mice. *Journal of Nutrition.* 2015; 145(3): 434–441.

330. Levy SM, Warren JJ, Broffitt B, Hillis SL, Kanellis MJ. Fluoride, beverages and dental caries in the primary dentition. *Caries Research.* 2003; 37(3): 157–165.

331. Hamasha AA-H, Warren JJ, Levy SM, Broffitt B, Kanellis MJ. Oral health behaviors of children in low and high socioeconomic status families. *Pediatric Dentistry.* 2006; 28(4): 310–315.

332. Burt BA, Kolker JL, Sandretto AM, Yuan Y, Sohn W, Ismail AI. Dietary patterns related to caries in a low-income adult population. *Caries Research.* 2006; 40(6): 473–480.

333. Singh GM, Micha R, Khatibzadeh S, Lim S, Ezzati M, Mozaffarian D. Estimated global, regional, and national disease burdens related to sugar-sweetened beverage consumption in 2010. *Circulation.* 2015; 132(8): 639–666.

334. Maloney J. Soda loses its U.S. crown: Americans now drink more bottled water. *Wall Street Journal.* March 9, 2017.

335. Al-Madi EM, AlJamie M, Al-Dukhail S, Mohammed Z, Abubakr NH. Dietary habits and oral hygiene practice amongst dental students at the College of Dentistry, Princess Nourah University. *Open Journal of Stomatology.* 2016; 6(1): 28–35.

336. Al-Majed I, Maguire A, Murray JJ. Risk factors for dental erosion in 5–6 year old and 12–14 year old boys in Saudi Arabia. *Community Dentistry and Oral Epidemiology.* 2002; 30(1): 38–46.

337. Jensdottir T, Arnadottir IB, Thorsdottir I, Bardow A, Gudmundsson K, Theodors A, Holbrook WP. Relationship between dental erosion, soft drink consumption, and gastro-esophageal reflux among Icelanders. *Clinical Oral Investigations.* 2004; 8(2): 91–96.

338. Reddy A, Norris DF, Momeni SS, Waldo B, Ruby JD. The pH of beverages in the United States. *Journal of the American Dental Association.* 2016; 147(4): 255–263.

339. Ireland AJ, McGuinness N, Sherriff M. An investigation into the ability of soft drinks to adhere to enamel. *Caries Research.* 1995; 29(6): 470–476.

340. Hara AT, Zero DT. Analysis of the erosive potential of calcium-containing acidic beverages. *European Journal of Oral Sciences.* 2008; 116(1): 60–65.

341. Jensdottir T, Holbrook P, Nauntofte B, Buchwald C, Bardow A. Immediate erosive potential of cola drinks and orange juices. *Journal of Dental Research.* 2006; 85(3): 226–230.

342. Aykut-Yetkiner A, Wiegand A, Bollhalder A, Becker K, Attin T. Effect of acidic solution viscosity on enamel erosion. *Journal of Dental Research.* 2013; 92(3): 289–294.

343. Doores S. "pH Control Agents and Acidulants." AL Branen, PM Davidson, S Salminen, JH Thorngate III (Eds.), In: *Food Additives, 2nd Edition, Revised and Expanded.* New York: Marcel Dekker Inc., 2002, 621–661.

344. Davidson PM, Juneja VK, Branen JK. "Antimicrobial Agents." AL Branen, PM Davidson, S Salminen, JH Thorngate III (Eds.), In: *Food Additives, 2nd Edition, Revised and Expanded.* New York: Marcel Dekker Inc., 2002, 563–620.

345. Lampila LE, Godber JP. "Food Phosphates." AL Branen, PM Davidson, S Salminen, JH Thorngate III (Eds.), In: *Food Additives, 2nd Edition, Revised and Expanded.* New York: Marcel Dekker Inc., 2002, 809–896.

346. Perrier® Bottled Water Quality Report. Nestlé Waters North America Inc. 2015. Available from: https://www.nestle-watersna.com/asset-library/documents/p_eng.pdf

347. S. Pellegrino® Bottled Water Quality Report. Nestlé Waters North America Inc. 2015. Available from: https://www.nestle-watersna.com/asset-library/documents/sp_eng.pdf

348. Copeland R. LaCroix fizzy water is everyone's favorite. Nobody knows what's in it. *Wall Street Journal.* September 13, 2017.

349. McDonald Jr. JL, Stookey GK. Laboratory studies concerning the effect of acid-containing beverages on enamel dissolution and experimental dental caries. *Journal of Dental Research.* 1973; 52(2): 211–216.

350. Mato I, Huidobro JF, Simal-Lozano J, Sancho MT. Simultaneous determination of organic acids in beverages by capillary zone electrophoresis. *Analytica Chimica Acta.* 2006; 565(2): 190–197.

351. Amelin VG, Podkolzin IV, Tretiakov AV. Determination of organic acids in alcoholic and non-alcoholic beverages by reserved-phase high-performance liquid chromatography. *Journal of Analytical Chemistry.* 2012; 67(3): 262–268.

352. Milosevic A. Sports drinks hazard to teeth. *British Journal of Sports Medicine.* 1997; 31(1): 28–30.

353. Coombes JS. Sports drinks and dental. *American Journal of Dentistry.* 2005; 18(2): 101–104.

354. Mathew T, Casamassimo PS, Hayes JR. Relationship between sports drinks and dental erosion in 304 university athletes in Columbus, Ohio, USA. *Caries Research.* 202; 36(4): 281–287.

355. Milosevic A, Kelly MJ, McLean AN. Sports supplement drinks and dental health in competitive swimmers and cyclists. *British Dental Journal.* 1997; 182(8): 303–308.

356. Shirreffs SM. Hydration in sport and exercise: water, sports drinks and other drinks. *Nutrition Bulletin.* 2009; 34(4): 374–379.

357. Taylor AA. What are sports drinks, and do regular athletes need them? *Chemical & Engineering News.* February 21, 2017.

358. Mettler S, Rusch C, Colombani PC. Osmolality and pH of sport and other drinks available in Switzerland. *Schweizerische Zeitschrift für Sportmedizin und Sporttraumatologie.* 2006; 54(3): 92–95.

359. Pottier A, Bouckaert J, Gilis W, Roels T, Derave W. Mouth rinse but not ingestion of a carbohydrate solution improves 1-h cycle time trial performance. *Scandinavian Journal of Medicine & Science in Sports.* 2010; 20(1): 105–111.

360. Jeukendrup AE. Oral carbohydrate rinse: placebo or beneficial? *Current Sports Medicine Reports.* 2013; 12(4): 222–227.

361. Beaven CM, Maulder P, Pooley A, Kilduff L, Cook C. Effects of caffeine and carbohydrate mouth rinses on repeated sprint

performance. *Applied Physiology, Nutrition, and Metabolism.* 2013; 38(6): 633–637.

362. Hutchinson A. When and why to swish-n-spit your sports drink. *Runners World.* July 17, 2013. Available from: http://www. runnersworld.com/sweat-science/when-and-why-to-swish-n-spit-your-sports-drink

363. Sinclair J, Bottoms L, Flynn C, Bradley E, Alexander G, McCullagh S, Finn T, Hurst HT. The effect of different durations of carbo-hydrate mouth rinse on cycling performance. *European Journal of Sports Science.* 2014; 14(3): 259–264.

364. Thomas K, Morris P, Stevenson E. Improved endurance capacity following chocolate milk consumption compared with 2 com-mercially available sports drinks. *Applied Physiology, Nutrition, and Metabolism.* 2009; 34(1): 78–82.

365. Watson P, Love TD, Maughan RJ, Shirreffs SM. A comparison of the effects of milk and a carbohydrate-electrolyte drink on the restoration of fluid balance and exercise capacity in a hot, humid environment. *European Journal of Applied Physiology.* 2008; 104(4): 633–642.

366. Cockburn E, Bell PG, Stevenson E. Effect of milk on team sport performance after exercise-induced muscle damage. *Medicine & Science in Sports & Exercise.* 2013; 45 (August 1): 1585–1592.

367. James LJ, Clayton D, Evans GH. Effect of milk protein addition to a carbohydrate-electrolyte rehydration solution ingested after exercise in the heat. *British Journal of Nutrition.* 2011; 105(3): 393–399.

368. López EF, Gómez EF. Simultaneous determination of the major organic acids, sugars, glycerol, and ethanol by HPLC in grape musts and white wines. *Journal of Chromatographic Science.* 1996; 34(5): 254–257.

369. Edelmann A, Diewok J, Rodriguez Baena J, Lendl B. High-performance liquid chromatography with diamond ATR-FTIR detection for the determination of carbohydrates, alcohols and organic acids in red wine. *Analytical and Bioanalytical Chemistry.* 2003; 376(1): 92–97.

370. Castiñeira A, Peña RM, Herrero C, García-Martín S. Analysis of organic acids in wine by capillary electrophoresis with direct UV detection. *Journal of Food Composition and Analysis.* 2002; 15(3): 319–331.

371. Obreque-Slier E, Espínola-Espínola V, López-Solís R. Wine pH prevails over buffering capacity of human saliva. *Journal of Agricultural and Food Chemistry.* 2016; 64(43): 8154–8159.

372. Mulic A, Tveit AB, Hove LH, Skaare AB. Dental erosive wear among Norwegian wine tasters. *Acta Odontologica Scandinavica.* 2011; 69(1): 21–26.

373. Mandel L. Dental erosion due to wine consumption. *Journal of the American Dental Association.* 2005; 136(1): 71–75.

374. Winslow C-EA, Broadhurst J, Buchanan RE, Krumwiede Jr. C, Rogers LA, Smith GH. The families and genera of the bacteria: Final report of the committee of the society of American bacteriologists on characterization and classification of bacterial types. *Journal of Bacteriology.* 1920; 5(3): 191–229.

375. Shahidi F, McDonald J, Chandrasekara A, Zhong Y. Phytochemicals of foods, beverages and fruit vinegars: chemistry and health effects. *Asia Pacific Journal of Clinical Nutrition.* 2008; 17(S1): 380–382.

376. White AM, Johnston, CS. Vinegar ingestion at bedtime moderates waking glucose concentrations in adults with well-controlled Type 2 diabetes. *Diabetes Care.* 2007; 30(11): 2814–2815.

377. do Nascimento RF, Cardoso DR, Lima Neto BS, Franco DW. Determination of acids in Brazilian sugar cane spirits and other

alcoholic beverages by HRGC-SPE. *Chromatographia*. 1998; 48(11/12): 751–757.

378. Montanari L. Perretti G, Natella F, Guidi A, Fantozzi P. Organic and phenolic acids in beer. *LWT—Food Science and Technology*. 1999; 32(8): 535–539.

379. Bekatorou A, Psarianos C, Koutinas AA. Production of food grade yeasts. *Food Technology and Biotechnology*. 2006; 44(3): 407–415.

380. Legras J-L, Merdinoglu D, Cornuet J-M, Karst F. Bread, beer and wine: *Saccharomyces cerevisiae* diversity reflects human history. *Molecular Ecology*. 2007; 16(1): 2091–2102.

381. Verstrepen KJ, Derdelinckx G, Dufour J-P, Winderickx J, Thevelein JM, Pretorius IS, Delvaux FR. Flavor-active esters: adding fruitiness to beer. *Journal of Bioscience and Bioengineering*. 2003; 96(2): 110–118.

382. Mäkinen OE, Wanhalinna V, Zannini E, Arendt EK. Foods for special dietary needs: Non-dairy plant based milk substitutes and fermented dairy type products. *Critical Reviews in Food Science and Nutrition*. 2016; 56(3): 339–349.

383. Souci SW, Fachmann W, Kraut H. *Food Composition and Nutrition Tables, 8th Edition*. Stuttgart: MedPharm Scientific Publishers, 2016.

384. Lodi CS, Sassaki KT, Fraiz FC, Delbem ACB, Rodrigues Martinhon CC. Evaluation of some properties of fermented milk beverages that affect the demineralization of dental enamel. *Brazilian Oral Research*. 2010; 24(1): 95–101.

385. Thomson ME, Thomson CW, Chandler NP. In vitro and intra-oral investigations into the cariogenic potential of human milk. *Caries Research*. 1996; 30(6): 434–438.

386. Sharp PF, Powell CK. Increase in the pH of the white and yolk of hens' eggs. *Industrial & Engineering Chemistry.* 1931; 23(2): 196–199.

387. Thomson ME. Effects of cheese, breadcrumbs, and a breadcrumb and cheese mixture on microhardness of bovine dental enamel in intraoral experiments. *Caries Research.* 1988; 22(4): 246–249.

388. Gedalia I, Ionat-Bendat D, Ben-Mosheh S, Shapira L. Tooth enamel softening with a cola type drink and rehardening with hard cheese or stimulated saliva *in situ. Journal of Oral Rehabilitation.* 1991; 18(6): 501–506.

389. Fasoli E, D'Amato A, Kravchuk AV, Citterio A, Righetti PG. In-depth proteomic analysis of non-alcoholic beverages with peptide ligand libraries: I: Almond milk and orgeat syrup. *Journal of Proteomics.* 2011; 74(7): 1080–1090.

390. Nielsen SJ, Kit BK, Ogden CL. Nut consumption among U.S. adults, 2009–2010. National Center for Health Statistics. 2014, NCHS data brief no. 176.

391. Abou-Dobara MA, Ismail MM, Refaat NM. Chemical composition, sensory evaluation and starter activity in cow, soy, peanut and rice milk. *Journal of Nutritional Health & Food Engineering.* 2016; 5(3): 00175.

392. Bernat N, Cháfer M, Chiralt A, Laparra JM, González-Martínez C. Almond milk fermented with different potentially probiotic bacteria improves iron uptake by intestinal epithelial (Caco-2) cells. *International Journal of Food Studies.* 2015; 4(1): 49–60.

393. Bernat Pérez N, Cháfer Náacher MT, Rodriguez Garcia J, Chiralt A, González Martínez MC. Effect of high pressure homogenization and heat treatment on physical properties and stability of almond and hazelnut milks. *Food Science and Technology.* 2015; 62(1): 488–496.

394. Belewu MA, Belewu KY. Comparative physico-chemical evaluation of tiger-nut, soybean and coconut milk sources. *International
Journal of Agriculture & Biology.* 2007; 9(5): 785–787.

395. Pedialyte® Mixed Fruit website. Accessed August 8, 2017; Available
from: https://pedialyte.com/products/classic/mixed-fruit

396. DuFrêne B. Global tea consumption remains robust. *Tea & Coffee
Trade Journal.* 2012; 184(10): 24–30.

397. Kosińska A, Andlauer W. "Antioxidant capacity of tea: effect
of processing and storage." VR Preedy (Ed.), In: *Processing and
Impact on Antioxidants in Beverages.* Amsterdam: Elsevier, 2014,
109–120.

398. Lin S-D, Udompornmongkol P, Yang J-H, Chen S-Y, Mau J-L.
Quality and antioxidant property of three types of tea infusions.
Journal of Food Processing and Preservation. 2014; 39(4): 1401–1408.

399. Santana-Rios G, Orner GA, Amantana A, Provost C, Wu S-Y,
Dashwood RH. Potent antimutagenic activity of white tea in comparison with green tea in the *Salmonella* assay. *Mutation Research.*
2001; 495(1): 61–74.

400. Ferrazzano GF, Amato I, Ingenito A, De Natale A, Pollio A. Anticariogenic effects of polyphenols from plant stimulant beverages
(cocoa, coffee, tea). *Fitoterapia.* 2009; 80(5): 255–262.

401. Chan EWC, Lim YY, Chong KL, Tan JBL, Wong SK. Antioxidant
properties of tropical and temperate herbal teas. *Journal of Food
Composition and Analysis.* 2010; 23(2): 185–189.

402. Narotzki B, Reznick AZ, Aizenbud D, Levy Y. Green tea: A
promising natural product in oral health. *Archives of Oral Biology.*
2012; 57(5): 429–435.

403. Cheng L, Li J, He L, Zhou X. Natural products and caries prevention. *Caries Research.* 2015; 49(Suppl 1): 38–45.

404. Chaudhuri KN. *The Trading World of Asia and the English East India Company, 1660–1760.* London: Cambridge University Press, 1978.

405. WG Clarence-Smith & S Topik (Eds.). *The Global Coffee Economy in Africa, Asia and Latin America, 1500–1989.* Cambridge: Cambridge University Press, 2003.

406. Rodrigues CI, Marta L, Maia R, Miranda M, Ribeirinho M, Máguas C. Application of solid-phase extraction to brewed coffee caffeine and organic acid determination by UV/HPLC. *Journal of Food Composition and Analysis.* 2007; 20(5): 440–448.

407. Fujioka K, Shibamoto T. Chlorogenic acid and caffeine contents in various commercial brewed coffees. *Food Chemistry.* 2008; 106(1): 217–221.

408. Alcázar A, Fernández-Cáceres PL, Martín MJ, Pablos F, González AG. Ion chromatographic determination of some organic acids, chloride and phosphate in coffee and tea. *Talanta.* 2003; 61(2): 95–101.

409. Lunkes LBF, Hashizume LN. Evaluation of the pH and titratable acidity of teas commercially available in Brazilian market. *Revista Gaúcha de Odontologia.* 2014; 62(1): 59–64.

410. Amoras DR, Corona SAM, Rodrigues Jr. AL, Serra MC. Effect of beverages on bovine dental enamel subjected to erosive challenges with hydrochloric acid. *Brazilian Dental Journal.* 2012; 23(4): 367–372.

411. Kato MT, Magalhães AC, Rios D, Hannas AR, Attin T, Buzalaf MAR. Protective effect of green tea on dentin erosion and abrasion. *Journal of Applied Oral Science.* 2009; 17(6): 560–564.

412. Simpson A, Shaw L, Smith AJ. Tooth surface pH during drinking of black tea. *British Dental Journal.* 2001; 190(7): 374–376.

413. Street R, Száková J, Drábek O, Mládková L. The status of micro-nutrients (Cu, Fe, Mn, Zn) in tea and tea infusions in selected

samples imported to the Czech Republic. *Czech Journal of Food Sciences.* 2006; 24(2): 62–71.

414. Saha G, Choudhury SS, Bera B, Kumar PM. Biochemical and microbiological characterization of white tea. *IOSR Journal of Environmental Science, Toxicology and Food Technology.* 2017; 11(5): 74–80.

415. Akyuz S, Yarat A. The pH and neutralisable acidity of the most-consumed Turkish fruit and herbal teas. *Oral Health and Dental Management in the Black Sea Countries.* 2010; 9(2): 75–78.

416. Lussi A, Megert B, Shellis RP, Wang X. Analysis of the erosive effect of different dietary substances and medications. *British Journal of Nutrition.* 2012; 107(2): 252–262.

417. Rees JS, Loyn T, Rowe W, Kunst Q, McAndrew R. The ability of fruit teas to remove the smear layer: an in vitro study of tubule patency. *Journal of Dentistry.* 2006; 34(1): 67–76.

418. Jeszka-Skowron M, Krawczyk M, Zgola-Grześkowiak A. Determination of antioxidant activity, rutin, quercetin, phenolic acids and trace elements in tea infusions: Influence of citric acid addition on extraction of metals. *Journal of Food Composition and Analysis.* 2015; 40(6): 70–77.

419. Malinowska E, Inkielewicz I, Czarnowski W, Szefer P. Assessment of fluoride concentration and daily intake by human from tea and herbal infusions. *Food and Chemical Toxicology.* 2008; 46(3): 1055–1061.

420. Yuwono M. Determination of fluoride in black, green and herbal teas by ion-selective electrode using a standard-addition method. *Dental Journal (Majalah Kedokteran Gigi).* 2005; 38(2): 91–95.

421. Hodge HC. The concentration of fluorides in drinking water to give the point of minimum caries with maximum safety. *Journal of the American Dental Association.* 1950; 40(4): 436–439.

422. Patrick H, Nicklas TA. A review of family and social determinants of children's eating patterns and diet quality. *Journal of the American College of Nutrition.* 2005; 24(2): 83–92.

423. James WPT, Nelson M, Ralph A, Leather S. The contribution of nutrition to inequalities in health. *British Medical Journal.* 1997; 314(7093): 1545–1549

424. Zagorsky JL, Smith PK. The association between socioeconomic status and adult fast-food consumption in the U.S. *Economics & Human Biology.* 2017; 27(A): 12–25.

425. Close MA, Lytle LA, Viera AJ. Is frequency of fast food and sit-down restaurant eating occasions differentially associated with less healthful eating habits? *Preventive Medicine Reports.* 2016; 4(December): 574–577.

426. Belcher WH. The candy situation. *Confectioners Gazette.* 1919; 41(457): 15.

427. Lazzaris M, Farias MMAG, de Araújo SM, Schmitt BHE, Silveira EG. Erosive potential of commercially available candies. *Brazilian Research in Pediatric Dentistry and Integrated Clinic.* 2015; 15(1): 7–12.

428. Farias MMAG, Lazzaris de Oliveira MM, Schmitt BHE, da Silveira EG, de Araújo SM. Erosive potential of sugar-free hard candies dissolved in water and artificial saliva. *Brazilian Journal of Oral Science.* 2016; 15(1): 75–78.

429. Gambon DL, Brand HS, van Nieuw Amerongen A. The erosive potential of candy sprays. *British Dental Journal.* 2009; 2016(10): E20.

430. Lussi A, Carvalho TS. Analyses of the erosive effect of dietary substances and medications on deciduous teeth. *PLoS ONE.* 2015; 10(12): e0143957. https://www.ncbi.nlm.nih.gov/pmc/articles/PMC4689448/

431. Wagoner SN, Marshall TA, Qian F, Wefel JS. In vitro enamel erosion associated with commercially available original-flavor and

sour versions of candies. *Journal of the American Dental Association.* 2009; 140(7): 906–913.

432. Loewen RR, Marolt RJ, Ruby JD. Pucker Up: The effects of sour candy on your patients' oral health. *Northwest Dentistry.* 2007; 87(2): 20–33.

433. Brand HS, Gambon DL, van Dop LF, van Liere LE, Veerman ECI. The erosive potential of jawbreakers, a type of hard candy. *International Journal of Dental Hygiene.* 2010; 8(4): 308–312.

434. Larsen MJ, Nyvad B. Enamel erosion by some soft drinks and orange juices relative to their pH, buffering effect and contents of calcium phosphate. *Caries Research.* 1999; 33(1): 81–87.

435. Jensdottir T, Nauntofte B, Buchwald C, Bardow A. Effects of calcium on the erosive potential of acidic candies in saliva. *Caries Research.* 2007; 41(1): 68–73.

436. Deis RC, Kearsley MW. "Sorbitol and Mannitol." K O'Donnell & MW Kearsley (Eds.), In: *Sweeteners and Sugar Alternatives in Food Technology, 2nd Edition.* Oxford: Wiley-Blackwell, 2012, 331–346.

437. Burt BA. The use of sorbitol- and xylitol-sweetened chewing gum in caries control. *Journal of the American Dental Association.* 2006; 137(2): 190–196.

438. Maguire A. "Dental Health." K O'Donnell & MW Kearsley (Eds.), In: *Sweeteners and Sugar Alternatives in Food Technology, 2nd Edition.* Oxford: Wiley-Blackwell, 2012, 27–61.

439. Zacharis C. "Xylitol." K O'Donnell & MW Kearsley (Eds.), In: *Sweeteners and Sugar Alternatives in Food Technology, 2nd Edition.* Oxford: Wiley-Blackwell, 2012, 347–377.

440. de Cock P. "Erythritol." K O'Donnell & MW Kearsley (Eds.), In: *Sweeteners and Sugar Alternatives in Food Technology, 2nd Edition.* Oxford: Wiley-Blackwell, 2012, 215–241.

441. Kawanabe J, Hirasawa M, Takeuchi T, Oda T, Ikeda T. Noncariogenicity of erythritol as a substrate. *Caries Research.* 1992; 26(5): 358–362.

442. Mäkinen KK. Sugar alcohol sweeteners as alternatives to sugar with special consideration of xylitol. *Medical Principles and Practice.* 2011; 20(4): 303–320.

443. Birkhed D, Svensäter G, Edwardsson S. Cariological studies of individuals with long-term sorbitol consumption. *Caries Research.* 1990; 24(3): 220–223.

444. Loesche WJ, Grossman NS, Earnest R, Corpron R. The effect of chewing xylitol gum on the plaque and saliva levels of Streptococcus mutans. *Journal of the American Dental Association.* 1984; 108(4): 587–592.

445. Mäkinen KK. The rocky road of xylitol to its clinical application. *Journal of Dental Research.* 2000; 79(6): 1352–1355.

446. Salminen S, Salminen E, Koivistoinen P, Bridges J, Marks V. Gut microflora interactions with xylitol in the mouse, rat and man. *Food and Chemical Toxicology.* 1985; 23(11): 985–990.

447. Sutter VL. Anaerobes as normal flora. *Reviews of Infectious Diseases.* 1984; 6(Supplement 1): S62-S66.

448. Ritter AV, Bader JD, Leo MC, Preisser JS, Shugars DA, Vollmer WM, Amaechi BT, Holland JC. Tooth-surface-specific effects of xylitol: Randomized trial results. *Journal of Dental Research.* 2013; 92(6): 512–517.

449. Bader JD, Vollmer WM, Shugars DA, Gilbert GH, Amaechi BT, Brown JP, Laws RL, Funkhouser KA, Makhija SK, Riter AV, Leo MC. Results from the xylitol for adult caries trial (X-ACT). *Journal of the American Dental Association.* 2013; 144(1): 21–30.

450. Machiulskiene V, Nyvad B, Baelum V. Caries preventive effect of sugar-substituted chewing gum. *Community Dentistry and Oral Epidemiology.* 2001; 29(4): 278–288.

451. Dodds MWJ. The oral health benefits of chewing gum. *Journal of the Irish Dental Association.* 2012; 58(5): 253–261.

452. Rumessen JJ, Gudmand-Høyer E. Functional bowel disease: Malabsorption and abdominal distress after ingestion of fructose, sorbitol, and fructose-sorbitol mixtures. *Gastroenterology.* 1988; 95(3): 694–700.

453. Röytiö H, Tiihonen K, Ouwehand AC. "Digestive Health." K O'Donnell & MW Kearsley (Eds.), In: *Sweeteners and Sugar Alternatives in Food Technology, 2nd Edition.* Oxford: Wiley-Blackwell, 2012, 63–76.

454. Honkala S, Runnel R, Saag M, Olak J, Nõmmela, R, Russak S, Mäkinen P-L, Vahlberg T, Falony G, Mäkinen K, Honkala E. Effect of erythritol and xylitol on dental caries prevention in children. *Caries Research.* 2014; 48(5): 482–490.

455. Falony G, Honkala S, Runnel R, Olak J, Nõmmela, R, Russak S, Saag M, Mäkinen P-L, Mäkinen K, Vahlberg T, Honkala E. Long-term effect of erythritol on dental caries development during childhood: A posttreatment survival analysis. *Caries Research.* 2016; 50(6): 579–588.

456. Buzalaf MAB, Pessan JP, Honório HM, ten Cate JM. "Mechanisms of action of fluoride for caries control." MAR Buzalaf (Ed.), In: *Fluoride and the Oral Environment.* Basel: Karger Publishers, 2011, Vol 22, 97–114.

457. Ganss C, Klimek J, Brune V, Schürmann A. Effects of two fluoridation measures on erosion progression in human enamel and dentine *in situ. Caries Research.* 2004; 38(6): 561–566.

458. Magalhães AC, Wiegand A, Rios D, Buzalaf MAB, Lussi A. "Fluoride in dental erosion." MAR Buzalaf (Ed.), In: *Fluoride and the Oral Environment*. Basel: Karger Publishers, 2011, Vol 22, 158–170.

459. Huysmans M-C, Young Z, Ganss C. "The role of fluoride in erosion therapy." A Lussi & C Ganss (Eds.), In: *Erosive Tooth Wear: A Phenomenon of Clinical Significance*. Basel: Karger Publishers, 2014, Vol 25, 230–243.

460. Gedalia I, Anaise J, Westreich V, Fuks A. Predisposition to caries in hamsters following the erosive effect of a commercial citrus beverage administered with and without supplemental fluoride. *Journal of Dental Research*. 1975; 54(3): 496–499.

461. Segrave K. *America Brushes Up*. London: McFarland & Company, 2010.

462. Paget S. *Ambroise Paré and His Times, 1510–1590*. New York: The Knickerbocker Press, 1897.

463. Fauchard P. *Le Chirurgien Dentiste Ou Traite' Des Dents*. Paris: C. Pierre-Jean Mariette, 1746.

464. Pasteur L. "The Germ Theory and Its Applications to Medicine and Surgery." CW Elliot (Ed.), In: *Scientific Papers: Physiology, Medicine, Surgery, Geology*. New York: P.F. Collier & Son, 1910, 382–389.

465. Lister J. On the antiseptic principle in the practice of surgery. *British Medical Journal*. 1867; 2(351): 246–248.

466. Lister JB. *The Collected Papers of Josef Baron Lister, Volume II*. Oxford: Clarendon Press, 1909.

467. Barker GT. Carbolic acid as a therapeutic agent in dentistry. *Dental Cosmos*. 1862; 4(1): 189–190.

468. Listerine advertisements from the 20th century. Available from: http://www.vintageadbrowser.com/beauty-and-hygiene-ads-1910s/7

469. Blodgett SS. What are our dentifrices? *Dental Cosmos.* 1859; 1(1): 240–242.

470. Latimer JS. Dentifrice. *Dental Cosmos.* 1862; 4(1): 423–425.

471. American Dental Association. Minutes from the 13th Annual Meeting in Ohio: Third Day—Afternoon Session. *Dental Cosmos.* 1873; 15(11): 589–604.

472. Sozodont advertisement. *American Quarterly Church Review.* 1866; 17(1): 9.

473. Sozodont advertisement. *Harper's Hand-Book for Travellers in Europe and the East.* New York: Harper & Brothers, 1878, Vol 2.

474. Dr. Lyon's Tooth Powder 1891 advertisement. Available from: https://www.periodpaper.com/collections/vintage-advertising-art/dental.

475. Doctor Sheffield's Crème Dentifrice advertisement. *The Theatre.* 1886; 1(1): 31.

476. RSC. Sheffield's cream dentifrice. *The Dental Office and Laboratory.* 1892; 6(2): 62.

477. Lloyd Manufacturing Cocaine Tooth Drops 1885 advertisement. Available from: http://www.bonkersinstitute.org/medshow/cocainedrops.html

478. CF Boehringer & Soehne chemical advertisement. *American Druggist and Pharmaceutical Record.* 1895; 27(8).

479. Leggo WA. Local anaesthetics. *Dominion Dental Journal.* 1895; 7(7): 187–191.

480. 1912 Colgate ribbon dental cream image. Available from: http://knickoftime.net/?b2w=http://knickoftimeinteriors.blogspot.com/2012/07/antique-graphics-wednesday-1912-colgate.html

481. Colgate advertisement. *Collier's*. 1919; 64(15): 31.

482. Kolynos advertisement. *Saturday Evening Post*. 1917; 190(16): 88.

483. Johnson RW. How Kolynos turned the corner in sixteen months. *Printers' Ink*. 1913; 84(10): 17–19.

484. RPR. Kolynos. *The Druggists Circular*. 1913; 58(9): 526.

485. Kolynos advertising puts over a container improvement. *Printers' Ink*. 1920; 111(2): 17–18.

486. Pebeco advertisement. *Good Housekeeping*. 1920; 70(5): 201.

487. Pepsodent advertisement. *Good Housekeeping*. 1920; 70(6): 108.

488. Taylor JM, Greeley H, Limerick V, Merritt AH, Stillman PR, Hyatt TP, Buckley JP, Carney MF. Highfalutin dupery: Comment on the falsity of various published claims for certain dentifrices. *Journal of Dental Research*. 1919; 1(4): 497–506.

489. Franke EC, Gies WJ. Experimental studies of the validity of advertised claims for products of public importance in relation to oral hygiene or dental therapeutics. 2. The advertised claim that Pepsodent, when used as a dentifrice, removes mucin plaques from teeth, by digesting such plaques, is wholly unwarranted. *Journal of Dental Research*. 1919; 1(4): 511–513.

490. Veader L, Frier WA. Oral hygiene. *Dental Cosmos*. 1927; 69(6): 559–567.

491. Moss HV, Schilb TW. "Dentifrice base." US Patent 2,359,326. Issued October 3, 1944.

492. Prinz H. The relationship of oral secretions to dental caries. I. Methods of determining the amylolytic index of human saliva. *Dental Cosmos*. 1918; 60(2): 140–147.

493. Hansen HL, Fosdick LS, Epple CF. The action of mouth organisms on certain carbohydrates. *Journal of the American Dental Association*. 1937; 24(10): 1611–1617.

494. Fosdick LS. Carbohydrate degradation by mouth organisms. I. *Journal of the American Dental Association.* 1939; 26(3): 415–417.

495. Muntz JA. Production of acids from glucose by dental plaque material. *Journal of Biological Chemistry.* 1943; 148(1): 225–236.

496. Fosdick LS, Campaigne EE. Some chemical differences between the saliva of caries-immune and that of caries-susceptible patients. *Journal of the American Dental Association.* 1939; 26(6): 954–957.

497. Fancher OE, Calandra JC, Fosdick LS. The effect of vitamins on acid formation in saliva. *Journal of Dental Research.* 1944; 23(1): 23–29.

498. Calandra JC, Fancher OE, Fosdick LS. The effect of synthetic vitamin K and related compounds on the rate of acid formation in saliva. *Journal of Dental Research.* 1944; 23(1): 31–37.

499. Fosdick LS, Rapp GW. The effect of proteolytic enzymes on acid formation in the mouth. *Journal of Dental Research.* 1944; 23(2): 81–83.

500. Fosdick LS, Rapp GW. The effect of amylolytic enzymes on acid production in saliva. *Journal of Dental Research.* 1944; 23(2): 85–87.

501. Muntz JA, Miller BF. Factors influencing penetration of synthetic detergents and certain other compounds into dental plaque material. *Journal of Dental Research.* 1943; 22(1): 73–83.

502. Fosdick LS. The degradation of sugars in the mouth and the use of chewing gum and vitamin K in the control of dental caries. *Journal of Dental Research.* 1948; 27(2): 235–241.

503. Fosdick LS, Calandra JC, Blackwell RQ, Burrill JH. A new approach to the problem of dental caries control. *Journal of Dental Research.* 1953; 32(4): 486–496.

504. King WJ. "Oral preparation for inhibition of dental caries." US Patent 2,689,170. Issued September 14, 1954.

505. Baum HM. "Dehydroacetic acid dental compositions." US Patent 2,746,905. Issued May 22, 1956.

506. Zipkin I, McClure FJ. The effect of sodium lauroyl sarcosinate (SLS), sodium lauryl sulfate (SLSO$_4$), and dehydroacetic acid (DHA) on occlusal and smooth surface caries in the rat. *Journal of Dental Research*. 1955; 34(5): 768–769.

507. Teitelbaum MJ. The dentifrice battle. *TIC*. 1959; 18(3): 12–16.

508. Ipana with WD-9 advertisement. *LIFE*. 1953; 35(15): 183. Available from: https://www.pics4life.net/collections/drug-store/products/ipana-toothpaste-page-life-october-12-1953

509. GLEEM with GL-70 advertisement. *TIME*. 1958; 71(13). Available from: https://en.wikipedia.org/wiki/File:Gleem_with_GL-70_ad_from_TIME.png

510. Listerine with antizyme advertisement. *LIFE*. 1955; 38(8): 10. Available from: https://books.google.com/books?id=LFQEAA AAMBAJ&pg=PA10&lpg=PA10&dq=Listerine+antizyme&sou rce=bl&ots=BkvCgQ0Jjn&sig=5bwJFAfAX9Yf8RwODO8eMF mVR4g&hl=en&sa=X&ved=0ahUKEwiL_5OPgfrVAhUm9IM KHSK5Dvk4ChDoAQgtMAM#v=onepage&q=Listerine%20 antizyme&f=false

511. Colgate with Gardol advertisement. *LIFE*. 1957; 42(9): 173. Available from: https://books.google.com/books?id=rUEEAAAMBAJ&pg= RA1-PA173&dq=Colgate+cleans+cleans+cleans+gardol&hl=en &sa=X&ved=0ahUKEwiIsPagqfrVAhUq64MKHeROAs0Q6 AEIKDAA#v=onepage&q=Colgate%20cleans%20cleans%20 cleans%20gardol&f=false

512. Colgate with Gardol 1950s television advertisement. Available from: https://www.youtube.com/watch?v=FY5HdJIPhk8

513. American Dental Association statement on dentifrice advertising claims. *Journal of the American Dental Association.* 1958; 57(5): 745–752.

514. Clarke JK. On the bacterial factor in the aetiology of dental caries. *British Journal of Experimental Pathology.* 1924; 5(3): 141–147.

515. Bunting RW, Palmerlee F. The role of bacillus acidophilus in dental caries. *Journal of the American Dental Association.* 1925; 12(4): 381–413.

516. Jay P. Bacillus acidophilus and dental caries. *Journal of the American Dental Association.* 1929; 16(2): 230–235.

517. Jay P, Crowley M, Hadley FP, Bunting RW. Bacteriologic and immunologic studies on dental caries. *Journal of the American Dental Association.* 1933; 20(12): 2130–2148.

518. Bowen WH. Vaccine against dental caries—A personal view. *Journal of Dental Research.* 1996; 75(8): 1530–1533.

519. Williams NB. Immunization of human beings with oral lactobacilli. *Journal of Dental Research.* 1944; 23(6): 403–411.

520. Parsons EI, McCollum EV, Frobisher Jr. M. The effect of immunization against lactobacilli and acidogenic cocci on the tooth flora of the rat. *American Journal of Epidemiology.* 1946; 43(1): 41–48.

521. Sweeney EA, Shaw JH, Childs EL. Effect of passive immunization on the dental caries incidence of caries-susceptible rats. *Journal of Dental Research.* 1966; 45(4): 993–997.

522. Kesel RG. Dental caries: Etiology, control and activity tests. *Journal of the American Dental Association.* 1943; 30(1): 25–39.

523. Stephan RM. Changes in hydrogen-ion concentration on tooth surfaces and in carious lesions. *Journal of the American Dental Association.* 1940; 27(5): 718–723.

524. Stephan RM. Two factors of possible importance in relation to the etiology and treatment of dental caries and other dental diseases. *Science*. 1940; 92(2399): 578–579.

525. Stephan RM. The effect of urea in counteracting the influence of carbohydrates on the pH of dental plaques. *Journal of Dental Research*. 1943; 22(1): 63–71.

526. Bowen GHW, Hamilton IR. Survival of oral bacteria. *Critical Reviews in Oral Biology and Medicine*. 1998; 9(1): 54–85.

527. Kesel RG, O'Donnell JF, Kirch ER. Deamination of amino acids by the human oral flora; its role in dental caries immunity. *Science*. 1945; 101(2618): 230–231.

528. Kesel RG, O'Donnell JF, Kirch ER, Wach EC. The amino acids and their deaminating systems present in human saliva. *American Journal of Orthodontics and Oral Surgery*. 1947; 33(2): B68-B79.

529. Moncada G, Maureira J, Neira M, Reyes E, Oliveira Junior OB, Faleiros S, Palma P, Corsini G, Ugalde C, Gordan VV, Yevenes I. Salivary urease and ADS enzymatic activity as endogenous protection against dental caries in children. *Journal of Clinical Pediatric Dentistry*. 2015; 39(4): 358–363.

530. Morou-Bermudez E, Elias-Boneta A, Billings RJ, Burne RA, Garcia-Rivas V, Brigoni-Nazario V, Suarez-Perez E. Urease activity in dental plaque and saliva of children during a three-year study period and its relationship with other caries risk factors. *Archives of Oral Biology*. 2011; 56(11): 1282–1289.

531. Kesel RG, O'Donnell JF, Kirch ER, Wach EC. The biological production and therapeutic use of ammonia in the oral cavity in relation to dental caries prevention. *Journal of the American Dental Association*. 1946; 33(11): 695–714.

532. Ayers SH, Rupp P, Mudge CS. The production of ammonia and carbon dioxide by streptococci. *Journal of Infectious Diseases.* 1921; 29(3): 235–260.

533. Niven Jr. CF, Smiley KL, Sherman JM. The hydrolysis of arginine by streptococci. *Journal of Bacteriology.* 1942; 43(6): 651–660.

534. Kesel RG, O'Donnell JF, Kirch ER, Wach EC. Ammonia production in the oral cavity and the use of ammonium salts for the control of dental caries. *American Journal of Orthodontics and Oral Surgery.* 1947; 33(2): B80-B101.

535. Kesel RG. The effectiveness of dentifrices, mouthwashes, and ammonia-urea compounds in the control of dental caries. *Journal of Dental Research.* 1948; 27(2): 244–258.

536. Kleinberg I. "Means and method for improving natural defences against caries." US Patent 4,154,813. Issued May 15, 1979.

537. Acevedo AM, Machado C, Rivera LE, Wolff M, Kleinberg I. The inhibitory effect of an arginine bicarbonate/calcium carbonate (CaviStat®)-containing dentifrice on the development of dental caries in Venezuelan school children. *Journal of Clinical Dentistry.* 2005; 16(3): 63–70.

538. Kraivaphan P, Amornchat C, Triratana T, Mateo LR, Ellwood R, Cummins D, DeVizio W, Zhang Y-P. Two-year caries clinical study of the efficacy of novel dentifrices containing 1.5% arginine, an insoluble calcium compound and 1,450 ppm fluoride. *Caries Research.* 2013; 47(6): 582–590.

539. Zheng X, Cheng X, Wang L. Qiu W, Wang S, Zhou Y, Li M, Li Y, Cheng L, Li J, Zhou X, Xu S. Combinatorial effects of arginine and fluoride on oral bacteria. *Journal of Dental Research.* 2015; 94(2): 344–353.

540. Ástvaldsdór Á, Naimi-Akbar A, Davidson T, Brolund A, Lintamo L, Granath AA, Tranaeus S, Östlund P. Arginine and caries

prevention: A systematic review. *Caries Research*. 2016; 50(4): 383–393.

541. Poboży E, Czarkowska W, Trojanowicz M. Determination of amino acids in saliva using capillary electrophoresis with fluorimetric detection. *Journal of Biochemical and Biophysical Methods*. 2006; 67(1): 37–47.

542. U.S. District Court for the Eastern District of Illinois. 133 F. Supp. 580. The University of Illinois Foundation vs. Block Drug Co., Amm-i-dent, Inc., F.W. Woolworth Co., and Chester J. Henschel. July 12, 1955. Available at: http://law.justia.com/cases/federal/district-courts/FSupp/133/580/1981555/

543. Lehn & Fink's PEB-AMMO ammoniated dentifrice advertisement. *The Pittsburgh Press*. August 17, 1949; 173.

544. Burk NF, Greenberg DM. The physical chemistry of the proteins in non-aqueous and mixed solvents. I. The state of aggregation of certain proteins in urea-water solutions. *Journal of Biological Chemistry*. 1930; 87(2): 197–238.

545. Anson ML, Mirsky AE. The effect of denaturation on the viscosity of protein systems. *Journal of General Physiology*. 1932; 15(3): 341–350.

546. Henschel CJ, Lieber L. Caries incidence reduction by unsupervised use of 27.5 per cent ammonium therapy dentifrice. *Journal of Dental Research*. 1949; 28(3): 248–257.

547. Slanetz LW, Brown EA. Studies on the numbers of bacteria in the mouth and their reduction by the use of oral antiseptics. *Journal of Dental Research*. 1950; 28(3): 313–323.

548. Pearlman S, Hill TJ. Influence of ammonia and of urea upon *L. acidophilus* 4646. I. Studies on growth. *Journal of Dental Research*. 1951; 30(4): 542–557.

549. MacLeod RA, Snell EE. The effect of related ion on the potassium requirement of lactic acid bacteria. *Journal of Biological Chemistry.* 1948; 176(1): 39–52.

550. MacLeod RA, Snell EE. Some mineral requirement of lactic acid bacteria. *Journal of Biological Chemistry.* 1947; 170(1): 351–365.

551. Morou-Bermudez E, Rodriguez S, Bello AS, Dominguez-Bello MG. Urease and dental plaque microbial profiles in children. *PLoS ONE.* 2015; 10(9): e0139315. http://journals.plos.org/plosone/article?id=10.1371/journal.pone.0139315

552. 1915 Nobel Prize in Chemistry: Richard Willstätter. Available from: https://www.nobelprize.org/nobel_prizes/chemistry/laureates/1915/

553. Willstätter R, Stoll A. *Untersuchungen über chlorophyll.* Berlin: Verlag Von Julius Springer, 1913.

554. Fulton Jr. JF. *Animal Chlorophyll: Its Relation To Haemoglobin And To Other Animal Pigments.* No. 137. Cambridge: Bermuda Biological Station for Research, 1922.

555. Gruskin B. "Therapeutic agent for use in the treatment of infection." US Patent 2,120,667. Issued June 14, 1938.

556. Gruskin B. Chlorophyll—its therapeutic place in acute and suppurative disease. *American Journal of Surgery.* 1940; 49(1): 49–55.

557. Medicine: Chlorophyll For Colds. *TIME.* 1940; 36(4): 56–57.

558. Diamond HW, Smith RA. "Soluble compound of chlorophyll and synthesis thereof." US Patent 2,476,358. Issued July 19, 1949.

559. Esten MM, Dannin AG. Chlorophyll therapy and its relation to pathogenic bacteria. *Butler University Botanical Studies.* 1950; 9(1): 212–217.

560. Smith LW. The present status of topical chlorophyll therapy. *New York State Journal of Medicine.* 1955; 55(14): 2041–2050.

561. Big EJ. Nature's mystery: Chlorophyll and photosynthesis. *Bios.* 1943; 14(1): 44–48.

562. Bowler C, Van Montagu M, Inzé D. Superoxide dismutase and stress tolerance. *Annual Review of Plant Physiology and Plant Molecular Biology.* 1992; 43(1): 83–116.

563. Azizullah A, Rehman ZU, Ali I, Murad W, Muhammad N, Ullah W, Häder D-P. Chlorophyll derivatives can be an efficient weapon in the fight against dengue. *Parasitology Research.* 2014; 113(12): 4321–4326.

564. Mowbray S. The antibacterial activity of chlorophyll. *British Medical Journal.* 1957; 1(5013): 268–270.

565. Gruskin B. "Acid neutralizing abrasive chlorophyll dentifrice." US Patent Reissue 24,573. Reissued December 9, 1958.

566. The Era of Good Smelling. *LIFE.* 1952; 32(18): 133–134.

567. Rapp GW. The effect of water soluble chlorophyll "A" on Lactobacillus Acidophilus counts of saliva. *Journal of Dental Research.* 1949; 28(6): 633 (Abstract 1).

568. Griffiths B, Rapp GW. The effect of water soluble chlorophyll on mouth organisms. *Journal of Dental Research.* 1950; 29(5): 690 (Abstract 98).

569. Nevin TA, Bibby BG. The effect of sodium copper chlorophyllin on pure cultures of oral-type organisms. *Journal of Dental Research.* 1954; 33(4): 571–579.

570. Chlorodent chlorophyll dentifrice advertisement. *LIFE.* 1952; 33(18): 12. Available from: https://books.google.com/books?id =1IEAAAAMBAJ&pg=PA12&dq=1952+Chlorodent+Toothpas te+Ad&hl=en&sa=X&ved=0ahUKEwiikcDCiJvWAhVH2SYK HceZDvIQ6AEIQzAG#v=onepage&q&f=false

571. Retail Trade: Green Gold. *TIME.* 1952; 59(15): 102.

572. Colgate chlorophyll dentifrice advertisement. *LIFE*. 1952; 33(7): 40. Available from: https://books.google.com/books?id=Y1YEA AAAMBAJ&pg=PA40&dq=1952+colgate+chlorophyll+Toothpast e&hl=en&sa=X&ved=0ahUKEwjpoofwiZvWAhVM6yYKHRG nChEQ6AEINDAC#v=onepage&q&f=false

573. Amm-i-dent chlorophyll dentifrice advertisement. *LIFE*. 1952; 32(24): 57. Available from: http://gogd.tjs-labs.com/ show-picture?id=1126032351&size=NORM

574. Bureau of economic research and statistics. The ILWU-PMA dental program: first year statistics. IV. The nine dental plans. *Journal of the American Dental Association*. 1958; 57(6): 754–760.

575. American Dental Association statement on dentifrice advertising claims. *Journal of the American Dental Association*. 1958; 57(4): 546–561.

576. Procter & Gamble advertisement for Crest with Fluoristan. Available from: https://www.youtube.com/watch?v=v72NHYp8KD4

577. American Dental Association statement on dentifrice advertising claims. *Journal of the American Dental Association*. 1958; 57(3): 430–433.

578. Pfarrer AM, Karlinsey RL. Challenges of implementing new remineralization technologies. *Advances in Dental Research*. 2009; 21(1): 79–82.

579. Pessan JP, Toumba KJ, Buzalaf MAR. "Topical Use of Fluorides for Caries Control." Buzalaf MAR (Ed.), In: *Fluoride and the Oral Environment*. Basel: Karger Publishers, 2011, Vol 22, 115–132.

580. Dana JD. *A Manual of Mineralogy*. London: Delf & Trübner, 1852.

581. Harvey FL. *The Minerals and Rocks of Arkansas*. Philadelphia: Grant & Faires, 1886.

582. Ulrich EO, Tangier Smith WS. *The Lead, Zinc, and Fluorspar Deposits of Western Kentucky.* Washington: Government Printing Office, 1905.

583. Landes KK. Colorado pegmatites. *The American Mineralogist.* 1935; 20(5): 319–333.

584. McKay FS, Black GV. Mottled teeth: An endemic developmental imperfection of the teeth, heretofore unknown in the literature of dentistry. *Dental Cosmos.* 1916; 58(2): 129–156.

585. Eager JM. Denti di Chiaie (Chiaie teeth). *Public Health Reports.* 1901; 16(44): 284–285.

586. Kempf GA, McKay FS. Mottled enamel in a segregated population. *Public Health Reports.* 1930; 45(48): 2923–2940.

587. Williams JL. Mottled enamel, and other studies of normal and pathological conditions of this tissue. *Journal of Dental Research.* 1923; 5(3): 117–195.

588. Schüssler DM, O'Conner JT. *The Biochemical Treatment of Disease, New Translation of 12th German Edition.* Philadelphia: F.E. Boericke, 1885.

589. Wilson T. On the presence of fluorine as a test for the fossilization of animal bones. *The American Naturalist.* 1895; 29(340): 301–317.

590. Wilson T. On the presence of fluorine as a test for the fossilization of animal bones. *The American Naturalist.* 1895; 29(341): 439–456.

591. Iyengar V, Woittiez J. Trace elements in human clinical specimens: Evaluation of literature data to identify reference values. *Clinical Chemistry.* 1988; 34(3): 474–481.

592. Iyengar GV, Tandon L. Minor and trace elements in human bones and teeth. No. NAHRES-39. International Atomic Energy Agency, 1999.

593. The Chemistry of Life: The Human Body. April 16, 2009. Available from: http://www.livescience.com/3505-chemistry-life-human-body.html

594. Buzalaf MAR, Whitford, GM. "Fluoride Metabolism." Buzalaf MAR (Ed.), In: *Fluoride and the Oral Environment*. Basel: Karger Publishers, 2011, Vol 22, 20–36.

595. Monier-Williams GW. The distribution of fluorine in animal and vegetable tissues, and its estimation in minute quantities. *The Chemical World*. 1912; 1(8): 255–257.

596. Van Burkalow A. Fluorine in United States waters supplies: Pilot project for the atlas of diseases. *Geographical Review*. 1946; 36(2): 177–193.

597. McCollum EV, Simmonds N, Becker JE, Bunting RW. The effect of additions of fluorine to the diet of the rat on the quality of the teeth. *Journal of Biological Chemistry*. 1925; 63(3): 553–562.

598. Whitford, GM. "Acute Toxicity of Ingested Fluoride." Buzalaf MAR (Ed.), In: *Fluoride and the Oral Environment*. Basel: Karger Publishers, 2011, Vol 22, 66–80.

599. Turneaure CE, Russel HL. *Public Water-Supplies. Requirements, Resources, and the Construction of Works*. New York: John Wiley & Sons, 1901.

600. Thresh JC. *The Examination of Waters and Water Supplies*. Philadelphia: P. Blakiston's Son & Co, 1904.

601. Allen TF. *Effects of Lead Upon Healthy Individuals*. Philadelphia: Sherman & Co., 1878.

602. Buonocore MG, Bibby BG. The effects of various ions on enamel solubility. *Journal of Dental Research*. 1945; 24(2): 103–108.

603. Asgar K. Chemical analysis of human teeth. *Journal of Dental Research*. 1956; 35(5): 742–748.

604. Verbeeck RMH, Lassuyt CJ, Heijligers HJM, Driessens FCM, Vrolijk JWGA. Lattice parameters and cation distribution of solid solutions of calcium and lead hydroxyapatite. *Calcified Tissue International*. 1981; 33(1): 243–247.

605. Churchill HV. The occurrence of fluorides in some waters of the United States. *Journal of Dental Research*. 1932; 12(1): 141–148.

606. Elvove E. Estimation of fluorides in waters. *Public Health Reports*. 1933; 48(40): 1219–1222.

607. Dean HT, McKay FS. Production of mottled enamel halted by a change in common water supply. American Journal of Public Health and the Nations Health. 1939; 29(6): 590–596.

608. Dean HT, Elvove E. Some epidemiological aspects of chronic endemic dental fluorosis. *American Journal of Public Health and the Nations Health*. 1936; 26(6): 567–575.

609. Dean HT. Some reflections on the epidemiology of fluorine and dental health. *American Journal of Public Health and the Nations Health*. 1953; 43(6): 704–709.

610. Smith MC, Lantz E, Smith HV. The cause of mottled enamel. *Journal of Dental Research*. 1932; 12(1): 149–159.

611. Dean HT, Jay P, Arnold Jr. FA, Elvove E. Domestic water and dental caries: II. A study of 2,832 white children, aged 12–14 years, of 8 suburban Chicago communities, including Lactobacillus Acidophilus studies of 1,761 children. *Public Health Reports*. 1941; 56(15): 761–792.

612. Sampaio FC, Levy SM. "Systemic Fluoride." Buzalaf MAR (Ed.), In: *Fluoride and the Oral Environment*. Basel: Karger Publishers, 2011, Vol 22, 133–145.

613. Den Besten P, Li W. "Chronic Fluoride Toxicity: Dental Fluorosis." Buzalaf MAR (Ed.), In: *Fluoride and the Oral Environment*. Basel: Karger Publishers, 2011, Vol 22, 81–96.

614. Schamschula RG, Barmes DE. Fluoride and health: Dental caries, osteoporosis and cardiovascular disease. *Annual Review of Nutrition*. 1981; 1(1): 427–435.

615. Whitford GM, Sampaio FC, Pinto CS, Maria AG, Cardoso VE, Buzalaf MA. Pharmacokinetics of ingested fluoride: lack of effect of chemical compound. *Archives of Oral Biology*. 2008; 53(11): 1037–1041.

616. Horowitz HS. The future of water fluoridation and other systemic fluorides. *Journal of Dental Research*. 1990; 68(Spec Iss): 760–764.

617. Platteborze PL. Fluoridation. Making tooth decay go away. *Michigan History*. 2014; May/June: 39–44.

618. Council on Dental Therapeutics. Changes in drugs, chemicals and devices during the war period. *Journal of the American Dental Association*. 1946; 33(1): 44–48.

619. Armstrong WD, Brekhus PJ. Possible relationship between the fluorine content of enamel and resistance to dental caries. *Journal of Dental Research*. 1938; 17(5): 393–399.

620. Cheyne VD. Human dental caries and topically applied fluorine: A preliminary report. *Journal of the American Dental Association*. 1942; 29(5): 804–807.

621. Bibby BG. Preliminary report on the use of sodium fluoride applications in caries prophylaxis. *Journal of Dental Research*. 1942; 21(Abstract 45): 314.

622. Largent EJ, Moses JB. Topical application of fluoride and fluoride absorption. *Journal of the American Dental Association*. 1943; 30(15): 1246–1249.

623. Knutson JW, Armstrong WD. The effect of topically applied sodium fluoride on dental caries experience. *Public Health Reports*. 1943; 58(47): 1701–1715.

624. Bibby BG. The use of fluorine in the prevention of dental caries. I. Rationale and approach. *Journal of the American Dental Association.* 1944; 31(3): 228–236.

625. Bibby BG. The use of fluorine in the prevention of dental caries. II. Effect of sodium fluoride applications. *Journal of the American Dental Association.* 1944; 31(5): 317–321.

626. Bibby BG. The use of fluorine in the prevention of dental caries. III. A consideration of the effectiveness of various fluoride mixtures. *Journal of the American Dental Association.* 1947; 34(1): 26–32.

627. Galagan DJ, Knutson JW. The effect of topically applied sodium fluoride on dental caries experience. V. Report of findings with two, four and six applications of sodium fluoride and of lead fluoride. *Public Health Reports.* 1947; 62(41): 1477–1483.

628. Bibby BG. A test of the effect of fluoride-containing dentifrices on dental caries. *Journal of Dental Research.* 1945; 24(6): 297–303.

629. Jay P. Fluorine and dental caries. *Journal of the American Dental Association.* 1946; 33(7): 489–495.

630. Phillips RW. Effect of fluorides on hardness of tooth enamel. *Journal of the American Dental Association.* 1948; 37(1): 1–13.

631. Shaner EO, Smith RR. Clinical and bacteriological studies of the use of a fluoride dentifrice. *Journal of Dental Research.* 1946; 25(3): 121–126.

632. Bibby BG. Fluoride mouthwashes, fluoride dentifrices, and other uses of fluorides in control of caries. *Journal of Dental Research.* 1948; 27(3): 367–375.

633. Muhler JC, Radike AW, Nebergall WH, Day HG. The effect of a stannous fluoride-containing dentifrice on caries reduction in children. *Journal of Dental Research.* 1954; 33(5): 606–612.

634. Nebergall WH. "Dentifrice Preparations." US Patent 2,876,166. Issued March 3, 1959.

635. Muhler JC, Radike AW, Nebergall WH, Day HG. The effect of a stannous fluoride-containing dentifrice on caries reduction in adults. *Journal of Dental Research*. 1959; 35(1): 49–53.

636. Brudevold F, McCann HG, Nilsson R, Richardson B, Coklica V. The chemistry of caries inhibition problems and challenges in topical treatments. *Journal of Dental Research*. 1967; 46(1): 37–45.

637. Brudevold F, Hein JW, Bonner JF, Nevin RB, Bibby BG, Hodge HC. Reaction of tooth surfaces with one ppm of fluoride as sodium fluoride. *Journal of Dental Research*. 1957; 36(5): 771–779.

638. Gerould CH. Electron microscope study of the mechanism of fluorine deposition in teeth. *Journal of Dental Research*. 1945; 24(5): 223–233.

639. McCann HG. Reactions of fluoride ion with hydroxyapatite. *Journal of Biological Chemistry*. 1953; 201(1): 247–259.

640. McCann HG, Bullock FA. Reactions of fluoride ion with powdered enamel and dentin. *Journal of Dental Research*. 1955; 34(1): 59–67.

641. Fischer RB, Muhler JC. The effect of sodium fluorine upon the surface structure of powdered enamel. *Journal of Dental Research*. 1952; 31(6): 751–755.

642. Jeansonne BG, Feagin FF. Effects of various topical fluorides on subsequent mineralization and dissolution of enamel. *Journal of Dental Research*. 1972; 51(3): 767–772.

643. Phantumvanit P, Feagin FF, Koulourides T. Strong and weak acid sampling for fluoride of enamel remineralized in sodium fluoride solutions. *Caries Research*. 1977; 11(1): 52–61.

644. Rathje W. The formation of hydroxyfluor-apatite in tooth enamel under influence of drinking water containing fluoride. *Journal of Dental Research*. 1952; 31(6): 761–766.

645. Chow LC, Brown WE. Reaction of dicalcium phosphate dihydrate with fluoride. *Journal of Dental Research*. 1973; 52(6): 1220–1227.

646. Fischer RB, Muhler JC, Wust CJ. Effects of several fluoride reagents on the surface structure of powdered dental enamel. *Journal of Dental Research*. 1954; 33(1): 50–54.

647. Stookey GK, Hudson JT, Muhler JC. Laboratory studies concerning the effectiveness and safety of various fluoride and fluoride-phosphate systems. *Journal of Dental Research*. 1967; 46(3): 503–513.

648. Stookey GK. Critical evaluation of the composition and use of topical fluorides. *Journal of Dental Research*. 1990; 69(Spec Iss): 805–812.

649. Featherstone JDB. Remineralization, the natural caries repair process—the need for new approaches. *Advances in Dental Research*. 2009; 21(1): 4–7.

650. Karlinsey RL, Pfarrer AM. Fluoride plus functionalized β-TCP: A promising combination for robust remineralization. *Advances in Dental Research*. 2012; 24(2): 48–52.

651. Richardson B. Fixation of topically applied fluoride in enamel. *Journal of Dental Research*. 1967; 46(1): 87–93.

652. Rølla G, Saxegaard E. Critical evaluation of the composition and use of topical fluorides, with emphasis on the role of calcium fluoride in caries inhibition. *Journal of Dental Research*. 1990; 69(Spec Iss): 780–785.

653. Øgaard B. CaF_2 formation: Cariostatic properties and factors of enhancing the effect. *Caries Research*. 2001; 35(Suppl 1): 40–44.

654. Larsen MJ, Richards A. The influence of saliva on the formation of calcium fluoride-like material on human dental enamel. *Caries Research*. 2001; 35(1): 57–60.

655. Margalit D, Gedalia I. Release of fluoride into saliva after topical fluoride application. *Journal of Dental Research.* 1969; 48(1): 93–96.

656. Arends J, Schuthof J. Fluoride content in human enamel after fluoride application and washing—an in vitro study. *Caries Research.* 1975; 9(5): 363–372.

657. Petersson LG, Pakhomov GN, Twetman S. "Fluoride varnish for community-based caries prevention in children." Geneva: World Health Organization, 1997, 1–18.

658. Karlinsey RL. Fluoride varnishes: Why they work & what to look for. *EC Dental Science.* 2016; 5(6): 1220–1223.

659. Chow LC, Brown WE. Formation of $CaHPO_4 \bullet 2H_2O$ in tooth enamel as an intermediate product in topical fluoride treatments. *Journal of Dental Research.* 1975; 54(1): 65–76.

660. Tung MS, Chow LC, Brown WE. Hydrolysis of dicalcium phosphate dihydrate in the presence or absence of calcium fluoride. *Journal of Dental Research.* 1985; 64(1): 2–5.

661. Vogel GL, Chow LC, Carey CM. Calcium pre-rinse greatly increases overnight salivary fluoride after a 228 ppm fluoride rinse. *Caries Research.* 2008; 42(5): 401–404.

662. Vogel GL. "Oral fluoride reservoirs and the prevention of dental caries." Buzalaf MAR (Ed.), In: *Fluoride and the Oral Environment.* Basel: Karger Publishers, 2011, Vol 22, 146–157.

663. Tung MS. "Methods And Compositions For Mineralizing And Fluoridating Calcified Tissues." US Patent 5,268,167. Issued December 7, 1993.

664. Winston AE, Usen N. "Stable Single-Part Compositions And The Use Thereof For Remineralization Of Lesions in Teeth." US Patent 5,571,502. Issued November 5, 1996.

665. Winston AE, Usen N. "Processes And Compositions For The Remineralization Of Teeth." US Patent 5,603,922. Issued February 18, 1997.

666. Schemehorn BR, Winston AE. Laboratory enamel solubility reduction and fluoride uptake from Enamelon dentifrice. *Journal of Clinical Dentistry*. 1999; 10(1): 9–12.

667. Tung MS, Eichmiller FC. Amorphous calcium phosphates for tooth mineralization. *Compendium of Continuous Education in Dentistry*. 2004; 25(9): 9–13.

668. Schemehorn BR, Wood GD, McHale W, Winston AE. Comparison of fluoride uptake into tooth enamel from two fluoride varnishes containing different calcium phosphate sources. *Journal of Clinical Dentistry*. 2011; 22(2): 51–54.

669. Karlinsey RL. Benefits of functionalized tricalcium phosphate. *EC Dental Science*. 2016; 7(1): 41–42.

670. Karlinsey RL, Mackey AC. Solid-state preparation and dental application of an organically modified calcium phosphate. *Journal of Materials Science*. 2009; 44(1): 346–349.

671. Karlinsey RL, Mackey AC, Walker ER, Frederick KE. Surfactant-modified β-TCP: structure, properties, and in vitro remineralization of subsurface enamel lesions. *Journal of Materials Science: Materials in Medicine*. 2010; 21(7): 2009–2020.

672. Karlinsey RL, Mackey AC, Walker ER, Frederick KE. Preparation, characterization and in vitro efficacy of an acid-modified β-TCP material for dental hard-tissue remineralization. *Acta Biomaterialia*. 2010; 6(3): 969–978.

673. de Oliveira AFB, Mathews SM, Ramalingam K, Amaechi B. The effectiveness of an NaF rinse containing fTCP on eroded enamel remineralization. *Journal of Public Health*. 2016; 24(2): 147–152.

674. Karlinsey RL, Mackey AC, Walker ER, Amaechi BT, Karthikeyan R, Najibfard K, Pfarrer AM. Remineralization potential of 5,000 ppm fluoride dentifrices evaluated in a pH cycling model. *Journal of Dentistry and Oral Hygiene*. 2010; 2(1): 1–6. doi: http://www.academicjournals.org/journal/JDOH/article-full-text-pdf/A316A40869

675. Amaechi BT, Ramalingam K, Mensinkai PK, Chedjieu I. *In situ* remineralization of early caries by a new high-fluoride dentifrice. *General Dentistry*. 2012; 60(4): 186–192.

676. Food and Drug Administration. Topical fluoride preparations for reducing incidence of dental caries. *Federal Register*. 1974; 39(94): 1724.

677. Griffin SO, Regnier E, Griffin PM, Huntley V. Effectiveness of fluoride in preventing caries in adults. *Journal of Dental Research*. 2007; 86(5): 410–415.

678. Do LG, Spencer AJ. Risk-benefit balance in the use of fluoride among young children. *Journal of Dental Research*. 2007; 86(8): 723–728.

679. Radnai M, Fazekas A. Caries prevalence in adults seven years after previous exposure to fluoride in domestic salt. *Acta Medica Dentica Helvetica*. 1999; 4(10): 163–166.

680. Yengopal V, Chikte UM, Mickenautsch S, Oliveira LB, Bhayat A. Efficacy of salt fluoridation. *South African Dental Journal*. 2010; 65(2): 60–67.

681. Newbrun E. Finn Brudevold: Discovery of acidulated phosphate fluoride in caries prevention. *Journal of Dental Research*. 2011; 90(8): 977–980.

682. Marinho VC, Higgins JP, Sheiham A, Logan S. Fluoride mouth-rinses for preventing dental caries in children and adolescents. *Cochrane Database of Systematic Reviews*. 2003; 3: Article CD002284.

683. Marinho VC, Higgins JPT, Sheiham A, Logan S. Combinations of topical fluoride (toothpastes, mouthrinses, gels, varnishes) versus single topical fluoride for preventing dental caries in children and adolescents. *Cochrane Database of Systematic Reviews*. 2004; 1: CD002781.

684. Benson PE, Parkin N, Millett DT, Dyer FE, Vine S, Shah A. Fluorides for the prevention of white spots on teeth during fixed brace treatment. *Cochrane Database of Systematic Reviews*. 2004; 3: CD003809.

685. Marinho VC, Higgins JPT, Sheiham A, Logan S. One topical fluoride (toothpastes, or mouthrinses, or gels, or varnishes) versus another for preventing dental caries in children and adolescents. *Cochrane Database of Systematic Reviews*. 2004; 1: CD002780.

686. Mellberg JR. Evaluation of topical fluoride preparations. *Journal of Dental Research*. 1990; 69(Spec Iss): 771–779.

687. Ekstrand J. Pharmacokinetic aspects of topical fluorides. *Journal of Dental Research*. 1987; 66(5): 1061–1065.

688. Whitford GM. Fluoride in dental products: Safety considerations. *Journal of Dental Research*. 1987; 66(5): 1056–1060.

689. Rojas Zelad KG. Thesis: Fluoride concentration in urine after topical fluoride application in pediatric patients in educational institution No. 80706—Miramar. Universidad Nacional de Trujillo, Peru. 2017; doi: http://dspace.unitru.edu.pe/handle/UNITRU/7532.

690. Stookey GK, Schemehorn BR, Drook CA, Cheetham BL. The effect of rinsing with water immediately after a professional fluoride gel application on fluoride uptake in demineralized enamel: an in vivo study. *Pediatric Dentistry*. 1996; 8(2): 153–157.

691. Garcia RI, Gregorich SE, Ramos-Gomez F, Braun PA, Wilson A, Albino J, Tiwari T, Harper M, Batliner TS, Rasmussen M, Cheng NF, Santo W, Geltman PL, Henshaw M, Gansky SA. Absence of fluoride varnish-related adverse events in caries prevention trials

in young children, United States. *Preventing Chronic Disease.* 2017; 14(E17): 160372. doi: http://dx.doi.org/10.5888/pcd14.160372.

692. Ramos-Gomez FJ, Crystal YO, Domejean S, Featherstone JDB. Minimal intervention dentistry: Part 3. Paediatric dental care—prevention and management protocols using caries risk assessment for infants and young children. *British Dental Journal.* 2012; 213(10): 501–508.

693. Weyant RJ, Tracy SL, Anselmo T, Beltrán-Aguilar ED, Donly KJ, Frese WA, Hujoel PP, Iafolla T, Kohn W, Kumar J, Levy SM, Tinanoff N, Wright JT, Zero D, Aravamudhan K, Frantsve-Hawley J, Meyer DM. Topical fluoride for caries prevention: Executive summary of the updated clinical recommendations and supporting systematic review. *Journal of the American Dental Association.* 2013; 144(11): 1279–1291.

694. American Academy of Pediatric Dentistry, Liaison with other Groups Committee. Policy on use of fluoride. Reference Manual. 2008; 33(6): 40–41.

695. Centers for Disease Control and Prevention. Recommendations for using fluoride to prevent and control dental caries in the United States. *MMWR.* 2001; 50(RR14): 1–42.

696. Moyer VA, on behalf of U.S. Preventive Services Task Force. Prevention of dental caries in children from birth through age 5 years: U.S. Preventive Services Task Force Recommendation Statement. *Pediatrics.* 2014; 133(5): 1–10.

697. Swigonski NL, Yoder KM, Maupome G, Ofner S. Dental providers' attitudes regarding the application of fluoride varnish by pediatric health care providers. *Journal of Public Health Dentistry.* 2009; 69(4): 242–247.

698. Hendrix KS, Downs SM, Brophy G, Doebbeling CC, Swignoski NL. Threshold analysis of reimbursing physicians for the

application of fluoride varnish in young children. *Journal of Public Health Dentistry*. 2013; 73: 297–303.

699. Brudevold F, Gardner DE, Smith FA. The distribution of fluoride in human enamel. *Journal of Dental Research*. 1956; 35(3): 420–429.

700. Stearns RI. Incorporation of fluoride by human enamel: I. Solid-state diffusion process. *Journal of Dental Research*. 1970; 49(6): 1444–1451.

701. Brudevold F, McCann HG. Enamel solubility tests and their significance in regard to dental caries. *Annals of the New York Academy of Sciences*. 1968; 153: 20–51.

702. 3M Oral Care Vanish™ 5% NaF White Varnish with Tri-Calcium Phosphate. Available from: http://www.3m.com/3M/en_US/company-us/all-3m-products/~/vanish-Vanish-5-Sodium-Fluoride-White-Varnish-with-Tri-Calcium-Phosphate?N=5002385+3294768932&rt=rud

703. 3M Oral Care Clinpro™ White Vanish with TCP. Available from: http://solutions.3m.co.uk/wps/portal/3M/en_GB/3M_ESPE/Dental-Manufacturers/Products/Preventive-Dentistry/Dental-Prevention/Tooth-Desensitiser/

704. Kolb V, Klaiber P, Pfarrer A, Farlee R. *In vivo* study: Migration and salivary fluoride after varnish application. *Journal of Dental Research*. 2010; 89(Spec Iss A): Abstract 312.

705. Kolb V, Klaiber P, Pfarrer A. *In vivo* study: Fluoride varnish migration and salivary fluoride. *Journal of Dental Research*. 2010; 89(Spec Iss B): Abstract 4013.

706. Cochrane NJ, Shen P, Yuan Y, Reynolds EC. Ion release from calcium and fluoride containing dental varnishes. *Australian Dental Journal*. 2014; 59(1): 100–105.

707. Karlinsey RL. "Hybrid Organic/Inorganic Chemical Hybrid Systems, Including Functionalized Calcium Phosphate Hybrid

Systems, And A Solid-State Method For Producing The Same." US Patent 8,556,553. Issued October 15, 2013.

708. Pitchika V, Kokel C, Andreeva J, Crispin A, Hickel R, Kühnisch J, Heinrich-Weltzien R. Effectiveness of a new fluoride varnish for caries prevention in pre-school children. *Journal of Clinical Pediatric Dentistry*. 2013; 38(1): 7–12.

709. Damyanova D, Ivanova K. The effect of mineralizing fluorine varnish on the progression of initial caries of enamel in temporary dentition by laser fluorescence. *American Journal of Engineering Research*. 2017; 6(9): 39–43.

710. Damyanova D. Evaluation of the effect of mineralization varnish on the progression of D1 and D2 enamel caries lesions in temporary dentition. *Varna Medical Forum*. 2017; 6(2): 66–70.

711. Damyanova D, Angelova S, Targova-Dimitrova T. Clinical study remineralization effect of mineralization varnish. *IOSR Journal of Dental and Medical Sciences*. 2016; 15(8): 134–146.

712. Kolb V, Burgio P, Klaiber P, Neuenfeldt E, Klutzke R, Pfarrer A. Migration of fluoride varnish after application: An *in vivo* study. *Journal of Dental Research*. 2009; 88(Spec Iss A): Abstract 1170.

713. Flanigan P-J, Vang F, Pfarrer A. Remineralization and acid resistance effects of 5% NaF varnishes. *Journal of Dental Research*. 2010; 89(Spec Iss B): Abstract 383.

714. Al Amoudi SA, Pani SC, Al Omari M. The effect of the addition of tricalcium phosphate to 5% sodium fluoride varnishes on the microhardness of enamel of primary teeth. *International Journal of Dentistry*. 2013; Article ID 486358.

715. Elkassas D, Arafa A. Remineralizing efficacy of different calcium-phosphate and fluoride based delivery vehicles on artificial caries like enamel lesions. *Journal of Dentistry*. 2014; 42(4): 466–474.

716. Ulkur F, Ekçi ES, Nalbantgil D, Sandalli N. *In vitro* effects of two topical varnish materials and Er:YAG laser irradiation on enamel demineralization around orthodontic brackets. *The Scientific World Journal.* 2014; Article ID 490503.

717. Karlinsey RL, Mackey AC, Dodge LE, Schwandt CS. Noncontact remineralization of incipient lesion treated with a 5% sodium fluoride varnish in vitro. *Journal of Dentistry* for Children. 2014; 81(1): 7–13.

718. Flanigan P-J, Klaiber P, Vang F, Haeberlein I, Stein C. High fluoride content alone in varnishes does not guarantee high surface microhardness remineralization. *Caries Research.* 2014; 48(5): 407.

719. Darshana D, Mithra HN, Fayaz G, Pushparaj S. Compartive evaluation of effect of a remineralizing agent on bleached tooth surface: An *in-vitro* study. *Journal of Pharmaceutical and Scientific Innovation.* 2014; 3(4): 371–374.

720. Al-Ajlan S. Functional tricalcium-phosphate influence on remineralization process of fluoridated enamel surface. *Journal of Dental Research.* 2015; 94(Spec Iss A): Abstract 3915.

721. Zhu Y-T, Liu J-F, Li X-X, Huang J-Y, Li Y-L. Clinical study on the effect of Clinpro™ White Varnish fluoride protective coating on tooth surface demineralization in orthodontic treatment. *International Journal of Stomatology.* 2015; 42(3): 306–309. doi: 10.7518/gjkq.2015.03.015

722. Arafa A. Synergistic remineralization effectiveness of calcium, phosphate and fluoride based systems in primary teeth. *Pediatric Dental Journal.* 2017; 27(1): 65–71.

723. Cho H-J, Lee H-C, Lee J-Y, Jin B-H. Tricalcium phosphate: Remineralization ability of fluoride varnish containing tricalcium phosphate by time. *Journal of Korean Academy of Oral Health.* 2017; 41(1): 3–8.

724. Al Dehailan L, Lippert F, González-Cabezas C, Eckert GJ, Martinez-Mier EA. Fluoride concentration in saliva and biofilm fluid following the application of three fluoride varnishes. *Journal of Dentistry*. 2017; 50(5): 87–93.

725. Pamir T, Ercan E, Ergücü Z, Önal B. Clinical effect of a fluoride varnish including tri-calcium phosphate on relieving dentin sensitivity. *Turkish Clinics Journal of Dental Science*. 2015; 21(1): 18–24.

726. Oliveira BH, Salazar M, Carvalho DM, Falcão A, Campos K, Nadanovsky P. Biannual fluoride varnish applications and caries incidence in pre-schoolers: A 24-month follow-up randomized placebo-controlled clinical trial. *Caries Research*. 2014; 48(3): 228–236.

727. Gao SS, Zhang S, Mei ML, Lo EC-M, Chu C-H. Caries remineralisation and arresting effect in children by professionally applied fluoride treatment—a systematic review. *BMC Oral Health*. 2016; 16:12. https://bmcoralhealth.biomedcentral.com/articles/10.1186/s12903-016-0171-6

728. Rosenblatt A, Stamford TCM, Niederman R. Silver diamine fluoride: A caries "silver-fluoride bullet." *Journal of Dental Research*. 2009; 88(2): 116–125.

729. Yee R, Holmgren C, Mulder J, Lama D, Walker D, van Palenstein Helderman W. Efficacy of silver diamine fluoride for arresting caries treatment. *Journal of Dental Research*. 2009; 88(7): 644–647.

730. Gluzman R, Katz RV, Frey BJ, McGowan R. Prevention of root caries: A literature review of primary and secondary preventive agents. *Special Care in Dentistry*. 2013; 33(3): 133–140.

731. Chen A, Cho M, Kichler S, Lam J, Liaque A, Sultan S. Silver diamine fluoride: An alternative to topical fluorides. *Journal of the Canadian Dental Association*. 2012; 78(1): 1–14.

732. American Dental Association. Silver diamine fluoride in caries management. July 12, 2016. Available from: http://

www.ada.org/en/science-research/science-in-the-news/
silver-diamine-fluoride-in-caries-management

733. Crystal YO, Janal MN, Hamilton DS, Niederman R. Parental perceptions and acceptance of silver diamine fluoride staining. *Journal of the American Dental Association*. 2017; 148(7): 510–518.

734. Zero DT. Dentifrices, mouthwashes, and remineralization/caries arrestment strategies. *BMC Oral Health*. 2006; 6(Suppl 1): S9. https://www.ncbi.nlm.nih.gov/pmc/articles/PMC2147065/

735. Lippert F. "An introduction to toothpaste—its purpose, history and ingredients." van Loveren C (Ed.), In: *Toothpastes*. Basel: Karger Publishers, 2013, Vol 23, 1–14.

736. Marinho VC, Higgins JPT, Logan S, Sheiham A. Fluoride toothpastes for preventing dental caries in children and adolescents. *Cochrane Database of Systematic Reviews*. 2003; 1: CD002278.

737. Tavss EA, Mellberg JR, Joziak M, Gambogi RJ, Fisher SW. Relationship between dentifrice fluoride concentration and clinical caries reduction. *American Journal of Dentistry*. 2003; 16(6): 369–374.

738. Walsh T, Worthington HV, Glenny AM, Appelbe P, Marinho VCC, Shi X. Fluoride toothpastes of different concentrations for preventing dental caries in children and adolescents. *Cochrane Database of Systematic Reviews*. 2010; 1: CD007868.

739. Vani G, Babu G, Panchanatham N. Toothpaste brands—A study of consumer behaviour in Bangalore city. *Journal of Economics and Behavioral Studies*. 2010; 1(1): 27–39.

740. Lee H-S, O'Mahony M. Sensory evaluation and marketing: measurement of a consumer concept. *Food Quality and Preference*. 2005; 16(3): 227–235.

741. Gutierrez BPB. Determinants of toothpaste brand choice in urban Philippines. *Philippine Management Review*. 2005; 12(1): 45–71.

742. Amaechi BT, van Loveren C. "Fluorides and non-fluoride remineralization systems." van Loveren C (Ed.), In: *Toothpastes*. Basel: Karger Publishers, 2013, Vol 23, 15–26.

743. 3M Clinpro™ Tooth Crème. Available from: http://www.3m.com/3M/en_US/company-us/all-3m-products/~/Clinpro-Tooth-Cr%C3%A8me-0-21-NaF-Anticavity-Toothpaste-Vanilla-Mint-12117?N=5002385+3293403768&rt=rud

744. 3M Clinpro™ 5000. Available from: http://www.3m.com/3M/en_US/company-us/all-3m-products/~/clinpro-5000-Clinpro-5000-1-1-Sodium-Fluoride-Anti-Cavity-Toothpaste?N=5002385+3294768934&rt=rud

745. NIH RePORTER. Award search for 'Karlinsey Robert'. Available from: https://projectreporter.nih.gov/reporter_pisummary.cfm?pi_id=8449750&map=y; or, see www.indianananotech.com for summary information.

746. Karlinsey RL, Mackey AC, Stookey GK, AM Pfarrer. *In vitro* assessments of experimental NaF dentifrices containing a prospective calcium phosphate technology. *American Journal of Dentistry*. 2009; 22(3): 180–184.

747. Karlinsey RL, Mackey AC, Stookey GK. *In vitro* remineralization efficacy of NaF systems containing unique forms of calcium. *American Journal of Dentistry*. 2009; 22(3): 185–188.

748. Patil N, Choudhari S, Kulkarni S, Joshi SR. Comparative evaluation of remineralizing potential of three agents on artificially demineralized human enamel: An *in vitro* study. *Journal of Conservative Dentistry*. 2013; 16(2): 116–120.

749. Babu V, Dave PN, Bhanushali PV, Moureen A, Shah S, Kiran YC. Comparative analysis of remineralizing potential of three commercially available agents—An in vitro study. *IOSR Journal of Dental and Medical Sciences*. 2017; 16(2): 1–5.

750. Singla MG, Relhan N, Tangri T. An in vitro study to evaluate and compare the effects of various commercially available remineralizing agents on surface microhardness of artificially produced enamel lesions. *IOSR Journal of Dental and Medical Sciences.* 2017; 13(2): 67–72.

751. Bolin KA, Karlinsey RL, Mackey A, Bitouni A, Jones D, Skur P. *In situ* evaluation of 950 and 1100 ppm dentifrices. *Journal of Dental Research.* 2013; 92(Spec Iss A): Abstract 2030.

752. Karlinsey, Mackey AC, Walker ER. Cross-sectional microhardness assessment of enamel remineralization from calcium-containing NaF formulations. *Caries Research.* 2009; 43(3): 221.

753. Buckshey S, Anthonappa R, King N, Itthagarun A. Remineralizing action of CPP-ACP reagents on artificial carious lesions. *International Journal of Paediatric Dentistry.* 2011; 21(Suppl 1): 31.

754. Sri-Aularawat W, Nakornchai S, Thaweboon S, Korsuwannawong S. Effect of tricalcium phosphate, casein phosphopeptide—amorphous calcium phosphate and sodium fluoride products on demineralization of artificial advanced enamel lesions. *International Journal of Oral Research.* 2012; 3(e2): 1–8.

755. Hamba H, Nakamura K, Nikaido T, Tagami J. Effect of remineralization of enamel subsurface lesions by toothpaste containing fTCP and NaF: a micro-CT analysis. *Journal of the Japanese Society for Dental Materials and Devices.* 2015; 34(2): 129.

756. Vanichvatana S, Auychai P. Efficacy of two calcium phosphate pastes on the remineralization of artificial caries: a randomized controlled double-blind *in situ* study. *International Journal of Oral Science.* 2013; 5(4): 224–228.

757. Linlin H, Masayoshi F. *In vitro* assessment of enamel acid resistance, dentin tubule occlusion and element incorporation with

fluoride and *f*TCP-containing toothpaste. *Japanese Journal of Conservative Dentistry.* 2016; 59(2): 228–235.

758. Karlinsey RL, Mackey AC, Schwandt CS, Walker TJ. SEM evaluation of demineralized dentin treated with professional-strength NaF topical pastes. *American Journal of Dentistry.* 2011; 24(6): 357–362.

759. Naoum SJ, Lenard A, Martin FE, Ellakwa A. Enhancing fluoride mediated dentine sensitivity relief through functionalised tri-calcium phosphate activity. *International Scholarly Research Notes.* 2015; Article ID 905019. doi: https://www.hindawi.com/journals/isrn/2015/905019/

760. Marquis RE. Inhibition of streptococcal adenosine triphosphatase by fluoride. *Journal of Dental Research.* 1977; 56(6): 704.

761. Dreizen S, Brown LR, Daly TE, Drane JB. Prevention of xerostomia-related dental caries in irradiated cancer patients. *Journal of Dental Research.* 1977; 56(2): 99–104.

762. Brown LR, Handler SF, Horton IM, Streckfuss JL, Dreizen S. Effect of sodium fluoride on the viability and growth of *Streptococcus mutans. Journal of Dental Research.* 1980; 59(2): 159–167.

763. Domon-Tawaraya H, Nakajo K, Washio J, Ashizawa T, Ichino T, Sugawara H, Fukumoto S, Takahashi N. Divalent cations enhance fluoride binding to *Streptococcus mutans* and *Streptococcus sanguinis* cells and subsequently inhibit bacterial acid production. *Caries Research.* 2013; 47(2): 141–149.

764. Featherstone JDB, Rapozo-Hilo M, Le C. Inhibition of demineralization and promotion of remineralization by 5000 ppm F dentifrices. *Journal of Dental Research.* 2010; 89(Spec Iss B): Abstract 386.

765. White V. Evidences for hypersensitivity management. *Journal of Dental Research.* 2012; 91 (Spec Iss A): Abstract 134.

766. Amaechi BT, Gugnani S, Gugnani N, Pandit N, Vishwanat L, Gelfond J. Clinical trial of toothpastes for treating dentin hypersensitivity. *Journal of Dental Research*. 2015; 94(Spec Iss A): Abstract 4257.

767. Brown LR, Dreizen S, Daly TE, Drane JB, Handler S, Riggan LJ, Johnston DA. Interrelations of oral microorganisms, immunoglobulins, and dental caries following radiotherapy. *Journal of Dental Research*. 1978; 57(9–10): 882–893.

768. Joziak MT, Fisher SW, Schemehorn B. Comparison of enamel fluoride uptake and fluoride release from liquid and paste dentifrices. *Journal of Dental Research*. 2003; 82(Spec Iss): Abstrct 1355.

769. Mannaa A, Campus G, Carlén A, Lingström P. Caries-risk profile variations after short-term use of 5000 ppm fluoride toothpaste. *Acta Odontologica Scandinavica*. 2013; 72(3): 228–234.

770. Mannaa A, Carlén A, Zaura E, Bujis MJ, Bukhary S, Lingström P. Effects of high-fluoride dentifrice (5,000-ppm) on caries-related plaque and salivary variables. *Clinical Oral Investigations*. 2014; 18(5): 1419–1426.

771. Wefel JS. Effects of fluoride on caries development and progression using intra-oral models. *Journal of Dental Research*. 1990; 69(Spec Iss): 626–633.

772. Amaechi BT. Remineralization—the buzzword for early MI caries management. *British Dental Journal*. 2017; 223(3): 173–182.

773. Jenkins GN, Speirs RL. Some observations on the fluoride concentration of dental tissues. *Journal of Dental Research*. 1954; 33(5): 734.

774. Ferretti GA, Tanzer JM, Tinanoff N. The effect of fluoride and stannous ion on *Streptococcus mutans*. Viability, growth, acid, glucan production and adherence. *Caries Research*. 1982; 16(4): 298–307.

775. Hamilton IR. Effects of fluoride on enzymatic regulation of bacterial carbohydrate metabolism. *Caries Research*. 1977; 11(Suppl. 1): 262–291.

776. Hamilton IR, Bowden GH. Response of freshly isolated strains of *Streptococcus mutans* and *Streptococcus mitior* to change in pH in the presence and absence of fluoride during growth in continuous culture. *Infection and Immunity*. 1982; 36(1): 255–262.

777. Luoma H. Potassium content of cariogenic streptococci influenced by pH, fluoride, molybdenum, and ethanol. *European Journal of Oral Sciences*. 1972; 80(1): 18–25.

778. Luoma H, Tuompo H. The relationship between sugar metabolism and potassium translocation by caries-inducing streptococci and the inhibitory role of fluoride. *Archives of Oral Biology*. 1975; 20(11): 749–755.

779. Greger JEG, Izaguirre-Fernández EJ, Eisenberg AD. Adenosine 5'-triphosphate content of *Streptococcus mutans* GS-5 during fluoride-mediated death at low pH. *Caries Research*. 1985; 19(4): 307–313.

780. Whitford GM, Schuster GS, Pashley DH, Venkateswarlu P. Fluoride uptake by *Streptococcus mutans* 6715. *Infection and Immunity*. 1977; 18(3): 680–687.

781. Bowden GHW, Odlum O, Nolette N, Hamilton IR. Microbial populations growing in the presence of fluoride at low pH isolated from dental plaque of children living in an area with fluoridated water. *Infection and Immunity*. 1982; 36(1): 247–254.

782. Rosen S, Frea JI, Hsu SM. Effect of fluoride-resistant microorganisms on dental caries. *Journal of Dental Research*. 1978; 57(2): 180.

783. Baker JL, Sudarsan N, Weinberg Z, Roth A, Stockbridge RB, Breaker RR. Widespread genetic switches and toxicity resistance proteins for fluoride. *Science*. 2012; 335(6065): 233–235.

784. Breaker RR. New insight on the response of bacteria to fluoride. *Caries Research*. 2012; 46(1): 78–81.

785. Streckfuss JL, Perkins D, Horton IM, Brown LR, Dreizen S, Graves L. Fluoride resistance and adherence of selected strains of *Streptococcus mutans* on smooth surfaces after exposure to fluoride. *Journal of Dental Research*. 1980; 59(2): 151–158.

786. Rose RK, Shellis RP, Lee AR. The role of cation bridging in microbial fluoride binding. *Caries Research*. 1996; 30(6): 458–464.

787. Rose RK, Hogg SD, Shellis RP. A quantitative study of calcium binding and isolated streptococcal cell walls and lipoteichoic acid: Comparison with whole cells. *Journal of Dental Research*. 1994; 73(11): 1742–1747.

788. Burchard RP, Dworkin M. Light-induced lysis and carotenogenesis in *Myxococcus xanthus*. *Journal of Bacteriology*. 1966; 91(2): 535–545.

789. Saier Jr. MH. Bacterial phosphoenolpyruvate:sugar phosphotransferase systems: Structural, functional, and evolutionary interrelationships. *Bacteriological Reviews*. 1977; 41(4): 856–871.

790. Aranha H, Evans SL, Arceneaux JEL, Byers BR. Calcium modulation of growth of *Streptococcus mutans*. *Journal of General Microbiology*. 1986; 132(9): 2661–2663.

791. Sitthisettapong T, Phantumvanit P, Huebner C, DeRouen T. Effect of CPP-ACP paste on dental caries in primary teeth: A randomized trial. *Journal of Dental Research*. 2012; 91(9): 847–825.

792. Li J, Xie X, Wang Y, Yin W, Antoun JS, Farella M, Mei L. Long-term remineralizing effect of casein phosphopeptide-amorphous calcium phosphate (CPP-ACP) on early caries lesions in vivo: A systematic review. *Journal of Dentistry*. 2014; 42(7): 769–777.

793. Bowen WH. The effects of calcium, magnesium and manganese on dextran production by a cariogenic streptococcus. *Archives of Oral Biology*. 1971; 16(1): 115–119.

794. Guggenheim B. Streptococci of dental plaque. *Caries Research.* 1968; 2(2): 147–163.

795. Schachtele CF, Leung W-LS. Effect of sugar analogues on growth, sugar utilization, and acid production by *Streptococcus mutans. Journal of Dental Research.* 1975; 54(3): 433–440.

796. Stratul S, Didilescu A, Hanganu C, Greabu M, Totan A, Spinu T, Onisei D, Rusu D, Jentsch H, Sculean A. On the molecular basis of biofilm formation. Oral biofilms and systemic infections. *Timisoara Medical Journal.* 2008; 58(1–2): 118–123. doi: http://tmj. ro/article.php?art=1614054605124487

797. Marsh PD. Dental plaque as a microbial biofilm. *Caries Research.* 2004; 38(3): 204–211.

798. Gibbons RJ, Banghart SB. Synthesis of extracellular dextran by cariogenic bacteria and its presence in human dental plaque. *Archives of Oral Biology.* 1967; 12(1): 11–24.

799. Bowen WH, Hewitt MJ. Effect of fluoride on extracellular polysaccharide. *Journal of Dental Research.* 1974; 53(3): 627–629.

800. Newesely H. Changes in crystal types of low solubility calcium phosphates in the presence of accompanying ions. *Archives of Oral Biology.* 1961; 6(Spec Suppl): 174–180.

801. Feagin FF, Gonzalez M, Jeansonne BG. Kinetic reactions of calcium, phosphate, and fluoride ions at the enamel surface-solution interface. *Calcified Tissue Research.* 1972; 10(1): 113–127.

802. Moreno EC, Kresak M, Zahradnik RT. Physicochemical aspects of fluoride-apatite systems relevant to the study of dental caries. *Caries Research.* 1977; 11(Suppl 1): 142–171.

803. Brečević LJ, Füredi-Milhofer H. Precipitation of calcium phosphates from electrolyte solutions. II. The formation and transformation of the precipitates. *Calcified Tissue International.* 1972; 10(1): 82–90.

804. Brown WE, Eidelman N, Tomažič B. Octacalcium phosphate as a precursor in biomineral formation. *Advances in Dental Research.* 1987; 1(2): 306–313.

805. Tung MS. "Calcium phosphates: Structure, composition, solubility, and stability." Amjad Z (Ed.), In: *Calcium Phosphates in Biological and Industrial Systems.* Norwell: Kluwer Academic Publishers, 1998, Vol 23, 1–19.

806. Eanes ED, Meyer JL. The influence of fluoride on apatite formation from unstable supersaturated solutions at pH 7.4. *Journal of Dental Research.* 1978; 57(4): 617–624.

807. Eanes ED. The influence of fluoride on the seeded growth of apatite from stable supersaturated solutions at pH 7.4. *Journal of Dental Research.* 1980; 59(2): 144–150.

808. Koulourides T. Summary of session II: Fluoride and the caries process. *Journal of Dental Research.* 1990; 69(2 Supplement): 558.

809. Bansal R, Bolin KA, Abdellatif HM, Shulman JD. Knowledge, attitude and use of fluorides among dentists in Texas. *Journal of Contemporary Dental Practice.* 2012; 13(3): 375–379.

810. Yoder KM, Maupome G, Ofner S, Swignoski NL. Knowledge and use of fluoride among Indiana dental professionals. *Journal of Public Health Dentistry.* 2007; 67(3): 140–147.

811. Aljafari AK, Gallagher JE, Hosey MT. Failure on all fronts: general dental practitioners' views on promoting oral health in high caries risk children—a qualitative study. *BMC Oral Health.* 2015; 15: 45. https://bmcoralhealth.biomedcentral.com/articles/10.1186/s12903-015-0032-8

812. Duijster D, de Jong-Lenters M, Verrips E, van Loveren C. Establishing oral health promoting behaviors in children—parents' views on barriers, facilitators and professional support: a qualitative study. *BMC Oral Health.* 2015; 15: 157. https://www.ncbi.nlm.nih.gov/pmc/articles/PMC4676163/

813. Becks H, Wainwright WW. Human Saliva. XVI. Relationship of total calcium to inorganic phosphorus of resting saliva. *Journal of Dental Research*. 1946; 25(4): 275–283.

814. Dawes C, Jenkins GN. The effects of different stimuli on the composition of saliva in man. *Journal of Physiology*. 1964; 170(1): 86–100.

815. Dawes C. The composition of human saliva secreted in response to a gustatory stimulus and to pilocarpine. *Journal of Physiology*. 1966; 183(2): 360–368.

816. Dawes C. Rhythms in salivary flow rate and composition. *International Journal of Chronobiology*. 1974; 2(3): 253–279.

817. Hara AT, Karlinsey RL, Zero DT. Dentine remineralisation by simulated saliva formulations with different Ca and Pi contents. *Caries Research*. 2008; 42(1): 51–56.

818. Walser M. Ion association. VI. Interactions between calcium, magnesium, inorganic phosphate, citrate and protein in normal human plasma. *Journal of Clinical Investigation*. 1961; 40(4): 723–730.

819. Posner AS. Crystal chemistry of bone mineral. *Physiological Reviews*. 1969; 49(4): 760–792.

820. Wilson RM, Elliott JC, Dowker SEP, Smith RI. Rietveld structure refinement of precipitated carbonate apatite using neutron diffraction data. *Biomaterials*. 2004; 25(11): 2205–2213.

821. Antonakos A, Liarokapis E, Leventouri T. Micro-Raman and FTIR studies of synthetic and natural apatites. *Biomaterials*. 2007; 28(19): 3043–3054.

822. Beniash E, Metzler RA, Lam RSK, Gilbert PUPA. Transient amorphous calcium phosphate in forming enamel. *Journal of Structural Biology*. 2009; 166(2): 133–143.

823. Wopenka B, Pasters JD. A mineralogic perspective on the apatite in bone. *Materials Science and Engineering C.* 2005; 25(2): 131–143.

824. Jiang H, Liu X-Y. Principles of mimicking and engineering the self-organized structure of hard tissues. *Journal of Biological Chemistry.* 2004; 279(40): 41286–41293.

825. Van Kemenade MJJM, De Bruyn PL. A kinetic study of precipitation from supersaturated calcium phosphate solutions. *Journal of Colloid and Interface Science.* 1987; 118(2): 564–585.

826. Ostwald W, McGowan G. *The Scientific Foundations of Analytical Chemistry Treated In An Elementary Manner, 2nd Edition.* New York: The Macmillan Company, 1900.

827. Eanes ED, Posner AS. Division of Biophysics: Kinetics and mechanism of conversion of noncrystalline calcium phosphate to crystalline hydroxyapatite. *Transactions of the New York Academy of Sciences.* 1965; 28(2): 233–241.

828. Pan H, Liu XY, Tang R, Xu HY. Mystery of the transformation from amorphous calcium phosphate to hydroxyapatite. *Chemical Communications.* 2010; 46(39): 7415–7417.

829. Albee FH. Studies in bone growth. *Annals of Surgery.* 1920; 71(1): 32–39.

830. Nancollas GH, Mohan MS. The growth of hydroxyapatite crystals. *Archives of Oral Biology.* 1970; 15(8): 731–745.

831. Nancollas GH, Tomažič B. Growth of calcium phosphate on hydroxyapatite crystals. Effect of supersaturation and ionic medium. *Journal of Physical Chemistry.* 1974; 78(22): 2218–2225.

832. Jiang H, Liu X-Y, Zhang G, Li Y. Kinetics and template nucleation of self-assembled hydroxyapatite nanocrystallites by chondroitin sulfate. *Journal of Biological Chemistry.* 2005; 280(51): 42061–42066.

833. Tomažič B, Tomson M, Nancollas GH. Growth of calcium phosphates on hydroxyapatite crystals: The effect of magnesium. *Archives of Oral Biology.* 1975; 20(12): 803–909.

834. Rapp GW, Prapuolenis A, Madonia J. Pyrophosphate: A factor in tooth erosion. *Journal of Dental Research.* 1960; 39(2): 372–376.

835. Nancollas GK. The involvement of calcium phosphates in biological mineralization and demineralization processes. *Pure and Applied Chemistry.* 1992; 64(11): 1673–1678.

836. Matsunaga K. First-principles study of substitutional magnesium and zinc in hydroxyapatite and octacalcium phosphate. *Journal of Chemical Physics.* 2008; 128(24): 245101.

837. Koulourides T, Feagin F, Pigman W. Remineralization of dental enamel by saliva *in vitro. Annals of the New York Academy of Sciences.* 1965; 131(2): 751–757.

838. Melia TP, Moffitt WP. Secondary nucleation from aqueous solution. *Industrial and Engineering Chemistry Fundamentals.* 1964; 3(4): 313–317.

839. Amjad Z, Koutsoukos P, Tomson MB, Nancollas GH. The growth of hydroxyapatite from solution. A new constant composition method. *Journal of Dental Research.* 1978; 57(9–10): 909.

840. Amjad Z, Nancollas GH. A kinetic and morphological study of mineralization of bovine tooth enamel surfaces. *Archives of Oral Biology.* 1980; 25(2): 95–101.

841. Johansson B. Remineralization of slightly etched enamel. *Journal of Dental Research.* 1965; 44(1): 64–70.

842. Featherstone JDB, Rodgers BE, Smith MW. Physicochemical requirements for rapid remineralization of early carious lesions. *Caries Research.* 1981; 15(3): 221–235.

843. Pan H-B, Darvell BW. Solubility of TTCP and β-TCP by solid titration. *Archives of Oral Biology.* 2009; 54(7): 671–677.

844. Larsen MJ, Pearce EIF. Saturation of human saliva with respect to calcium salts. *Archives of Oral Biology.* 2003; 48(4): 317–322.

845. Collys K, Cleymaet R, Coomans D, Michotte Y, Slop D. Rehardening of surface softened and surface etched enamel in vitro and by intraoral exposure. *Caries Research.* 1993; 27(1): 15–20.

846. ten Cate JM, Arends J. Remineralization of artificial enamel lesions *in vitro.* II. Determination of activation energy and reaction order. *Caries Research.* 1978; 12(4): 213–222.

847. Jardim JJ, Pagot MA, Maltz M. Artificial enamel dental caries treated with different topical fluoride regimens: An *in situ* study. *Journal of Dentistry.* 2008; 36(6): 296–401.

848. Gelhard TBFM, ten Cate M, Arends J. Rehardening of artificial enamel lesions *in vivo. Caries Research.* 1979; 13(2): 80–83.

849. Ganss C, Klimek J, Brune V, Schürmann A. Effects of two fluoridation measures on erosion progression in human enamel and dentine *in situ. Caries Research.* 2004; 38(6): 561–566.

850. Huysmans M-C, Young Z, Ganss C. "The role of fluoride in erosion therapy." A Lussi & C Ganss (Eds.), In: *Erosive Tooth Wear: A Phenomenon of Clinical Significance.* Basel: Karger Publishers, 2014, Vol 25, 230–243.

851. Ganss C, Lussi A, Schlueter N. "The histological features and physical properties of eroded dental hard tissues." A Lussi & C Ganss (Eds.), In: *Erosive Tooth Wear: A Phenomenon of Clinical Significance.* Basel: Karger Publishers, 2014, Vol 25, 99–107.

852. Wang X, Megert B, Hellwig E, Neuhaus KW, Lussi A. Preventing erosion with novel agents. *Journal of Dentistry.* 2011; 39(2): 163–170.

853. Cummins D. Clinical evidence for the superior efficacy of a dentifrice containing 8.0% arginine and calcium carbonate in providing instant and lasting relief of dentin hypersensitivity. *American Journal of Dentistry*. 2011; 22(Spec Iss): 97–99.

854. West NX, He T, Macdonald EL, Seong J, Hellin N, Barker ML, Eversole SL. Erosion protection benefits of stabilized SnF_2 dentifrice versus an arginine-sodium monofluorophosphate dentifrice: results from *in vitro* and *in situ* clinical studies. *Clinical Oral Investigations*. 2017; 21(2): 533–540.

855. Stookey GK, DePaola PF, Featherstone JDB, Fejerskov O, Möller IJ, Rotberg S, Stephen KW, Wefel JS. A critical review of the relative anticaries efficacy of sodium fluoride and sodium monofluorophosphate dentifrices. *Caries Research*. 1993; 27(4): 337–360.

856. Burwell AK, Litkowski LJ, Greenspan DC. Calcium sodium phosphosilicate (NovaMin®): Remineralization potential. *Advances in Dental Research*. 2009; 21(1): 35–39.

857. Wefel JS. NovaMin®: Likely clinical success. *Advances in Dental Research*. 2009; 21(1): 40–43.

858. Hench LL. The story of Bioglass®. *Journal of Materials Science: Materials in Medicine*. 2006; 17(11): 967–978.

859. Gendreau L, Barlow APS, Mason SC. Overview of the clinical evidence for the use of Novamin® in providing relief from the pain of dentin hypersensitivity. *Journal of Clinical Dentistry*. 2011; 22(Spec Iss): 90–95.

860. Acharya AB, Surve SM, Thakur SL. A clinical study of the effect of calcium sodium phosphosilicate on dentin hypersensitivity. *Journal of Clinical and Experimental Dentistry*. 2013; 5(1): 18–22.

861. Jones JR. Review of bioactive glass: From Hench to hybrids. *Acta Biomaterialia*. 2013; 9(1): 4457–4486.

862. Morgan A, Joziak MT, Prencipe M. Fluoride availability of professional products with 5000 ppm F-. *Journal of Dental Research*. 2012; 91(Spec Iss A): Abstract 1081.

863. Sensodyne® Repair & Protect. Available from: https://www.sensodyne.co.nz/products/repair-and-protect.html.

864. Sensodyne® Repair & Protect in US. Available from: https://us.sensodyne.com/products/repair-and-protect-whitening-toothpaste/

865. Summary of FDA 510k approval (#K040473) for Novamin® in the Oravive™ paste as tubule occlusion agent. March 10, 20104. Available from: https://www.accessdata.fda.gov/cdrh_docs/pdf4/K040473.pdf

866. Larsen MJ. Chemical events during tooth dissolution. *Journal of Dental Research*. 1990; 69(Spec Iss): 575–580.

867. U.S. Environmental Protection Agency Exposure Assessment Models. Available from: https://www.epa.gov/exposure-assessment-models/minteqa2

868. Moreno EC, Gregory TM, Brown WE. Preparation and solubility of hydroxyapatite. *Journal of Research of the National Bureau of Standards—A. Physics and Chemistry*. 1968; 72A(6): 773–782.

869. Reynolds EC. Remineralization of enamel subsurface lesions by casein phosphopeptide-stabilized calcium phosphate solutions. *Journal of Dental Research*. 1997; 76(9): 1587–1595.

870. Reynolds EC. Calcium phosphate-based remineralization systems: scientific evidence? *Australian Dental Journal*. 2008; 53(3): 268–273.

871. Eanes ED, Meyer JL. The maturation of crystalline calcium phosphates in aqueous suspensions at physiologic pH. *Calcified Tissue Research*. 1977; 23(3): 259–269.

872. Zhang F, Chang J, Lu J, Lin K, Ning C. Bioinspired structure of bioceramics for bone regeneration in load-bearing sites. *Acta Biomaterialia*. 2007; 3(6): 896–904.

873. Ghosh SK, Nandi SK, Kundu B, Datta S, De DK, Roy SK, Basu D. *In vivo* response of porous hydroxyapatite and β-tricalcium phosphate prepared by aqueous solution combustion method and comparison with bioglass scaffolds. *Journal of Biomedical Materials Research Part B: Applied Biomaterials.* 2008; 86(1): 217–227.

874. Yashima M, Sakai A, Kamiyama T, Hoshikawa A. Crystal structure analysis of β-tricalcium phosphate $Ca_3(PO_4)_2$ by neutron powder diffraction. *Journal of Solid State Chemistry.* 2003; 175(2): 272–277.

875. Dorozhkin SV. Calcium orthophosphates and human beings. A historical perspective from the 1770s until 1940. *Biomatter.* 2012; 2(2): 53–70.

876. Bell A (Proprietor). *Encyclopaedia Britannica; or, a dictionary of arts, sciences, and miscellaneous literature, 4th Edition, Volume V.* Edinburgh: Archibald Constable and Company, 1810.

877. Food and Drug Administration. Dental devices: Reclassification of tricalcium phosphate granules and classification of other bone grafting material for dental bone repair. *Federal Register.* 2005; 70(81): 21947–21950.

878. Gustafsson JP. Visual MINTEQ 3.1. Available from: https://vminteq.lwr.kth.se/

879. Shen P, Manton DJ, Cochrane NJ, Walker GD, Yuan Y, Reynolds C, Reynolds EC. Effect of added calcium phosphate on enamel remineralization by fluoride in a randomized controlled *in situ* model. *Journal of Dentistry.* 2011; 39(7): 518–525.

880. Damyanova D. In vitro studies with X-ray diffraction. *Varna Medical Forum.* 2016; 5(2): 19–22.

881. Damyanova D, Tachev D. X-ray micro-tomography examination of specimens of deciduous teeth. *Varna Medical Forum.* 2017; 6(1): 86–91.

882. Damyanova D, Atanasova S. Investigation of the remineralization effect through scanning electron microscopy. *International Journal of Engineering Research and Application*. 2016; 6(5): 73–76.

883. Shen P, Bagheri R, Walker GD, Yuan Y, Stanton, Reynolds C, Reynolds EC. Effect of calcium phosphate addition to fluoride containing dental varnishes on enamel demineralization. *Australian Dental Journal*. 2016; 61(3): 357–365.

884. Addadi L, Raz S, Weiner S. Taking advantage of disorder: amorphous calcium carbonate and its roles in biomineralization. *Advanced Materials*. 2003; 15(12): 959–970.

885. Mahamid J, Sharir A, Addadi L, Weiner S. Amorphous calcium phosphate is a major component of the forming fin bones of zebrafish: Indications for an amorphous precursor phase. *Proceedings of the National Academy of Sciences*. 2008; 105(35): 12748–12753.

886. Meyers MA, Chen P-Y, Lin AY-M, Seki Y. Biological materials: Structure and mechanical properties. *Progress in Materials Science*. 2008; 53(1): 1–206.

887. Sharma E, Vishwanathamurthy RA, Nadella M, Savitha AN, Gundannavar G, Hussain MA. A randomised study to compare salivary pH, calcium, phosphate and calculus formation after using anticavity dentifrices containing Recaldent® and functionalized tri-calcium phosphate. *Journal of Indian Society of Periodontology*. 2012; 46(4): 504–507.

888. Reynolds EC. Casein phosphopeptide-amorphous calcium phosphate: The scientific evidence. *Advances in Dental Research*. 2009; 21(1): 25–29.

889. Huang GJ, Roloff-Chiang B, Mills BE, Shalchi S, Spiekerman C, Korpak AM, Starrett JL, Greenlee GM, Drangsholt RJ, Matunas JC. Effectiveness of MI Paste Plus and PreviDent fluoride varnish for treatment of white spot lesions: A randomized controlled trial.

American Journal of Orthodontics and Dentofacial Orthopedics. 2013; 143(1): 31–41.

890. Singh S, Singh SP, Goyal A, Utreja AK, Jena AK. Effects of various remineralizing agents on the outcome of post-orthodontic white spot lesions (WSLs): a clinical trial. *Progress in Orthodontics.* 2016; 17(1): 25.

891. Rao SK, Bhat GS, Aradhya S, Devi A, Bhat M. Study of the efficacy of toothpaste containing casein phosphopeptide in the prevention of dental caries: a randomized controlled trial in 12- to 15-year-old high caries risk children in Bangalore, India. *Caries Research.* 2009; 43(6): 430–435.

892. Yengopal V, Mickenautsch S. Caries preventive effect of casein phosphopeptide-amorphous calcium phosphate (CPP-ACP): a meta-analysis. *Acta Odontologica Scandinavica.* 2009; 67(6): 321–332.

893. Li J, Xie X, Wang Y, Yin W, Antoun JS, Farella M, Mei L. Long-term remineralizing effect of casein phosphopeptide-amorphous calcium phosphate (CPP-ACP) on early caries lesions in vivo: A systematic review. *Journal of Dentistry.* 2014; 42(7): 769–777.

894. Azarpazhooh A, Limeback H. Clinical efficacy of casein derivatives: A systematic review of the literature. *Journal of the American Dental Association.* 2008; 139(7): 915–924.

895. Zero DT. Recaldent™ evidence for clinical activity. *Advances in Dental Research.* 2009; 21(1): 30–34.

896. Raphael S, Blinkhorn A. Is there a place for Tooth Mousse® in the prevention and treatment of early dental caries? A systematic review. *BMC Oral Health.* 2015; 15(1): 113. doi: https://bmcoralhealth. biomedcentral.com/articles/10.1186/s12903-015-0095-6

897. Ghassemi A, Hooper W, Winston AE, Sowinski J, Bowman JP, Sharma NC. Effectiveness of a baking-soda toothpaste delivering calcium and phosphate in reducing dentinal hypersensitivity. *Journal of Clinical Dentistry.* 2009; 20(7): 203–210.

898. Evans RW, Clark P, Jia N. The caries management system: are preventive effects sustained postclinical trial? *Community Dentistry and Oral Epidemiology.* 2016; 44(2): 188–197.

899. Newkirk G. Abstracts: Items of Interest. *Dominion Dental Journal.* 1895; 7(2): 35.

900. Black GV. *A Work on Operative Dentistry in Two Volumes. Volume 1, The Pathology of the Hard Tissues of the Teeth.* Chicago: Medico-Dental Publishing Company, 1920.

901. Taft J (Ed.). Operative dentistry: Preventive dentistry. *Dental Register.* 1895; 49(5): 237.

902. Ismail AI, Tellez M, Pitts NB, Ekstrand KR, Ricketts D, Longbottom C, Eggertsson H, Deery C, Fisher J, Young DA, Featherstone JDB, Evans W, Zeller GG, Zero D, Martignon S, Fontana M, Zandona A. Caries management pathways preserve dental tissues and promote oral health. *Community Dentistry and Oral Epidemiology.* 2013; 41(1): e12-e40.

903. Sheiham A. Minimal intervention in dental care. *Medical Principles and Practice.* 2012; 11(Suppl 1): 2–6.

904. Belstrøm D, Sembler-Møller ML, Grande MA, Kirkby N, Cotton SL, Paster BJ, Twetman S, Holmstrup P. Impact of oral hygiene discontinuation on supragingival and salivary microbiomes. *JDR Clinical & Translational Research.* 2017; Article ID: 2380084417723635.

905. Axelsson P, Lindhe J. The effect of a plaque control program on gingivitis and dental caries in schoolchildren. *Journal of Dental Research.* 1977; 56(Spec Iss C): 142–148.

906. Ito A, Hayashi M, Hamasaki T, Ebisu S. How regular visits and preventive programs affect onset of adult caries. *Journal of Dental Research*. 2012; 91(7): S52-S58.

907. Bakhshandeh A, Ekstrand K. Infiltration and sealing versus fluoride treatment of occlusal caries lesions in primary molar teeth. 2–3 years results. *International Journal of Paediatric Dentistry*. 2015; 25(1): 43–50.

908. White JM, Eakle S. Rationale and treatment approach in minimally invasive dentistry. *Journal of the American Dental Association*. 2000; 131: 13S-19S.

909. Murdoch-Kinch CA, McLean ME. Minimally invasive dentistry. *Journal of the American Dental Association*. 2003; 134(1): 87–95.

910. Hamilton JC, Dennison JB, Stoffers KW, Gregory WA, Welch KB. Early treatment of incipient carious lesions: a two-year clinical evaluation. *Journal of the American Dental Association*. 2002; 133(12): 1643–1651.

911. Wechsler LD. Simple dental treatments may reverse decay. *Wall Street Journal*. April 11, 2016.

912. Tickle M, O'Neill C, Donaldson M, Birch S, Noble S, Killough S, Murphy L, Greer M, Brodison J, Verghis R, Worthington HV. A randomized controlled trial of caries prevention in dental practice. *Journal of Dental Research*.

913. Frencken JE, Innes NPT, Schwendicke F. Managing carious lesions: Why do we need consensus on terminology and clinical recommendations on carious tissue removal? *Advances in Dental Research*. 2016; 28(2): 46–48.

914. Innes NPT, Frencken JE, Bjørndal L, Maltz M, Manton DJ, Ricketts D, Van Landuyt K, Banerjee A, Campus G, Doméjean S, Fontana M, Leal S, Lo E, Machiulskiene V, Schulte A, Splieth C, Zandona A, Schwendicke F. Managing carious lesions: Consensus

recommendations on terminology. *Advances in Dental Research*. 2016; 28(2): 49–57.

915. Wetselaar P, Faris A, Lobbezoo F. A plea for the development of an universally accepted modular tooth wear evaluation system. *BMC Oral Health*. 2016; 16(1): 115. doi: https://bmcoralhealth.biomedcentral.com/articles/10.1186/s12903-016-0309-6

916. Street Jr. RL, Makoul G, Arora NK, Epstein RM. How does communication heal? Pathways linking clinician-patient communication to health outcomes. *Patient Education and Counseling*. 2009; 74(3): 295–301.

917. Nakai Y, Hirakawa T, Milgrom P, Coolidge T, Heima M, Mori Y, Ishihara C, Yakushiji N, Yoshida T, Shimono T. The Children's Fear Survey Schedule-Dental Subscale in Japan. *Community Dentistry and Oral Epidemiology*. 2005; 33(3): 196–204.

918. Poulton R, Menzies RG. Non-associative fear acquisition: a review of the evidence from retrospective and longitudinal research. *Behaviour Research and Therapy*. 2002; 40(2): 127–149.

919. Yamada T, Kuwano S, Ebisu S, Hayashi M. Statistical analysis for subjective and objective evaluations of dental drill sounds. *PLoS ONE*. 2016; 11(7): e1059926. doi: http://journals.plos.org/plosone/article?id=10.1371/journal.pone.0159926

920. American Dental Association. Principles of Ethics and Code of Professional Conduct. Patient Autonomy. Available from: http://www.ada.org/en/about-the-ada/principles-of-ethics-code-of-professional-conduct/patient-autonomy

921. Misra S, Daly B, Dunne S, Millar B, Packer M, Asimakopoulou K. Dentist-patient communication: what do patients and dentists remember following a consultation? Implications for patient compliance. *Patient Preference and Adherence*. 2013; 7: 543–549.

922. Khan K, Ruby B, Goldblatt RS, Schensul JJ, Reisine S. A pilot study to assess oral health literacy by comparing a word recognition and comprehension tool. *BMC Oral Health*. 2014; 14(1): 135. doi: http://www.biomedcentral.com/1472–6831/14/135

923. Karlinsey RL. Emphasizing minimally invasive strategies for improved dental care of children. *Journal of Dentistry, Oral Disorders & Therapy*. 2017; 5(2): 1–3.

924. Anonymous. Abstracts: Items of Interest. *Dominion Dental Journal*. 1895; 7(3): 83.

925. Innes NPT, Schwendicke F. Restorative thresholds for carious lesions: Systematic review and meta-analysis. *Journal of Dental Research*. 2017; 96(5): 501–508.

926. Gordan VV, Riley III JL, Geraldeli S, Rindal DB, Qvist V, Fellows JL, Kellum HP, Gilbert GH, DPBRN Collaborative Group. Repair or replacement of defective restorations by dentists in the Dental PBRN. *Journal of the American Dental Association*. 2012; 143(6): 593–601.

927. Craig JS. Ethics and third-party payers. *Journal of the American Dental Association*. 2017; 148(9): 631.

928. Helgeson M. Economic models for prevention: making a system work for patients. *BMC Oral Health*. 2015; 15(Suppl 11): S11. doi: http://www.biomedcentral.com/1472–6831/15/S1/S11

929. Nash DA. Adding dental therapists to the health care team to improve access to oral health care for children. *Academic Pediatrics*. 2009; 9(6): 446–451.

930. American Dental Hygienists' Association. Transforming Dental Hygiene Education and the Profession for the 21st Century. October 26, 2015. Available at: http://tenndha.com/wp-content/uploads/2015/10/ADHA-White-Paper.pdf

931. Azad MB, Abou-Setta AM, Chauhan BF, Rabbani R, Lys J, Copstein L, Mann A, Jeyaraman MM, Reid AE, Fiander M, MacKay DS, McGavock J, Wicklow B, Zarychanksi R. Nonnutritive sweeteners and cardiometabolic health: a systematic review and meta-analyasis of randomized controlled trials and prospective cohort studies. *Canadian Medical Association Journal.* 2017; 189(28): E929-E939.

932. Krumholz H. Why one cardiologist has drunk his last diet soda. *Wall Street Journal.* September 14, 2017.

933. Levin GV, Zehner LR, Saunders JP, Beadle JR. Sugar substitutes: their energy values, bulk characteristics, and potential health benefits. *American Journal of Clinical Nutrition.* 1995; 62(5): 1161S-1168S.

934. Ruxton CHS, Gardner EJ, McNulty HM. Is sugar consumption detrimental to health? A review of the evidence 1995–2006. *Critical Reviews in Food Science and Nutrition.* 2009; 50(1): 1–19.

935. Gibson S, Gunn P, Wittekind A, Cottrell R. The effects of sucrose on metabolic health: A systematic review of human intervention studies in healthy adults. *Critical Reviews in Food Science and Nutrition.* 2013; 53(6): 591–614.

936. Lovegrove A, Edwards CH, De Noni I, Patel H, El SN, Grassby T, Zielke C, Ulmius M, Nilsson L, Butterworth PJ, Ellis PR, Shewry PR. Role of polysaccharides in food, digestion, and health. *Critical Reviews in Food Science and Nutrition.* 2017; 57(2): 237–253.

937. Rapsomaniki E, Timmis A, George j, Pujades-Rodriguez M, Shah AD, Denaxas S, White IR, Caulfied MJ, Deanfield JE, Smeeth L, Williams B, Hingorani A, Hemingway H. Blood pressure and incidence of twelve cardiovascular diseases: lifetime risks, healthy life-years lots, and age-specific associations in 1.25 million people. *Lancet.* 2014; 383(9932): 1899–1911.

938. Sukhabogi JR, Shekar CBR, Hameed IA, Ramana IV, Sandhu G. Oral health status among 12- and 15-year-old children from government and private schools in Hyderabad, Andhra Pradesh, India. *Annals of Medical and Health Sciences Research.* 2014; 4(3): 272–277.

939. Claudino D, Traebert J. Malocclusion, dental aesthetic self-perception and quality of life in a 18 to 21 year-old population: a cross section study. *BMC Oral Health.* 2013; 13: 3. doi: https://bmcoralhealth.biomedcentral.com/articles/10.1186/1472-6831-13-3

940. Cotrim ER, Vasconcelos Júnior ÁV, Santos Haddad ACS, Reis SAB. Perception of adults' smile esthetics among orthodontists, clinicians and laypeople. *Dental Press Journal of Orthodontics.* 2015; 20(1): 40–44.

941. Hujoel P. Dietary carbohydrates and dental-systemic diseases. *Journal of Dental Research.* 2009; 88(6): 490–502.

942. Slavkin HC, Baum BJ. Relationship of dental and oral pathology to systemic illness. *Journal of the American Medical Association.* 2000; 284(10): 1215–1217.

943. Ritchie CS, Joshipura K, Hung, H-C, Douglass CW. Nutrition as a mediator in the relation between oral and systemic disease: Associations between specific measures of adult oral health and nutrition outcomes. *Critical Reviews in Oral Biology and Medicine.* 2002; 13(3): 291–300.

944. Azarpazhooh A, Leake JL. Systematic review of the association between respiratory diseases and oral health. *Journal of Periodontology.* 2006; 77(9): 1465–1482.

945. Meurman JH, Sanz M, Janket S-J. Oral health, atherosclerosis, and cardiovascular disease. *Critical Reviews in Oral Biology and Medicine.* 2004; 15(6): 403–413.

946. DeStefano F, Anda RF, Kahn HS, Williamson DF, Russel CM. Dental disease and risk of coronary heart disease and mortality. *British Medical Journal.* 1993; 306(6879): 688–691.

947. Genco RJ, Genco FD. Common risk factors in the management of periodontal and associated systemic diseases: The dental setting and interprofessional collaboration. *Journal of Evidence Based Dental Practice.* 2014; 14(S): 4–16.

948. Pussinen PJ, Könönen E. Oral health: A modifiable risk factor for cardiovascular diseases or a confounded association? *European Journal of Preventive Cardiology.* 2016; 23(8): 834–838.

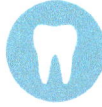

Index

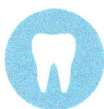

Acknowledgments

A number people have contributed indelibly to my involvement in dental research, especially Dr. Domenick Zero and Mr. Bruce Schemehorn: in accepting me under your research umbrella for the purposes of pursuing oral health research activities, you helped shape my initial foray into oral health research and for this I am forever grateful. With tremendous respect and gratitude, I thank Dr. George K. Stookey, whom I consider a godfather of fluoride toothpaste and of fluoride research in general, is an excellent mentor for all researchers (young and old alike!) and enabled my successful transition from an academic-scientist to scientist-entrepreneur on several fronts. Among many collaborators, colleagues and assistants, I want to highlight a few that stand out to me: Dr. Christabel Fowler, Dr. Bennett Amaechi, Dr. Makoto Asaizumi, Dr. Rajeev Thaper, Dr. Anderson Hara, Mr. Mike Brewer, and Mr. Stephen Langdon—each of you has shaped me in various capacities over the years and I humbly appreciate and admire your unique skillsets and, importantly, your friendship; and, to Mr. Allen C. Mackey, who was my right-hand in our research endeavors day-in and day-out. Dr. Bill Lyon was instrumental in facilitating my transition from postdoctoral studies to the dental school, and then again in formation of my company—thank you! For selecting a promising calcium phosphate technology and supporting its development, I humbly thank Mr. Aaron Pfarrer and 3M Oral Care; moreover, 3M Oral Care continues to be an excellent partner. As funding for scientific study is always a critical challenge especially for new ideas, I've been fortunate to receive critical funding from the National Institutes of Health and funding mechanisms from the states of Indiana and Texas. To my parents and brother, who have long-provided kind words of support. Tami, you are my champion, and Teegan, your energy is infectious: both of you are incredible and you inspire me more than you know. Finally, to you, dear reader, thank you for allowing me to share some of my insight with you.

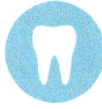

About the Author

Dr. Robert L. Karlinsey earned a BS in Physics and PhD in Chemical Physics, holds several patents, and has published in multiple fields including dentistry, chemistry, and materials science. His lifelong struggles with this own dental decay ultimately inspired his transition from studying various nonlife science systems to investigating the remineralization of teeth. After a faculty appointment at the Indiana University School of Dentistry, he made an entrepreneurial leap and, in collaboration with a legend in fluoride research, founded Indiana Nanotech, LLC in order to progress his remineralization discoveries. As a Principal Investigator, Dr. Karlinsey has procured significant, competitive grant funding from federal and state-level agencies, including the US National Institutes of Health. His tooth-strengthening inventions are found, for instance, in several 3M Oral Care dental products available worldwide.

rob@rlkphd.com
www.rlkphd.com

www.ingramcontent.com/pod-product-compliance
Lightning Source LLC
Chambersburg PA
CBHW041913190326
41458CB00023B/6250